A. A. Czitrom
and H. Winkler (eds.)

Orthopaedic
Allograft Surgery

SpringerWienNewYork

Andrei A. Czitrom, M.D., Ph.D.
Orthopaedic Center of Dallas, Texas, U.S.A.

Heinz Winkler, M.D.
Department of Orthopaedics, Donauspital, Vienna, Austria

© 1996 Springer-Verlag/Wien

Softcover reprint of the hardcover 1st edition 1996

Product Liability: The publisher can give no guarantee for information about drug dosage and application thereof contained in this book. In every individual case the respective user must check its accuracy by consulting other pharmaceutical literature. The use of registered names, trademarks, etc. in this publication does not imply, even in the absence of a specific statement, that such names are exempt from the relevant protective laws and regulations and therefore free for general use.

Typesetting: Thomson Press (India) Ltd., New Delhi 110001

Graphic design: Ecke Bonk

Printed on acid-free and chlorine free bleached paper

With 94 partly coloured Figures

Library of Congress Cataloging-in-Publication Data

Orthopaedic allograft surgery / Andrei Alexander Czitrom and Heinz
   Winkler (eds.).
      p. cm.
   Includes bibliographical references and index.

   ISBN-13: 978-3-7091-7423-4   e-ISBN-13: 978-3-7091-6885-1
   DOI: 10.1007/978-3-7091-6885-1

   1. Bone-grafting. I. Czitrom, Andrei A. II. Winkler, Heinz.
   [DNLM: 1. Transplantation, Homologous. WE 190 0765 1996]
   RD123.078   1996
   617.4′710592—dc20

Foreword

This volume is the work product of an international group of authors who are experienced in the field of musculoskeletal allografts. The chapters are written by experts in many differing areas of allografting and represents the current knowledge in this rapidly changing dynamic field. The reconstructive community and their patients owe a significant debt of gratitude to Doctors Czitrom and Winkler for this volume.

William F. Enneking, M.D.

Preface

What follows is the result of a timely project bringing together the newest ideas of top experts worldwide in a rapidly growing technology: Orthopaedic Allograft Surgery. The title of the book reflects a method rather than a speciality. It transgresses well established subspecialities of orthopaedic surgery such as joint replacement, oncology, spine, trauma and sports medicine. The technology encompasses knowledge of tissue banking, biology and biomechanics, both in a research and clinical sense. The common denominator for those interested is the need and ability to provide or use allogeneic tissues in orthopaedic applications. Inherent to a multiauthored text based on chapters written by authors from many parts of the world is a variety in format and style. While we tried to some extent reducing large discrepancies, there was no attempt made to eliminate dissimilarities. We did not aim for a homogeneous textbook. Rather, we asked for originality, novelty, individuality in the presentation of data and concepts. Consequently, chapters vary in format from that seen in a scientific article to that of a descriptive essay. The result is a compendium of world knowledge presented in a singular way by each authority.

We are indebted to those who sponsored this project, based on an international workshop on musculoskeletal allografts held in Vienna in October 7–9, 1994 under the auspices of IAEA: International Atomic Energy Agency, European Association of Tissue Banks, Musculoskeletal Transplant Foundation, Johnson & Johnson Orthopedics and Cryolife Inc.

Springer-Verlag's support and committment to scholars of orthopaedic transplantation have now become a tradition: Bone Transplantation (1989), Bone Implant Grafting (1992) and Orthopaedic Allograft Surgery (1996) are titles giving practicing surgeons regular updates in a topic that is undergoing fast change.

Dallas, Texas, U.S.A., and Vienna, Austria
June 3, 1996

Andrei Czitrom
Heinz Winkler

Contents

Spine and Trauma

Tendon, Meniscus and Osteochondral Grafts

Bone Banking, Biology and Biomechanics

Current Concepts in Bone Grafting

H. Burchardt

Pennsylvania Regional Tissue Bank, Pennsylvania, U.S.A.

The usual alternative to an autograft is the man-made implant device, or the use of allografts. Implants are readily available and produced with remarkable precision, yet they are not readily incorporated into the skeleton, and the attachment of soft-tissues remains a problem.

Allografts, or biological materials from donors with a different genetic background than the recipients', are not limited in supply, soft tissues can be attached or become biologically attached to them, and they can be used in conjunction with implants. Historically, allografts have achieved some success when measured against the "gold-standard" autograft. Occasional problems do occur with allogeneic materials including nonunions, fatigue, failure, and, infrequently, the complete resorption of the transplant. The attractive feature with the use of allografts is the capacity to perform a skeletal joint reconstruction which otherwise would have to be performed with implants.

Regardless of whether an autograft or an allograft is used to alleviate a skeletal problem, the vascular status of the site, the type of bone materials (cortical/cancellous), and the size, shape, and biomechanical properties associated with the site needs to be considered. Associated with these variables are the biodynamics of the host in response to the tissue that occurs from the time of transplantation to the time of incorporation and secondary remodeling.

It is the purpose of this review to describe the fate of the bones which have been transplanted, and the underlying biological mechanisms that influence their functional outcome.

Primary Histological Features of Autogenous Transplants

Axhausen and Barth [1] determined that bone transplants undergo necrosis, that a successful repair of a transplant depended on the intimate contact of the graft with a vascular host tissue, and that necrotic bone was replaced by new tissue moving along channels cleared by invasive blood vessels. For the purposes of this review, the phrase "creeping substitution" will be used to describe the temporal and spatial piecemeal repair activities whereby new viable bone replaces old necrotic bone.

Regardless of the origin of the donor transplant material, a common term used to describe repair of the bone transplant is "incorporation." Incorporation is the process of uniting the host tissue to the transplant material as well as the envelopment and admixture of necrotic and viable new bone. The mechanisms of incorporation for cancellous and cortical bone are similar, although some differences exist. Incorporation also varies between autogenous and allogeneic tissues.

The incidence of graft-to-host union and creeping substitution repair reflects a biologic acceptance of the transplant, while later remodeling of the template assures the subsequent functional usefulness of the transplant. The process of incorporation is primarily the function of the recipient bed and depends on the close contact with viable donor tissue. The inherent variables for incorporation are the proliferative activities of osteoconduction, and biomechanical properties of the graft and site. Incorporation is also somewhat dependent upon physiologic skeletal metabolism, and the age of the recipient [2].

The histology of autogenous cortical or cancellous transplant incorporation and repair has some definite similarities as well as some obvious differences. During the first two weeks post-transplantation, areas of coagulated blood or hematomas are evident in the transplant beds. Coagulated blood does not play a significant role in the transplant repair process. During the first week, the transplants are the focus of inflammation and vascular buds infiltrating the transplant bed [3, 4, 5]. The rapidity with which a graft will be revascularized depends somewhat on whether it is cancellous or cortical graft material.

Two weeks after transplantation, the transplant and its bed become increasingly dominated by fibrous granulation tissue. Osteoclasts, although seen as early as four days after transplantation, become conspicuous by the tenth day [6]. Within the transplant, cells which have not been maintained by diffusion of nutrients through adequate graft revascularization, undergo necrosis: osteocytic autolysis is delineated by vacant lacunae. The necrotic tissue in the Haversian and Volkmann spaces are gradually removed by macrophages [7, 8] which precedes the invasion of capillary ingrowth. Some cells at the periphery of the grafts are maintained by passive diffusion of nutrients from the surrounding host soft tissues and these cells may play a participatory role in graft repair [5].

Secondary Histologic Features of Autografts

The secondary events of graft repair are dictated by the microanatomy or architecture of the tissue. Thus, cancellous bone transplants differ from cortical bone transplants by the rate of revascularization, the mechanism of creeping substitutional repair, and the completeness of the repair. The porous architecture of cancellous bone permits more rapid and complete revascularization of the tissue then is usually seen with cortical grafts. The consequence of this revascularization is a more complete replacement of the grafted material. The entire revascularization process of cancellous grafts may be completed within two weeks [5].

As the vascular invasion of cancellous transplants proceeds, primitive mesenchymal cells differentiate into osteogenic cells. Unlike in cortical transplants, the osteogenic cells differentiate into osteoblasts, and deposit a seam of osteoid upon the necrotic trabecular surfaces [9]. Thus, an initial increase in the density of the material or increased radioopaqueness develops, as seen on an x-ray film. The entrapped necrotic trabecular cores are gradually resorbed by osteoclasts with concomitant decrease in radiodensity as incorporation is consolidated and stress is transmitted to the grafted site. In time, the cancellous material tends to be completely replaced by viable new bone for necrotic bone.

Cortical bone autografts revascularize slowly, with the cortical interior being penetrated no earlier than one week, or at least twice the span of time required for cancellous tissue. The delay in revascularization may be attributed to the cortical architecture since vascular penetration of the transplant is primarily the result of peripheral osteoclastic resorption concomitant with vascular endothelial cells migrating into

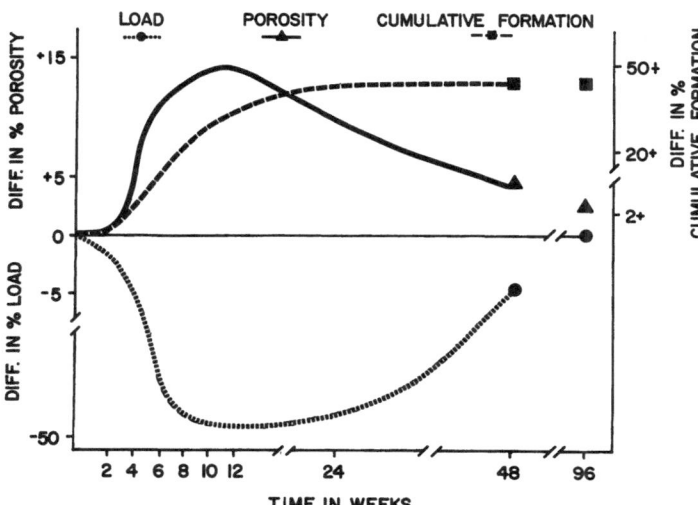

Fig. 1. The graph illustrates the quantitative and temporal relationship between the physical integrity and the biological processes of repair within a segmental cortical bone transplant. The initial persistence of strength (0–4 weeks after transplantation) indicates that the subsequent loss was due to reparative processes rather than to any intrinsic weakness in necrotic unrepaired bone. The sudden loss in strength in 6 weeks is caused by the increased internal porosity. From 6-12 weeks, the decrease in mechanical strength persists at approximately 50 percent less than normal. Porosity continues to increase until the 12th week due to the temporal lag in the apposition of new bone. At 24 weeks there is no real improvement in strength despite reduced porosity of the transplant and some maturation of the callus. At 48 weeks, however, the physical integrity of the transplant is normal because of decreased porosity. By 2 years, the physical integrity of the transplant and the internal porosity of the grafted material is normal. The biological incompleteness of repair (about 50 percent of the graft is viable) is insignificant because mechanical strength of the transplant is retained. The admixture of necrotic and viable bone will remain for years and probably for the life of the individual as a function of the individual's skeletal metabolic activity

peripheral Volkmann and Haversian canals. The pattern of cortical graft revascularization then follows pre-existing canals from the periphery into the interior [2, 3, 5, 10].

The revascularization pattern of cortical autografts influences the second histologic difference between cancellous and cortical bone repair. Unlike the initial osteoblastic new bone formation process seen in cancellous repair, the repair of cortical grafts is initiated by osteoclasts. In a temporal and spatial study (Fig. 1), resorptive activities followed the revascularization pattern of moving from the periphery towards the interior [2]. Thus, resorption of cortical autografts was initiated at its periphery as early as two weeks after transplantation with a preference to remove necrotic Haversian systems and interstitial lamellae. By the fourth week, resorption of the cortical interior was finally equivalent to the resorptive activities at the periphery. The resorptive process within the cortical interior enlarged Haversian canals, and proceeded with little removal of interstitial lamellae. When the appropriate cavity size was attained, somewhere between 75 and 250 microns, resorption ceased, and osteoblasts appeared and refilled the spaces.

The initiation of new bone formation in the cortical grafts seals off the remaining necrotic material from further osteoclastic encroachment. In the experimental temporal and spatial studies, significant bone formation usually occurred twelve weeks after transplantation and coincided with a consolidated graft-host junction, suggesting that physiologic stress may trigger bone formation via Wolff's Law. Additional studies suggested that creeping substitution of cortical bone grafts progressed transversely and parallel to the long axis of the transplanted segment [11].

The admixture of necrotic and viable bone in the cortical autograft remains basically unaltered once catabolic and anabolic stages of repair have been completed. In the experimental study (Fig. 1), the proportion of viable new bone to necrotic old bone increased from two weeks to six months. However, between six months and two years, the proportions remained static at roughly fifty percent [2]. Therefore, the third major difference between cortical and cancellous bone grafts is that cancellous grafts tend to be completely repaired, while cortical grafts tend to remain as admixtures of necrotic and viable bone.

A qualifying feature in any reparative process is the physiologic state of the individual. Thus, the rate, amount, and completeness of repair were found to be greater in the experimental animals that had more active physiologic remodeling than in those with less activity [2].

Two questions that remain to be answered with autogenous cortical grafts are: 1) What factors trigger the resorptive and appositional phases; and 2) What factors direct repair toward necrotic Haversian systems and not toward the interstitial lamellae?

Autograft Histology and Mechanical Properties

The strengths of a bone graft can be correlated with the process of repair [2]. Cancellous transplants are repaired by a process that first forms new bone onto the necrotic bony surfaces. The mere necrosis of bone does not alter the mechanical properties in a meaningful way. Thus, cancellous transplants tend first to be mechanically strengthened by the addition of new bone, and then, as the necrotic cores of bone are removed, the mechanical strength of transplanted areas tend to return to normal.

Conversely, cortical grafts are initially repaired by osteoclastic activity, which not only causes a loss of bone mass, but also induces mechanical weakening through stress risers with a concomitant decrease in the transplant's radiodensity. The weakening of the cortical transplant is therefore a function of the internal porosity (Fig. 1), which is caused by the cumulative effects of increased osteoclastic and decreased osteoblastic activities. Thus, experimental bone transplants are shown to be approximately 40 to 50 percent weaker than normal bone from 6 weeks to 6 months after transplantation as the porosity of the transplant increases approximately 15 percent [2]. By the end of 1 and 2 years following transplantation, the porosity is once again nearly normal, and mechanical strength and roentgenographic densities are equal to those of normal bone.

The importance of understanding the biodynamic effects of creeping substitutional repair by the clinician and patient is to protect the segmental transplants at the critical time when the resorptive phase has outstripped the appositional phase. It is not known precisely when these critical phases occur in humans, although the time of appearance probably varies as a function of age, physiologic repair capacity, and the type, size, and location of the transplant.

Bone Allograft Functional Result and Histology

The clinical and experimental superiority of an autograft over an allograft has been well documented. While autografts are regarded as the "Gold" standard, the comparison to allogeneic tissue can be argued to be spacious: 400–500,000 bone allografts are transplanted each year in the U.S. with apparent functional success equivalent to autografts. The autografts are recognized as "self", whereas the allograft and xenograft are recognized as "non-self" as a consequence of genetic disparity between the donor and the recipient [12, 13, 14]. Despite this lack of histocompatibility between the donor and the recipient, allografts generally proceed to a satisfactory clinical result, although at a slower rate than autogenous grafts [15, 16].

The historical experience with osteochondral, intercalary, and morsellized allografts indicates that the use of donar-allogeneic bone is a satisfactory approach to patient management. In 1925, Lexer described good clinical results in 50 percent of the cases studied, which included hemijoints and whole-joint transplants [17]. In 1966, Ottolenghi reported satisfaction with seven osteochondral allografts [18]. In 1973, Parrish reported that 70 percent of 21 patients with osteochondral allografts were satisfactory [19]. In 1969 and 1976, Spence and co-authors, and Schneider and Bright demonstrated the successful use of freeze-dried cancellous or cortical materials in treating cysts and promoting back fusion [20, 21]. In 1976 and 1983, Mankin and co-authors reported that 75 percent of over 200 large allograft cases were successful, with nonunion and infection rates between 10 and 15 percent [16, 22]. These clinical reports suggest the feasibility of allograft transplantation, despite genetic disparity between the donor and the recipient and, therefore, there are possible limitations to the use of allogeneic tissues.

The histologic features of allograft incorporation vary as a function of the genetic disparity and result in three possible alternatives according to experimental studies which are as follows: 1) accepted as an autogenous graft; 2) indolently accepted because of some genetic disparity; and 3) rejected because of strong genetic differences [23, 24]. In a six-month experimental study using the fibula as an allograft in a dog, three basic courses of allograft repair were observed. The first repair course reflected no apparent genetic transplantation differences between the donor and host and the allograft proceeded as if it were an autogenous graft. At the other end of the spectrum, the second repair course reflected strong genetic transplantation differences between the donor and the host as the allograft was rapidly and completely resorbed. Roentgenographic, microradiographic, and tetracycline fluorescence suggested that this vigorous rejection of an allograft occurs by continuous resorption at the periphery without any creeping substitutional repair.

The third allograft repair rests somewhere inbetween the two extremes to the spectrum and is characterized by a chronic and less marked genetic transplantation difference between the donor and the host. This repair course is characterized by: 1) nonunion or delayed graft-host union; 2) an increased incidence of fatigue fractures concomitant with the loss of the transplant's diameter; 3) considerably less internal repair than that seen for autografts; and 4) the formation of a callus that bridges the transplanted segments. Despite the formation of a bridging callus, the allografts are structurally weak since fatigue fractures and nonunions frequently occur.

The initial histologic response of the host to a fresh allograft, regardless of genetic disparity, is similar to that of an autograft. At the end of the first week post-transplantation, an inflammatory response is seen at the periphery of the graft [12, 25, 26, 27, 28]. The inflammatory reaction reaches peak activity toward the end of the second week. Lymphocytes may continue to predominate, and a fibrous tissue that encapsulates the allograft may develop during the next two months [29]. This inflammatory response, depending upon the genetic disparity between the donor and the recipient, may continue as a chronic inflammatory response for up to 8 months or longer [25, 29].

As a consequence of the initial histologic response, the regenerating vascular pattern around the allograft is less extensive than that for autografts [14]. By the end of the first week, the vessels become occluded because of inflammatory cells, with subsequent hyalinization being apparent [14, 12]. With the collapse of the vascular network, progressive necrosis of the periosteal cells may ensue [12, 25, 27], but a viable periosteal membrane is usually found.

The rate at which a transplant is incorporated into the host skeleton indicates, in part, whether the transplant is accepted or rejected. Successful incorporation includes the formation of callus around the transplant-host junction and internal repair of the transplant. New bone formation has been observed at the periphery of the autograft within the first week, with a maximal osteogenic peak near the end of the first week [30]. A similar process occurs in the allograft just prior to the immunologically driven vascular shutdown.

Once the allograft undergoes necrosis as a result of vascular insufficiency, a second phase of osteogenesis may be initiated by the host approximately 4 weeks after transplantation [10, 25, 31, 32]. This second osteogenic phase in allografts is not as prominent as the osteogenesis in fresh autografts since remodeling characteristics at 2 months are relatively inapparent throughout the allogeneic transplant [26, 27, 33, 34, 35].

The experimental histology previously described is not unlike the histology seen in patients having had deep-frozen allografts between 4 months and 3 years. Several prominent histologic characteristics were noted in recovered specimens: 1) union of the allograft to the host occurred routinely by callus formed both periosteally and endosteally; 2) the incorporative creeping substitution of necrotic bone with viable bone usually seen in autografts was strongly limited, if not absent, in the allografts; 3) the host-soft tissue attachment to the allografts is somewhat tenuous compared with that seen with autografts, and is accomplished by the formation of a thin zone (20 to 80 microns) of new bone.

The characteristics of allograft bony union to the host, limited remodeling, and modest periosteal new bone with soft tissue attachments suggest that the allograft is conditionally accepted by the host. The allograft appears to act more as a biologically inert material and may therefore be less able to respond to changing stresses (i.e. it is not a typical admixture of necrotic and viable new bone as seen with the autograft and the material may thus be more susceptible to fatiguing stresses). Conversely, if stress fractures should result in these grafts, fracture healing can occur because of a new viable host bone and periosteum encompassing the allograft. The features of graft-host union, limited graft remodeling, and a viable periosteum indicate the potential usefulness of allografts in appropriate clinical settings. The limitations of the graft material, however, still need to be identified.

References

1. Chase SN, Herndon CH (1955) The fate of autogenous and homogenous bone grafts: A historical review. J Bone Joint Surg 37A: 809
2. Enneking WF, Burchardt H, Puhl JJ, et al (1962) Physical and biological aspects of repair in dog cortical bone transplants. J Bone Joint Surg 57A: 232
3. Abbott LC, Schottstaedt ER, Saunders JB, et al (1947) The evaluation of cortical and cancellous bone as grafting material: A clinical and experimental study. J Bone Joint Surg 29: 381
4. Arora BK, Laskin DM (1964) Sex chromatin as a cellular label of osteogenesis by bone grafts. J Bone Joint Surg 46A: 1269

5. Deleu J, Trueta J (1965) Vascularization of bone grafts in the anterior chamber of the eye. J Bone Joint Surg 47B: 319

6. Heslop BF, Zeiss IM, Nisbet NW (1960) Studies on transference of bone: I. A comparison of autologous and homologous implants with reference to osteocyte survival, osteogenesis and host reaction. Br J Exp Pathol 41: 269

7. Anderson KJ, LeCocq JF, Akeson WH, et al (1964) End-point result of processed heterogenous, autogenous and homogenous bone transplants in the human: A histologic study. Clin Orthop 33: 220

8. Richany SF, Sprinz H, Kraner K, et al (1965) The role of the diaphyseal medulla in the repair and regeneration of the femoral shaft in the adult cat. J Bone Joint Surg 47A: 1565

9. Urist MR, McLean FC (1952) Osteogenic potency of new bone formation by induction in transplants to the anterior chamber of the eye. J Bone Joint Surg 34A: 443

10. Hammack BL, Enneking WF (1960) Comparative vascularization of autogenous and homogenous bone transplants. J Bone Joint Surg 42A: 811

11. Stevenson JS, Bright RW, Dunson GL, et al (1973) Technetium-99m phosphate bone imaging: A method for assessing bone graft healing. Radiology 110: 391

12. Enneking WF (1957) Histological investigation of bone transplants in immunologically prepared animals. J Bone Joint Surg 39A: 597

13. Langer F, Czitrom A, Pritzker KP, et al (1975) The immunogenicity of fresh and frozen allogeneic bone. J Bone Joint Surg 57A: 216

14. Zeiss IM, Nesbet NW, Heslop BF (1960) Studies on transference of bone. II. Vascularization of autologous and homologous implants of cortical bone in rats. Br J Exp Pathol 41: 345

15. Kruez FP, Hyatt GW, Turner TC, et al (1951) The preservation and clinical use of freeze-dried bone. J Bone Joint Surg 33A: 863

16. Mankin HJ, Doppelt SH, Tomford WW (1983) Clinical experience with allograft implantation. Clin Orthop 174: 69

17. Lexer E (1925) Joint transplantation and arthoplasty. Surg Gynecol Obstet 40: 782

18. Ottolenghi CE (1966) Massive osteoarticular bone grafts. J Bone Joint Surg 48B: 646

19. Parrish FF (1973) Allograft replacement of all or part of the end of a long bone following excision of a tumor: Report of twenty-one cases. J Bone Joint Surg 55A: 1

20. Schneider JR, Bright RW (1976) Anterior cervical fusion using preserved bone allografts. Transplant Proc S [Suppl 1]: 73

21. Spence KF, Bright PW, Fitzgerald SP, et al (1976) Solitary unicameral bone cyst: Treatment with freeze-dried crushed cortical bone allograft: a review of one hundred forty-four cases. J Bone Joint Surg 58A: 636

22. Mankin HJ, Fogelson FS, Trasher AZ, et al (1976) Massive resection and allograft transplantation in the treatment of malignant bone tumors. N Engl J Med 294: 1247

23. Bos GD, Goldbert VM, Powell AE, et al (1983) The effects of histocompatibility matching on canine frozen bone allografts. J Bone Joint Surg 65A: 89

24. Burchardt H, Glowczewskie FP, Enneking WF (1977) Allogenic segmental fibular transplants in azathioprine-immunosuppressed dogs. J Bone Joint Surg 59A: 881

25. Anderson KJ (1961) The behavior of autogenous and homogenous bone transplants in the anterior chamber of the rats' eye: A histological study of the effect of the size of the implant. J Bone Joint Surg 43A: 980

26. Bonfiglio M, Jeter WS (1972) Immunological responses to bone. Clin Orthop 87: 19–27

27. Bonfiglio M, Jeter WS Smith CL (1955) The immune concept: Its relation to bone transplantation. Ann NY Acad Sci 59: 417

28. Burwell RG, Gowland G (1962) Studies in the transplantation of bone: III. The immune responses of lymph nodes draining componants of fresh homologous cancellous bone and homologous bone treated by different methods. J Bone Joint Surg 44B: 131

29. Trentham DE, Townes AS, Kang AH, et al (1978) Humoral and cellular sensitivity to collagen in type II collagen induced arthritis in rats. J Clin Invest 61: 89

30. Anderson KJ, Schmidt J, Clawson DK (1959) The vascularization and cellular response induced by homogenous deproteinized bone transplants in the anterior chamber of the rat's eye. Plast Reconstr Surg 24: 97

31. Elves MW, Pratt LM (1975) The pattern of new bone formation in isografts of bone. Acta Orthop Scand 46: 549

32. Heiple KG, Chase SW, Herndon CH (1963) A comparative study of the healing process following different types of bone transplantation. J Bone Joint Surg 45A: 1593
33. Bonfiglio M, Jeter WS (1962) Further experimental studies on bone transplantation. J Bone Joint Surg 44A: 1029
34. Burwell RG (1963) Studies in the transplantation of bone: V. The capacity of fresh and treated homografts of bone to evoke transplantation immunity. J Bone Joint Surg 45B: 386
35. Goldberg VM, Lance EM (1972) Revascularization and accretion in transplantation: Quantitative study of the role of the allograft barrier. J Bone Joint Surg 54A: 807

Author's address: H. Burchardt, Ph.D., Executive Director, Pennsylvania Regional Tissue Bank, 814 Cedar Avenue, Scranton, Pennyslvania 18505, U.S.A.

Infectious Hazards of Bone Allograft Transplantation: Reducing the Risk*

T. Eastlund

Department of Laboratory Medicine and Pathology, University of Minnesota Hospitals and Clinic, Minneapolis, U.S.A.

Introduction

In recent years, due to the remarkable growth in cadaver tissue donation, the supply of donated bone and connective tissue allografts has greatly increased. The widened availability of these tissues has encouraged new clinical uses and has brought attention not only to their effectiveness and advantages over autografts but also to their drawbacks, side effects and complications. Infectious disease transmission is a serious concern for orthopedic surgeons and patients contemplating bone allograft use. Bacterial and viral diseases shown in Table 1 have been transmitted through the use of bone allografts [52, 62, 74]. Although bacteria and fungi can be introduced to the bone allograft during surgical removal from the donor or during bone processing, storage and implantation, this review will emphasize viral and bacterial diseases of donor origin and the important roles of donor screening and tissue processing, disinfection and sterilization for their prevention.

Bacterial Diseases

Bacterial infection due to a contaminated bone graft is rare. Lord et al. [83] observed one of 283 massive frozen bone allografts to be a cause of a postoperative infection. Tomford et al. [135] found one of 303 smaller freeze-dried bone grafts from the Navy Tissue Bank to be implicated in a recipient *Staphylococcus epidermidis* infection. These bacteria may have been donor-derived but were more likely acquired from the environment or surgeon at the time of procurement. Tomford et al. [136] reported an infection rate of about 5 percent in the use of 324 culture-negative, nonsterilized frozen bone allografts at the Massachusetts General Hospital. The bone allograft appeared responsible for infections in three patients, all of whom developed infection with *Serratia marcescens* and received bone from the same donor. They reported that postoperative bacterial infections following bone allograft use occurred at a rate that was not different from that observed following hip prosthesis surgery without the use of bone allograft. Others have reported bacterial infection as a complication of spinal surgery using bone allografts but, as a whole, the incidence was similar to that when using autograft [9, 79, 92, 137]. About

*This work was supported by funds from the American Red Cross.

Table 1. Infectious disease transmitted by bone allografts

Tissue	Infectious Disease	Reference
Cadaver Donor Bone	Bacteria	83, 135, 136
	HIV-1	126
	Hepatitis C Virus	43, 109
Living Donor Bone	HIV-1	38
	Hepatitis, unspecified	125
	Hepatitis C Virus	55
	Tuberculosis	72

40 years ago, several cases of tuberculosis infection of the spine were reported from the use of frozen rib allografts [72] in patients undergoing spinal fusion. The source of bone allograft was the rib resected during chest surgery from patients with active pulmonary tuberculosis who served as donors. Using current donor screening criteria, individuals with active or treated tuberculosis are excluded from donating [5, 31, 56, 86].

Viral Diseases

Hepatitis

Hepatitis has been caused by the use of refrigerated and frozen bone allografts, but not from bone grafts that were cleaned of cells and fat with water jetting and ethanol soaks prior to freeze drying or treated with sterilants such as gamma irradiation or ethylene oxide. In 1954, prior to the availability of viral hepatitis testing of donors, a Yale medical student received a refrigerated bone graft to treat a depressed fracture of the proximal tibia and developed viral hepatitis of unspecified type with jaundice 10 weeks later [125]. The bone graft was obtained from the amputated leg of a patient with occlusive vascular disease and gangrene. The donor had received blood transfusions three years previously. Otherwise, the donor was in good health, with normal liver function tests and without a history of jaundice or liver disease.

Three recent reports have documented that hepatitis C virus (HCV) can be transmitted from donor-to-recipient through the use of frozen, unprocessed bone allografts [43, 55, 109]. In a retrospective study using stored serum samples it was learned that HCV had been transmitted by the use of a frozen femoral head in orthopedic surgery two months after it had been donated by a patient undergoing hip arthroplasty [55]. This disease transmission was not preventable since testing of donors for HCV antibodies was not available at the time, a bone bank practice widespread since 1990. In another study, HCV was transmitted from an infected cadaveric tissue donor through frozen, unprocessed bone and tendon allografts, but not through freeze-dried bone allografts or frozen allografts that were treated with gamma irradiation [43]. In this study, the cadaver bone donor tested negative for HCV antibodies using a first generation test at the time of donation in 1990 but stored serum tested positive using a new, more sensitive test introduced two years later. In a report involving five HCV-infected organ and tissue donors, most of the recipients of frozen bone allografts did not become infected with HCV [109]. There have been no reports of hepatitis B virus transmission through bone transplantation.

Human Immunodeficiency Virus

It has been clearly demonstrated that viable HIV-1 can be recovered from bone, marrow and tendon of patients with acquired immunodeficiency syndrome (AIDS) [25, 94, 103, 117]. In 1984, a fatal HIV-1 infection was transmitted to a woman undergoing spinal fusion for scoliosis through the use of a frozen femoral head allograft. The femoral head had been donated during hip arthroplasty a few months earlier by a living donor who had a history of intravenous drug abuse and who had an enlarged lymph node that had been biopsied the previous year [38]. The donor and the bone recipient died of AIDS two years after the donation. A test for HIV-1 antibody was not available at the time of donation. This donor would not have been eligible to be a donor today due to this history of intravenous drug abuse.

A second case of HIV transmission through the use of frozen bone allografts involved a seronegative but HIV-infected cadaveric donor of multiple organs, corneas, bones, and connective tissues [126]. All three organ recipients and three of four recipients of frozen bone and tendon allografts became HIV infected. Follow-up testing of 34 recipients of other grafts from the donor showed they were all anti-HIV negative. This included the 25 recipients of freeze-dried bone and three recipients of freeze-dried fascia and tendon that had not been sterilized but had been cleansed of blood and marrow and treated with ethanol during processing. Similarly, the recipients of irradiated dura mater allografts did not become HIV infected. A test of the donor for HIV antibody was negative at the time of donation in October 1985, a few months after HIV test kits first became available. Between 1985 and 1991, there were several modifications which improved HIV antibody test kit sensitivity [129, 147]. Prior to 1989, HIV antibody was detectable a median of 63 days after initial infection [16, 69]. Using newer test kits in 1991, the seronegative interval was reported to be 45 days [110]. The HIV antibody test kits in use in 1991 detected twice as many infected individuals as did the 1985 test kits [101]. Today's HIV antibody test kits, introduced in 1992, are even more sensitive, detecting IgM, the earliest form of antibodies and shortening the seronegative interval by another 5 to 20 days to an estimated 20–25 days [30].

When donor medical history screening and selection processes are applied vigorously, the finding of HIV antibodies in bone donors is rare, with a prevalence not greatly different from that of voluntary blood donors [53, 63, 120, 121]. With the advent of excluding prospective donors with HIV risk factors and positive tests for HIV antibody, and especially with the addition of bone graft processing steps that include ethanol soaks and sterilization steps, the risk of HIV transmission by bone transplantation is now very remote, if not practically absent [8]. The risk of transmitting HIV through bone grafting has been calculated to be less than once in a million grafts, [26] and is even less if subjected to processing and sterilization steps using gamma irradiation or ethylene oxide.

Potential Transplant-transmitted Diseases

Syphilis

There have been no reports of syphilis being transmitted through bone grafts-probably due to the low prevalence in the screened donor population, absence of the organism in bone and low temperature storage of the graft which reduces infectivity. *Treponema pallidum*, the agent causing syphilis, does not survive when stored at 4°C beyond 72 hours [140]. However, the organism can remain viable if frozen with cryoprotectants such as dimethylsulfoxide or glycerol. Syphilis could possibly be transmitted if the graft is used immediately after donation and the donor is spirochetemic or if the bone contains the organism after the spirochete is cleared from the blood. During the incubation period and while a person is spirochetemic in the early stages of the illness, the syphilis screening test is negative. When testing becomes positive, the spirochetemia has resolved [11]. Thus, donor testing for syphilis, though commonly performed, is of dubious value. Donor screening tests, e.g., RPR and VDRL, are cardiolipin-based and are highly sensitive but nonspecific. Most reactive tests in donors are false-positives.

HTLV-I

Silent human T-lymphotropic virus (HTLV-I) infection has been transmitted from blood donors to transfusion recipients of cellular blood components but there have been no reports of HTLV-I transmission through bone allografts or other cadaveric organ and tissue grafts. HTLV-I is a retrovirus spread by routes somewhat similar to HIV-1 and if a person is infected it may be carried for life. However, infection doesn't usually cause clinically apparent disease and is common only in certain geographic locations such as Japan and the Caribbean. Infection may produce disease later in life. Approximately 0.25% of those infected have a life-time risk of developing tropical spastic paraparesis, also called HTLV-I associated myelopathy [75]. If infected at age 50, the life-time risk is 0.1%. The life-time risk of developing acute T-cell lymphoma-leukemia is approximately 2–4% in those infected as children [37]. While there have been few reports of these clinical disease transmitted by transfusion, HTLV-I screening of blood donors is routine in the USA but not in Europe [7]. National professional standards require HTLV-I testing of bone allograft donors in the U.S. [5, 31, 86] but it is not a requirement of federal regulations [6].

Creutzfeldt-Jakob Disease

Creutzfeldt-Jakob disease (CJD) occurs in the general population at a rate of one per million and is a fatal, rapidly-progressive dementing disease usually accompanied by myoclonus and characteristic electroencephalographic abnormalities. The disease is transmissible and is caused by a small infectious protein. There have been no reported cases of CJD from the use of bone allografts, but CJD has been transmitted from cadaveric tissue donors through use of pituitary-derived growth hormone and gonadotropin [23, 24], cornea, pericardium [122] and dura mater grafts [39, 85, 90, 133, 145]. Eight reports of CJD worldwide involved dura allografts obtained from a single German medical device manufacturer and transplanted in 1984 and 1985 [85, 145]. Several factors may have contributed to this outbreak: pooling of dura from multiple cadavers during processing and possibly obtaining dura from individuals who may have been demented. There is no diagnostic blood test for CJD; therefore, it is essential that tissue donor selection procedures exclude those who may have or suspected to have CJD. The importance of excluding prospective tissue donors with dementia is underscored by studies showing that 18% of patients with CJD initially presented with dementia as an isolated symptom [21] and 5% of those diagnosed with Alzheimer disease were shown to have CJD at autopsy [14]. Since national professional standards in the U.S. prohibit pooling of tissue from multiple donors during processing and do not allow donation by persons who have received pituitary-derived growth hormone or have dementia or other neurologic symptoms, it seems unlikely that CJD will pose a serious threat to the safety of bone allograft use.

The CJD infectious agent is surprisingly resistant to the usual sterilants and disinfectants but is susceptible to sodium hydroxide [20, 22]. Sodium hydroxide solubilizes proteins but if it were applied to bone it is uncertain whether it would impair the material properties or the osteoinductive function of bone allografts. It is also unknown whether sodium hydroxide can penetrate dense bone or can persist in the bone after processing [76]. Bone banks have not routinely adopted sodium hydroxide treatment of bone grafts since the prevalence of CJD is low in the general population and the risk is remote in carefully screened tissue donors, who are free of dementia or other neurologic symptoms and who have not received human pituitary growth hormone.

Other Potentially-Transmissible Diseases

Although rabies has been transmitted through transplantation of corneas [34, 35, 70] obtained from donors who had acute febrile and fatal neurologic illnesses, there have been no reports of transmission through bone, tendon or fascia allografts. Human organ transplants and human skin allografts have the capacity to transmit cytomegalovirus [1, 3, 41, 123] and parvovirus [48] infections, but there have been no reports of transmission to bone graft recipients. *Borellia burgdorfia* has been isolated from bone and articular cartilage of patients with Lyme disease but there have been no reports of transmission through bone transplantation. The granulomatous disease sarcoidosis involves bone in 10% of patients and is not generally considered an infectious illness. Although there was a report of transmission of sarcoidosis from donor-to-recipient through heart transplantation [28], there has been none reported through bone transplantation. Various protozoans (malaria, toxoplasmosis, Chagas' disease) have been transmitted through blood transfusion and organ transplantation but not through bone allografts.

Reducing the Risk by Donor Selection

To minimize the risk of transmission of infectious disease, several approaches taken by surgeons and bone banks have been important. An important initial approach by the surgeon is to use bone allografts judiciously, only when needed, and to consider the use of autografts, alternative nonhuman graft material, or sterilized bone allografts whenever possible. Bone transplantation is usually an elective, nonurgent surgical procedure using stored bone allografts. Storage prior to use permits further donor selection steps, blood infectious disease testing, a donor physical examination, and a review of autopsy results if an autopsy was performed (Table 2). Although there have been no carefully controlled prospective studies of bone allograft recipients to determine the true incidence of disease transmission, there is good reason to believe that these donor screening procedures and the effectiveness of processing and sterilization to reduce or eliminate bacteria and virus result in an extremely low risk of transmitting disease. Important initial steps are exercised by the bone bank by excluding those prospective cadaveric donors suspected to be at risk for HIV, hepatitis, or other viral or bacteriologic infections.

Cadaveric Bone Donor Selection

The final determination of suitability of a living or cadaveric bone donor to ensure that the donated bone allograft is safe and effective is made by the bone bank physician.

Table 2. Bone allograft donor screening steps

Medical and Social History-interview with next of kin

> Exclude those with infection, malignancy, HIV or hepatitis risk behaviors

Physical Examination

> IV drug abuse
> Signs of HIV infection
> Unexplained jaundice

Blood Tests

> anti-HIV-1/HIV-2[a,b,c]
> HbsAg[a,b,c]
> anti-HCV[a,b,c]
> syphilis[b,c]
> anti-HTLV-1[c]

Autopsy results, if performed

[a]Required by U.S. Federal regulation [6]
[b]Required by European Association of Tissue banks [56]
[c]Required by American Association of Tissue Banks [86]

Table 3. Medical history exclusions from bone allograft donation

Presence of infection
Presence or history of malignant disease
Presence of degenerative neurologic disease including dementia
Use of human pituitary-derived growth hormone
Connective tissue disorder or vasculitis
High dose corticosteroid use
Significant exposure to toxic substances
Irradiation to donated tissue
HIV or hepatitis risk behaviors

Minimum donor requirements have been set by national professional standards [5, 31, 56, 86], governmental guidelines [40], and federal regulation [6]. Donor eligibility is determined by means of medical and social history, blood tests, physical examination, and autopsy, if performed. Initial donor selection is based on the donor's medical history and circumstances surrounding the death. Donors are excluded if elements of the past medical and social history or recent hospitalization indicate a risk of infection, malignant disease, or inferior quality of tissue (Table 3). The legal consenting next of kin or life partner of a cadaveric bone donor or both must be directly interviewed to determine whether HIV and hepatitis risk behaviors (Table 4) were present [5, 31, 40, 56, 86]. Persons with HIV or hepatitis risk behaviors are excluded from donation. Age criteria are set to ensure skeletal maturity. The presence of other conditions, such as chronic corticosteroid use and advanced age which can weaken donated bone, will exclude bone donation particularly if the bone graft is for load-bearing applications.

The next screening step is a limited physical examination performed by bone bank staff at the time of cadaveric bone donation. The body is examined for signs of illegal drug use and signs of HIV infection, hepatitis and other infection or trauma over bodily sites that can affect the quality of donated bone.

Table 4. HIV and Hepatitis risk behaviors excluding bone allograft donation

Men who have had sex with other men in past five years
Nonmedical injection of drugs-intravenous, intramuscular, or subcutaneous in past five years
Exchanged sex for money or drugs in past five years
Receipt of coagulation factor concentrates
Persons with evidence of HIV infection*
Sex with any of the above in past 12 months
Diagnosis or treatment of syphilis or gonorrhea in the past 12 months
Explosure to known or potentially HIV-infected blood through percutaneous inoculation or
    through contact with an open wound, nonintact skin, or mucous membrane during the past
    12 months
Tattoo within past 12 months
Resident in penal institution
Clinical history of viral hepatitis

---

*Signs and symptoms are unexplained weight loss, night sweats, spots typical of Kaposi's sarcoma on
    or under the skin or mucous membranes, swollen lymph nodes lasting more than one month,
    persistent white spots or unusual blemishes in the mouth, fevers greater than 99 °F for more than 10
    days, persistent cough and shortness of breath, persistent diarrhea.

The minimum blood tests of cadaveric bone donors set by national professional standards include anti-HIV-1/HIV-2, HBsAg, anti-HTLV-I, anti-HCV and syphilis [31, 86]. U.S. federal regulation requires only HBsAg, anti-HIV and anti-HCV [6]. HIV antigen testing of the donor is not performed by most tissue banks. Large scale studies of low-risk [4] and high-risk [29] blood donor populations in the U.S. demonstrated a lack of utility for HIV antigen screening. Testing did not detect HIV-infected donors beyond those already detected by testing for HIV antibodies. However, in countries with a higher incidence of HIV infections, donor testing for HIV p24 antigen may be useful [102]. Studies are under way to determine whether testing donors for genomic HIV by polymerase chain reaction (PCR) has utility. One study of 1,424 cadaver bone donors showed that blood testing for HIV-1 antigen and genomic HIV by PCR did not detect additional HIV infected cadaveric bone donors [64]. All 1,424 donors negative for HIV-1 antibodies were also negative in testing for HIV DNA by PCR. No additional HIV infected donors could be confirmed using PCR testing. Although PCR is exquisitely sensitive, it may be premature to routinely apply it to cadaver donor testing in the U.S. due to the low HIV prevalence in the donor population, its uncertain positive utility, its false positive rate as well as its false negative rate due to hemoglobin contamination. Cadaveric blood samples are frequently contaminated by hemoglobin due to red cell hemolysis and this has interfered with blood test results [100, 108]. Testing for HIV DNA by PCR requires whole cells and reliance on results is hampered by the unreliability of cadaveric post mortem blood samples for extracting peripheral blood white cells immediately after collection or after frozen storage [2].

Many bone banks test donors for hepatitis B core antibodies, a test originally introduced for blood donors as a surrogate for detecting non-A, non-B hepatitis carriers. The utility of this test has been diminished since adding the test for antibodies to hepatitis C virus, the major cause of non-A, non-B hepatitis [13]. Blood cultures are often obtained to aid in determining whether the donor is infected, particularly if the donor was hospitalized with prolonged use of mechanically assisted ventilation or indwelling intravenous catheters, both of which increase the risk for bacteremia. Lastly, autopsies of donors are not generally required but, if performed, a final donor suitability determination is not made until the results of the autopsy have been reviewed by the bone bank physician [5, 31, 56, 86]. Autopsy findings that have disqualified donors include previously undiagnosed malignancy, widespread granulomas, abscess, and pneumonia.

Living Bone Donor Selection

Femoral heads can be donated by persons undergoing hip arthroplasty. Donor medical history screening and testing requirements are similar to those for cadaver bone donors, except that the donor medical history interview can be made directly and a retest for HIV and HCV antibodies is required 180 days following donation [31, 36, 86]. The retest permits identification of donors who were recently infected with HIV or HCV but seronegative at the time of donation. To date, this retest has not demonstrated utility.

Cadaveric Bone Collection

The collection of bone allografts from the cadaveric donor begins as soon as possible after death in order to reduce the risk of endogenous or exogenous bacterial contamination and to maximize the material and osteoinductive properties of the donated bone. National professional standards require bone recovery to be completed within 12 hours of death, or if the body is refrigerated, within 24 hours of death [5, 31, 56, 86]. Recovery of bone takes place in the hospital operating room or morgue, using careful aseptic technique after removing hair and cleansing the skin with antiseptics and covering non-operative sites with sterile drapes in the usual surgical fashion.

Quality of Cadaver Blood Samples

The testing of cadaveric tissue donor serum for infectious disease markers may be complicated by gross hemolysis of specimens [108] causing false positive results for hepatitis B surface antigen and HIV-1 p24 antigen depending upon the test kit used [100]. The presence of hemoglobin can also cause false-negative results when testing for HIV and HCV by PCR [2].

Reducing the Risk by Bone Processing and Sterilization

Bone allografts are usually heavily processed, soaked in antibiotics, purged of extraneous tissue, marrow and blood, exposed to ethanol, and often are sterilized. These processing steps further reduce if not eliminate the potential of infectious disease transmission [8].

Allograft Processing and Infectious Risk

The U.S.P.H.S./Centers for Disease Control recommends processing of bone and bone fragments and evacuation of all marrow components from whole bone wherever feasible to reduce the risk of HIV infection [40]. Most bone allografts are processed and freeze-dried with a moisture content less than 5% by weight. This permits convenient storage at room temperature. Freeze-drying itself does not inactivate microbes but indeed can preserve viability of infectious viruses and bacteria. However, prior to freeze-drying, bone undergoes other processing steps which reduce or eliminate viable organisms [8, 126]. Bone is debrided and water jetted to remove extraneous tissues, marrow and blood to a large extent. Following this most bone banks soak the bone in ethanol, which removes lipids and serves as a disinfectant. Ethanol has the capacity to kill HIV, other viruses and certain bacteria [15, 80, 116, 144]. Viruses such as hepatitis B, hepatitis C are inactivated by ethanol but those without a lipid soluble envelope such as parvovirus and hepatitis A virus are not [15, 80].

Bone Allograft Sterilization

Sterilization of bone allografts has been accomplished by several methods, including heat (boiling, autoclaving, pasteurizing), chemicals (ethylene oxide, glutaraldehyde, formaldehyde, iodophors), and gamma irradiation. In vitro antibiotic treatment prior to storage of bone in the frozen state is a surface decontaminant effective only against bacteria. Gamma irradiation and ethylene oxide are the most commonly used sterilants for bone allografts. The AATB surveyed bone bank practices during 1987 and 1988. Of those subjecting bone allografts to a sterilization process, two thirds reported using ethylene oxide, and one third, gamma irradiation [97]. A survey of AATB-accredited tissue banks in 1992 showed a trend away from the use of ethylene oxide, with sterilization by irradiation used twice as often as ethylene oxide [130]. Experimental studies have shown that HIV in bone can be inactivated during bone processing and exposure to sterilization steps such as heat, [54], ethylene oxide [54], gamma irradiation [32, 44, 45, 58, 67, 77, 128, 134], as well as ethanol [116, 144] and hydrochloric acid used during bone graft processing and demineralization [93].

Bone Allograft Sterilization by Gamma Irradiation-Effectiveness of Irradiation

The effectiveness of gamma irradiation for inactivating bacteria and viruses is well documented [17, 32, 44, 45, 58, 67, 77, 124, 128, 131] The minimum bacteriocidal level of gamma irradiation is 1 to 2 Mrads [19, 50, 139]. The minimum virucidal level for HIV is about 0.25 Mrads [128], but for other viruses, such as poliovirus, it may be up to 4 Mrads [50]. The dose required to eliminate all viable HIV-1 from bone depends on the amount of virus originally present. The dose of irradiation (the D_{10} value) needed to reduce the population of viable HIV by 90 percent (a one-log reduction) is 0.4 Mrad [44, 45]. Knowing this and the highest concentrations of HIV reported during the early acute infection [10, 46, 49, 51, 60, 68, 146], it can be estimated that 1.2 Mrad will bring the highest expected concentration of HIV to a single virion (a three-log reduction). Adding another 1.2 Mrad for a total dose of 2.4 Mrad (another three-log reduction) reduces the chance to one in a million of finding a single viable virion present, if the unprocessed bone was freshly derived from an acutely infected donor. Others have confirmed that 2.5 Mrad will reduce HIV concentrations by six logs [67, 77]. Campbell et al. [32] loaded dense bone with infectious HIV at concentrations 10 to 15 fold greater than that expected in human HIV infection and found that 2.5 Mrad was needed to eradicate infectivity. Fideler and associates [58] found that higher doses of irradiation (4 to 5 Mrad) are required to alter HIV DNA nucleic acid sequences sufficiently to render HIV in tendon undetectable by polymerase chain reaction (PCR). However, lower doses of irradiation can completely inactivate HIV despite leaving the nonviable, noninfectious HIV DNA detectable by PCR. Their study did not determine the dose required to render HIV nonviable and noninfectious.

Clinical Effectiveness of Irradiated Bone

Gamma irradiation of bone was introduced over 30 years ago [139] and is used widely. Uncontrolled human studies showed that irradiated calcified [12, 50, 66, 89, 139] and demineralized [61, 127] bone grafts are clinically effective. Numerous studies have shown that mineralized bone allografts irradiated at 2.5 to 3 Mrad are clinically effective. Clinical success rates of 85–92 percent are reported [83, 88, 89, 148]. In controlled studies, the clinical effectiveness of bone allografts subjected to 2.5 Mrad irradiation was comparable to nonirradiated bone allografts [88]. Irradiated demineralized bone has active osteoinductive activity and has been effective in nonstructural clinical applications.

Gamma Irradiation and Osteoinductive Properties

Irradiated bone allografts must promote new bone formation, incorporation and fusion with host bone to be clinically effective. Controlled studies of animals grafted with frozen [107] or freeze-dried [115] bone allografts subjected to 1 to 2.5 Mrad irradiation showed equal effectiveness and no reduction in bone formation when compared with autografts. In contrast, other controlled animal studies show that irradiation with 2.5 Mrad irradiation or greater causes a 20 percent [61] to 60 percent [27, 141] reduction in the capacity of demineralized bone grafts to induce ossification. Sherman and Hollinger [124] showed that irradiation with 1 to 4 Mrad caused a partial reduction of the osteoinductive capacity of demineralized bone in a dose-dependent fashion, whereas Weintroub and Reddi [143] showed that doses of 3 to 5 Mrad enhanced osteoinduction. In their study, the osteoinductive capacity of bone grafts was not reduced until doses of irradiation reached 5 to 15 Mrad. Ferraro and colleagues have also showed enhanced osteoinduction following bone allograft irradiation of 2 to 3 Mrad [57, 96]. Other recent studies have shown that irradiation at 1 to 1.5 Mrad does not reduce the osteoinductive capacity of demineralized bone powder [112] and that 1.6 to 1.9 Mrad does not diminish transforming growth factor-beta activity of demineralized bone [113].

Gamma Irradiation and Mechanical Properties

Several studies have shown that gamma irradiation at a dose of 3 Mrad or less has little deleterious effect on the mechanical properties of frozen bone [18, 19, 104–106, 138]. Above this, resistance to breaking by torsion and bending is reduced, with less effect on resistance to compression. Rutherford and Kateley found that 2 Mrad irradiation significantly reduced the strength of lyophilized dowels if irradiated after lyophilization, but not if irradiated during frozen storage prior to lyophilization [118]. Others have confirmed this effect if the allograft is lyophilized prior to irradiation [18, 19]. These data suggest that bone irradiated at high doses (>2.5 Mrad) might not be the best choice when the graft is primarily subjected to torsional loads, whereas the use of lyophilized or frozen bone irradiated at lower doses is acceptable when a graft is subjected to bending or compressive loads or if the graft is not subjected to mechanical stress.

Sterilization of Bone Allografts by Ethylene Oxide Gas

The introduction of ethylene oxide gas as an effective bone sterilant by Cloward [42] and Prolo and associates [114] over a decade ago simplified bone processing technology and facilitated the widespread use of sterilized air-dried and freeze-dried bone allografts. Ethylene oxide has an excellent track record as an effective sterilant in general and can inactivate HIV-1 within dense bone [54]. Ethylene oxide does not appear to have deleterious effects on bone mechanical properties; however, its impact, separated from the effects caused by lyophilization, has not been well studied. Although many studies have conflicting conclusions, ethylene oxide treatment does not seem to seriously reduce the clinical effectiveness of bone allografts. Uncontrolled studies in humans show that ethylene oxide-sterilized calcified bone grafts are clinically effective [42, 119] and are in wide use [97, 130]. Controlled studies in animals demonstrate that repair of bone defects with lyophilized calcified bone grafts is not affected by sterilization with ethylene oxide [114]. Bone grafts induce ossification more rapidly if they have been demineralized, exposing bone cell proliferation- and differentiation-promoting factors within bone matrix proteins [33, 65, 71, 95, 99]. Ethylene oxide-treated demineralized bone grafts have been effective in healing long bone segmental defects in rabbits [73], but had reduced effectiveness in rats [47]. A controlled dog study demonstrated that the osteoinductive capacity of demineralized bone grafts sterilized with ethylene oxide is the same as nonsterilized bone [115], whereas a study in rats by Sherman and Hollinger showed a reduction [124]. Munting and co-workers [98] reported that in vivo recalcification of sterilized, demineralized bone implants in rats was reduced by 83 percent using ethylene oxide and 60 percent using 2.5 Mrads of gamma irradiation.

Sterilization by Heat

Heat treatment is an effective sterilant but it has not been routinely applied to bone grafts. Exposure of bone allografts or autografts to autoclave temperatures, 121 °C for 20 minutes, is occasionally applied to eradicate accidental microbial contamination or to ablate a malignant bone tumor combined with reimplantation of the same bone [59]. Autoclaving has not been adopted as a routine sterilant of bone allografts because it impairs mechanical properties [78, 81, 84] and reduces incorporation [82, 142]. On the other hand, a lower dose of heat (pasteurization) at 60 °C for 10 hours or 56 °C to 80 °C for shorter time periods readily inactivates bacteria as well as at least a 6 log concentration of HIV-1, a 4.5 log concentration of hepatitis B virus and a 5 log concentration of non-A, non-B hepatitis virus [91, 111]. Although pasteurization has not been widely adopted for sterilizing bone allografts, it has been shown not to have significant deleterious effects on bone mechanical properties [122, 142, 149] or clinical effectiveness [142].

Summary

Bone allografts have been implicated in transmitting tuberculosis, HIV, hepatitis and bacterial infections to recipients. To prevent or at least minimize the risk of transmission of infectious disease, several steps are taken by surgeons and bone banks. An important initial approach is to judiciously use bone allografts only when needed and to consider use of autografts, alternative non-human graft material or sterilized bone allografts whenever possible. However, the most important approach is exercised by the tissue bank donor coordinator who carefully obtains a medical and social history excluding those suspected to be at risk for HIV, hepatitis or other viral or bacterial infections. Donor blood testing, physical examination, reviewing autopsy reports, the surgical removal of donated tissue using aseptic technique and processing the bone graft to remove blood and marrow are also important in providing tissue with a low risk of transmitting disease. Lastly, sterilization of tissues can be very effective but is not universally applicable because the clinical effectiveness of osteochondral allografts requiring chondrocyte viability are unable to withstand sterilization procedures. Although heat is an effective sterilant, the tissue disinfection and sterilization methods most often used by tissue banks are gamma irradiation and ethylene oxide. Application of these steps, beginning with a careful medical and social history evaluation of the prospective tissue donor, will assure a low risk of transmitting disease from the donor to the recipient.

Acknowledgement

I thank Robin Paulson and Peggy Stivers for manuscript preparation.

References

1. Abecassis MM, Welk JF, Bale J, et al (1994) Transmission of cytomegalovirus by skin allografts–a review. Tissue Cell Report 2: 14–17
2. Adam M, et al (1993) Rapid freezing of whole blood or buffy coat sample for polymerase chain reaction and cell culture analysis: Application to detection of human immunodeficiency virus in blood donor and recipient repositories. Transfusion 33: 504–508
3. Aguiar JW, Chang P, Rosenquist MD, et al (1994) Acquisition of cytomegalovirus infection through cadaver skin allograft in burn patients. Proceedings of the 26th Annual Meeting. American Burn Association, Orlando, Florida
4. Alter HJ, Epstein JS, Swenson SG, et al (1990) Prevalence of human immunodeficiency virus type 1 p24 antigen in U.S. blood donors – an assessment of the efficacy of testing in donor screening. N Engl J Med 323: 1312–1217
5. American Association of Tissue Banks (1992) Technical manual for tissue banking- musculoskeletal. McLean, Virginia: American Association of Tissue Banks
6. Anonymous (1993) 21 CFR 1270. Human tissue intended for transplantation. Federal Register 58: 65514–65521
7. Anonymous (editorial). HTLV-I. A screen too many? Lancet 2: 336
8. Asselmeier MA, Caspari RB, Bottenfield S (1993) A review of allograft processing and sterilization techniques and their role in transmission of human immunodeficiency virus. Am J Sports Med 21: 170–175
9. Aurori BF, Weierman RJ, Lowell HA, Nadel CI, Parsons JR (1985) Pseudoarthosis after spinal fusion for scoliosis. A comparison of autogeneic and allogeneic bone grafts. Clin Orthop 199: 153–158
10. Bankowski MJ, Landay AL, Staes B, et al (1992) Postmortem recovery of human immunodeficiency virus type 1 from plasma mononuclear cells. Arch Pathol Lab Med 116: 1124–1127
11. Barnes A (1991) Transfusion-transmitted treponemal infections. In: Smith D, Dodd RY (eds) Transfusion transmitted infections. Chicago: ASCP Press, pp 161–166
12. Basset CAL, Packard AG (1959) A clinical assay of cathode ray sterilized cadaver bone grafts. Acta Orthop Scand 28: 198–211
13. Blajchman M, Feinman S, Bull S (1993) Results of a prospective randomized multi-center trial to evaluate the non-A, non-B surrogate tests (ALT and anti-HBc) to prevent post-transfusion hepatitis. Blood 82 [Suppl I]: 204a
14. Boller F, Lopez O, Moosy J (1988) Diagnosis of dementia: Clinico-pathologic correlations. Neurology 38 [Suppl I]: 226
15. Bond WW, Favero MS, Peterson NJ, Ebert JW (1983) Inactivation of hepatitis B virus by intermediate-to-high level disinfectant chemical. J Clin Micro 18: 535–538
16. Bowen PA, Lobel SA, Caruana RJ, et al (1988) Transmission of human immunodeficiency virus (HIV) by transplantation: clinical aspects and time course analysis of viral antigenemia and antibody production. Ann Intern Med 108: 46–48

17. Bright RW, Friedlaender GE, Sell KW (1977) Tissue banking: The United States Navy tissue banks. Military Medicine 142: 503–510

18. Bright RW, Burchardt D (1983) The biomechanical properties of preserved bone grafts. In: Friedlaender GE, Mankin HJ, Sell KW (eds) Bone allografts-biology, banking and clinical applications. Boston: Little, Brown and Co, pp 241–247

19. Bright RW, Smarsh JD, Gambill VM (1983) Sterilization of human bone by irradiation. In: Friedlaender GE, Mankin HJ, Sell KW (eds) Osteochondral allografts-biology, banking and clinical applications. Boston: Little Brown and Co, pp 223–232

20. Brown P, Rowher RG, Gajdusek DC (1984) Sodium hydroxide decontamination of Creutzfeldt-Jakob disease virus. N Engl J Med 310: 727

21. Brown P, Cathala F, Castaigne P, Cajdusek DC (1986) Creutzfeldt-Jakob disease: Clinical analysis of a consecutive series of 230 neuropathologically verified cases. Ann Neurol 20: 597–602

22. Brown P, Gibbs CJ, Amyx HL, et al (1982) Chemical disinfection of Creutzfeldt-Jakob disease virus. N Engl J Med 306: 1279–1282

23. Brown P (1990) Iatrogenic Creutzfeldt-Jakob disease. Aust NZ J Med 20: 633–635

24. Brown P, Gajdusek DC, Gibbs CJ Asher DM (1985) Potential epidemic of Creutzfeldt-Jakob disease from human growth hormone therapy. N Engl J Med 313: 728–731

25. Buck BE, Resnick L, Shah SM, Malinin TI (1990) Human immunodeficiency virus cultured from bone. Implications for transplantation. Clin Orthop 251: 250–253

26. Buck BE, Malinin TI, Brown MD (1989) Bone transplantation and human immunodeficiency virus; an estimate of risk of acquired immunodeficiency syndrome (AIDS). Clin Orthop 240: 129–136

27. Buring K, Urist MR (1967) Effects of ionizing radiation on bone induction principle in the matrix of bone implants. Clin Orthop 55: 225–234

28. Burke W, Keogh A, Maloney P, et al (1990) Transmission of sarcoidosis via cardiac transplantation. Lancet 336: 1579

29. Busch MP, Taylor PE, Lenes BA, et al (1990) Screening of selected male blood donors for p24 antigen of human immunodeficiency virus type 1. N Engl J Med 323: 1308–1312

30. Busch MP (1994) HIV and blood transfusion: Focus on seroconversion. Vox Sang 67 [Suppl 3]: 13–18

31. Campagnari D, O'Malley J (eds), (1994) Standards of the American Red Cross Tissue Services, 6th edn. Washington, DC: American Red Cross Tissue Services

32. Campbell DG, Li P, Stephenson AJ, Oakeshott RD (1994) Sterilization of HIV by gamma irradiation. A bone allograft model. Int Orthop 18: 172–176

33. Canalis E, McCarthy TL, Centrella M (1989) Growth factors and the skeletal system. J Endocrinol Invest 12: 577–584

34. Centers for Disease Control (1981) Human-to-human transmission of rabies via corneal transplantation – Thailand. MMWR 30: 473–474

35. Centers for Disease Control (1979) Human-to-human transmission of rabies by a corneal transplant-Idaho. MMWR 28: 109–111

36. Centers for Disease Control (1988) Semen banking, organ and tissue transplantation, and HIV antibody testing. MMWR 37: 57–58, 63

37. Centers for Disease Control (1988) Licensure of screening tests for antibody to human T-lymphotropic virus MMWR 37: 736–740, 745–747

38. Centers for Disease Control (1988) Transmission of HIV through bone transplantation: Case report and public health recommendations. MMWR 37: 587–599

39. Centers for Disease Control (1989) Update: Creutzfeldt-Jakob disease in a patient receiving a cadaveric dura mater graft. MMWR 38: 37–43

40. Centers for Disease Control (1994) Guidelines for preventing transmission of human immunodeficiency virus through transplantation of human tissue and organs. MMWR 43 (RR-8): 1–17

41. Chou SW (1986) Acquisition of donor strains of cytomegalovirus by renal transplant recipients. N Engl J Med 314: 1418–1423

42. Cloward RB (1980) Gas-sterilized cadaver bone grafts for spinal fusion operations. A simplified bone bank. Spine 5: 4–10

43. Conrad EU, Gretch D, Obermeyer K, Moogk M, Sayers M, Wilson J, Strong DM (1995) The transmission of hepatitis C virus through tissue transplantation. J Bone Joint Surg 77-A: 214–224

24   T. Eastlund

44. Conroy B, Tomford W, Mankin H, Hirsch MS, Shooley RT (1992) Radiosensitivity of HIV-1. Potential application to sterilization of bone allografts. AIDS 5: 608–609

45. Conway B, Tomford WW (1992) Radiosensitivity of human immunodeficiency virus type 1. Clinical Infectious Diseases 14: 978–979

46. Coombs RW, Collier AC, Allian J-P, et al (1989) Plasma viremia in human immunodeficiency virus infection. N Engl J Med 321: 1626–1631

47. Cornell C, Lane JM, Nottebaert M, Klein C, Dowling C, Burnstein AH (1987) Effect of ethylene oxide sterilization upon bone inductive properties of demineralized bone matrix. Trans Orthop Res Soc 11: 74

48. Corral DA, Darras FS, Jensen CWB, et al (1993) Parvovirus B19 infection causing pure red cell aplasia in a recipient of pediatric donor kidneys. Transplantation 55: 427–430

49. Daar ES, Moudgli T, Meyer RD, et al (1991) Transient levels of viremia in patients with primary human immunodeficiency virus type 1 infection. N Engl J Med 324: 961–964

50. deVries PH, Badgley CE, Hartman JT (1958) Radiation sterilization of homogenous bone transplants utilizing radioactive cobalt. J Bone Joint Surg 40: 187–203

51. Dewar RL, Sarmiento ES, Lawton HM, et al (1992) Isolation of HIV-1 from plasma of infected individuals: An analysis of experimental conditions effecting successful virus propagation. J Acq Immune Defic Syndr 4: 822–828

52. Eastlund T (1995) Infectious disease transmission through cell, tissue and organ transplantation: Reducing the risk through donor selection. Cell Transplantation 4: 455–477

53. Eastlund T, Prather J, Stecker D, et al (1990) Infectious disease markers in surgical bone donations. Proceedings 14th Annual Meeting, American Association of Tissue Banks. Denver, Colorado

54. Eastlund T, Jackson B, Harvilla G, Sannerud K (1989) Inactivation of HIV within cortical bone by ethylene oxide or heat. Proceedings 13th Annual Meeting, American Association Tissue Banks. San Diego, Calif.

55. Eggen BM, Nordbo SA (1992) Transmission of HCV by organ transplantation (letter). N Engl J Med 326: 411

56. European Association of Tissue Banks (1995) General standards for tissue Banking. Vienna: OBIG Transplant

57. Ferraro SP, Moore-Ferraro SY, Moor TM (1991) Bactericidal gamma irradiation enhances rather than impairs osteoinduction by solid demineralized matrix in the rat. Trans Orthop Res Soc (Banff) 16: 288

58. Fideler B, Moore TM, Vanqsness CT, Rasheed S, Gendler E (1994) Effect of gamma irradiation on the human immunodeficiency virus. A study in frozen human bone-patellar ligament-bone grafts from infected cadavera. J Bone Joint Surg 76-A: 1032–1035

59. Freiberg A, Saltzman C, Smith W (1992) Replantation of an autoclaved, autogenous humerus in a patient who had chondrosarcoma. J Bone Joint Surg 74-A: 438–439

60. Gaines H, Albert J, Von Sydow M, et al (1987) HIV antigenemia and virus isolation from plasma during primary HIV infection. Lancet 1: 1317–1318

61. Glowacki J, Murray JE, Kaban LB, Folkman J, Mulliken JB (1981) Application of the biologic principle of induced osteogenesis for cranial facial defects. Lancet i: 959–962

62. Gottesdiener KM (1989) Transplanted infections: Donor-to-host transmission with the allograft. Ann Intern Med 110: 1001–1010

63. Hamilton J, Eastlund T, Steckler D, et al (1990) Low prevalence of human immunodeficiency virus seropositivity in surgical bone donors. A survey of 20 regional surgical bone banks. Proceedings 14th Annual Meeting, American Association of tissue Banks. Denver, Colorado

64. Harell J, McCreedy B, Johnston A (1993) PCR vs p24 antigen testing for detection of HIV-1 in cadaveric blood speciments. Proceedings 17th Annual Meeting, American Association of Tissue Banks. Boston, Mass.

65. Hauschka PV, Mavrakos AE, Iafrati MD, Doleman SE, Klagsbrun M (1986) Growth factors in bone matrix. Isolation of multiple types by affinity chromatography on heparin-seharose. J Biol Chem 261: 12665–12674

66. Hernigou P, Goutallier D (1988) Thirty massive allografts conserved by freezing and sterilized by irradiation. Trans Orthop Res Soc 12: 200

67. Hiemstra H, Tersmette M, Vos AH, et al (1992) Inactivation of HIV by gamma radiation and its effect on plasma and coagulation factors. Transfusion 31: 32–39

68. Ho DD, Moudgil T, Alam M (1989) Quantitation of human immunodeficiency virus type 1 in blood of infected persons. N Engl J Med 321: 1621–1625

69. Horsburgh CR Jr, Ou CY, Jason J, et al (1989) Duration of human immunodeficiency virus infection before defection of antibody. Lancet 2: 637–640

70. Houff SA, Burton RC, Wilson RW, et al (1979) Human-to-human transmission of rabies virus by corneal transplant. N Engl J Med 300: 603–604

71. Hulth A, Johnell O, Henricson A (1988) The implantation of demineralized fracture matrix yields more new bone formation than does intact matrix. Clin Orthop 234: 235–239

72. James JP (1953) Tuberculosis transmitted by banked bone. J Bone Joint Surg 35-B: 578

73. Janovec M, Dvorak K (1988) Autolyzed antigen-extracted allogeneic bone for bridging segmental diaphyseal bone defects in rabbits. Clin Orthop 229: 249–255

74. Kakaiya R, Miller WV, Gudino MD (1991) Tissue transplant transmitted infections. Transfusion 31: 277–284

75. Kaplan JE, Osame M, Kubota H, et al (1990) The risk of development of HTLV-I associated myelopathy/tropical spastic paraparesis among persons infected with HTLV-I. J Acquir Immune Defic Syndr 3: 1096–1101

76. Kearney JN, Johnson C (1991) Evaluation of NaOH treatment of human dura mater implants to obviate Creutzfeldt-Jakob transmission. Biomaterials 12: 431–432

77. Kitchen AD, Mann GF, Harrison JF, Zuckerman AJ (1989) Effect of gamma irradiation on the human immune deficiency virus and human coagulation proteins. Vox Sang 56: 223–229

78. Knaepler H, Garrel T, Seipp H, Aschere R, Gotzen L (1992) Autoklavierung von allogenen Knochentransplantaten als Alternative zur konventionellen Knochenbank. Orthopädische Praxis 28: 18–22

79. Knapp DR, Jones ET (1988) Use of cortical cancellous allograft for posterior spinal fusion. Clin Orthop 229: 99–106

80. Kobayashi H, Tsuzuki M, Koshimizu K, et al (1984) Susceptability of hepatitis B to disinfectants and heat. J Clin Micro 20: 214–216

81. Kohler P, Kreicbergs A, Stromberg L (1986) Structural properties of autoclaved bone. Acta Orthop Scand 57: 141–145

82. Kohler P, Kreicbergs A (1987) Incorporation of autoclaved allogeneic bone supplemented with allogeneic demineralized bone matrix. An experimental study in the rabbit. Clin Orthop 218: 247–258

83. Komender J, et al (1991) Therapeutic effects of transplantation of lyophilized and radiation-sterilized allogeneic bone. Clin Orthop 272: 38–49

84. Kreicbergs A, Kohler P (1989) Bone exposed to heat. In: Aebi M, Regazzoni P (eds) Bone transplantation. Berlin: Springer, pp 154–61

85. Lane KL, Brown P, Howell DN, et al (1994) Creutzfeldt-Jakob disease in a pregnant woman with an implanted dura mater graft. Neurosurgery 34: 737–740

86. Linden J (ed) (1996) American Association of Tissue Banks. Standards for Tissue Banking. McLean, Virginia: American Association Tissue Banks

87. Lord FC, Gebhardt MC, Tomford WW, Mankin HJ (1988) Infection in bone allografts. Incidence, nature and treatment. J Bone Joint Surg 70-A: 369–375

88. Loty B, Courpied JP, Tomeno B, Postel M, Forest M, Abelanet R (1990) Bone allografts sterilized by irradiation. Biological properties, procurement and results of 150 massive allografts. Intern Orthop 14: 237–242

89. Marmor L (1964) Irradiated bonegrafts. Am J Surg 107: 833–836

90. Masullo C, Pocchiari M, Macchi G, Alema G, Prazza G, Panzera MA (1989) Transmission of Creutzfeldt-Jakob disease by dural cadaveric graft. J Neurosurg 71: 954–955

91. Mauler R, Markle W, Hilfenhaus J (1987) Inactivation of HTLV-III/LAV, hepatitis B and non-A/non-B viruses by pasturization in human plasma preparations. Dev Biol Standard 67: 337–351

92. McCarthy RE, Peck RD, Morrissy RT, Hough AJ (1986) Allograft bone in spinal fusion for paralytic scoliosis. J Bone Joint Surg 68-A: 370–375

93. Mellonig JT, Prewett AB, Moyer MP (1992) HIV inactivation in a bone allograft. J Periodontol 63: 979–983

94. Merz H, Rytik G, Muller WEG, Roder W (1991) Bestimmung einer HIV-Infektion in menschlichen Knochen. Unfallchirurg 94: 47–49

95. Mohan S, Baylink DJ (1991) Bone growth factors. Clin Orthop 263: 30–48

96. Moore T, Gendler E, Moore-Ferraro S, Ferraro S (1992) Osteoinductive activity improved by 3 million Rads of gamma irradiation. Proceedings 16th Annual Meeting, American Association of Tissue Banks. San Diego, Calif. 39

97. Mowe J (1989) Survey of Tissue Banks-1988. American Association of Tissue Banks. McLean, Virginia

98. Munting E, Wilmart J-F, Wijne A, Hennebert P, Delloye C (1988) Effect of sterilization on osteoinduction. Comparison of five methods in demineralized rat bone. Acta Orthop Scand 58: 34

99. Muthukumaran N, Reddi AH (1985) Bone matrix-induced local bone formation. Clin Orthop 200: 159

100. Novick SL, Schrager JA, Nelson JA, Baskin BL (1993) A comparison of two HBsAg and two HIV-1 (p24) antigen EIA test kits with hemolyzed cadaveric blood specimens. Tissue Cell Report 1: 2–3

101. Nowicki MJ (1992) Re-evaluation of anti-HIV seroprevalence among blood donors with contemporary screening assays. Transfusion 32 [Suppl]: 32

102. Nuchprayoon C, Tanprasert S, Chumnijarakij T (1992) Is routine p24 HIV antigen screening justified in Thai blood donors? Lancet 340: 1041

103. Nyberg M, Suni J, Haltia M (1990) Isolation of human immunodeficiency virus (HIV at autopsy one to six days postmortem). Am J Clin Pathol 94: 422–425

104. Pelker RR, Friedlaender GE, Markham TC, et al (1984) Effects of freezing and freeze-drying on the biomechanical properties of rat bone. J Orthop Res 1: 405–411

105. Pelker RR, Fridelaender GE, Markham TC (1983) Biomechanical properties of bone allografts. Clin Orthop 174: 54–59

106. Pelker RR, Friedlaender GE (1987) Biomechanical aspects of bone autografts and allografts. Orthop Clin North Am 18: 235–239

107. Pellet S, Strong DM, Temesi A, Matthews JG (1983) Effects of irradiation on frozen corticocancellous bone allograft incorporation and immunogenicity. In: Friedlaender GE, Mankin HJ, Sell KW (eds) Osteochondral allografts-biology, banking and clinical applications. Boston: Little, Brown and Co, pp 353–361

108. Pepose JS, Buerger DG, Paul DA, Quinn TC, Darragh TM, Donegan E (1992) New developments in serologic screening of corneal donors for HIV-1 and hepatitis B virus infections. Ophthalmology 99: 879–888

109. Periera B, Milford E, Kirkman R, et al (1993) Low risk of liver disease in after tissue transplantation from donors with HCV. Lancet 341: 903–904

110. Peterson LR, Satten GA, Dodd R, et al (1992) Duration of time from onset of human immunodeficiency virus type 1 infectiousness to development of detectable antibody. Transfusion 34: 283–289

111. Piszkiewicz D, Apfelzweig R, Bourret L, et al (1988) Inactivation of HIV in antithrombin-III concentrate by pasteurization (letter). Transfusion 28: 198–199

112. Prewett AB, O'Leary RK, Damien CJ (1990) Investigation of the effect of low-dose gamma irradiation on the collagenous and non-collagenous proteins of bone matrix. Proceedings 12th Annual Meeting, American Society Bone Mineral Research, August 28–30, 1990

113. Puolakkainen PA, Ranchalis JE, Strong DM, Twardzik DR (1993) The effect of sterilization on transforming growth factor beta (TGF-beta) isolated from demineralized human bone. Transfusion 33: 679–685

114. Prolo DJ, Pedrotti PW, White DM (1980) Ethylene oxide sterilization of bone, dura mater and fascia lata for human transplantation. Neurosurgery 6: 529–539

115. Prolo DJ, Petrotti PW, Burres K, Oklunds S (1982) Superior osteogenesis in transplanted allogeneic canine skull following chemical sterilization. Clin Orthop 168: 230–242

116. Renik L, Veren K, Salahuddin SZ, Tondreau S, Markham PD (1986) Stability and inactivation of HTLV-III/LAV under clinical and laboratory environments. JAMA 225: 1887–1891

117. Roder W, Muller H, Muller WEG, Merz H (1992) HIV infection in human bone. J Bone Joint Surg 74-B: 179–180

118. Rutherford GW, Kateley JR (1988) The effects of irradiation and lyophilization on the mechanical properties of patellar-tendon and bone allografts. Proceeding of the Twelfth Annual Meeting, American Association of Tissue Banks 31

119. Salib R, Graber J (1996) Femoral cortical ring plus cancellous dowel: alternative in anterior lumbar interbody fusion. Tissue Cell Report 3: (in press)
120. Scofield C, Eastlund T, Steckler D, et al (1993) Prevalence of infectious disease markers in surgical bone donors. Proceedings 17th Annual Meeting, American Association of Tissue Banks. Boston, Mass.
121. Scofield C, Eastlund T, Larson N, et al (1993) Retesting of 1,608 living tissue donors for HIV and HCV. An evaluation of results. Proceedings 17th Annual Meeting, American Association of Tissue Banks. Boston, Mass.
122. Sharkey N, Hollstein S, Martin R (1991) Thermal inactivation of HIV in cadaveric specimens: biomechanical effects on bone. Proceeding Orthopaedic Research Society. Banff, Canada 279
123. Shelby J, Shanley J (1987) Transfer of murine cytomegalovirus by syngeneic skin grafts. Transplantation 44: 318–320
124. Sherman P, Hollinger P (1988) Bone implant sterilization – ethylene oxide versus cobalt 60 irradiation. Annual Meeting Proceedings, American Association Oral and Maxillofacial Surgery. Boston, Mass.
125. Shutkin NM (1954) Homologous-serum hepatitis following the use of refrigerated bone bank bone. J Bone Joint Surg 36-A: 160–162
126. Simonds RJ, Holmberg SD, Hurwitz RL, et al (1992) Transmission of human immunodeficiency virus type 1 from a seronegative organ snd tissue donor. N Engl J Med 326: 726–732
127. Sonis ST, Kaban LB, Glowacki J (1983) Clinical trial of demineralized bone powder in treatment of periodontal effectis. J Oral Med 38: 117–122
128. Spire B, Barre-Sinoussi F, Dormont D, Montagnier L, Chermann JC (1985) Inactivation of lymphadenopathy associated virus by heat, gamma rays and ultraviolet light. Lancet 1: 188–189
129. Stramer LS, Heller JS, Coombs RW, et al (1989) Markers of HIV infection prior to IgG antibody seropositivity. JAMA 262: 64–69
130. Strong DM, Eastlund T, Mowe J (1996) Tissue bank activity in the United States: 1992 survey of accredited tissue banks. Tissue Cell Report 3: (in press)
131. Sullivan R, Fassoletis AC, Larkin EP, Read BB, Peeler JT (1971) Inactivation of thirty viruses by gamma irradiation. Appl Microbiol 22: 61–65
132. Tange RA, Troost D, Limburg M (1990) Progressive fatal dementia (Creutzfeldt-Jakob disease) in a patient who received homograft tissue for tympanic membrane closure. Eur Arch Oto-rhinolaryngol 247: 199–201
133. Thadani V, Penar PL, Partington J, Kalb R, Janssen R, Schonberger LB, Rabkin CS, Prichard JW (1988) Creutzfeldt-Jakob disease probably acquired from a cadaveric dura mater graft. J Neurosurg 69: 766–769
134. Thomas FC, Ouwerkerk T, McKercher P (1992) Inactivation by gamma irradiation of animal viruses in simulated laboratory effluent. Appl Environ Micro 43: 1051–1056
135. Tomford WW, Starkweather RJ, Goldman MH (1981) A study of the clinical incidence of infection in the use of banked allograft bone. J Bone Joint Surg 63-A: 244–248
136. Tomford WW, Thongphasuk J, Mankin HJ, Ferraro MJ (1990) Frozen musculoskeletal allografts. A study of the clinical incidence and causes of infection associated with their use. J Bone Joint Surg 72-A: 1137–1143
137. Transfeldt E, Lonstein J, Winter R, et al (1985) Wound infections in reconstructive spinal surgery. Orthop Trans 9: 128–129
138. Triantafyllou N, Sotiorpoulo SE, Triantafyllou J (1973) The mechanical properties of lyophilized and irradiated bone grafts. Acta Orthop Belg 41: 35–44
139. Turner TC, Bassett CAL, Pate JW, Sawyer PN, Trump JG, Wright JG (1956) Sterilization of preserved bone grafts by high voltage cathode irradiation. J Bone Joint Surg 38: 862–884
140. Turner TB, Diseker TH (1941) Duration of infectivity of Treponema pallidum in citrated blood stored under conditions obtained in blood banks. Bull Johns Hopkins Hosp 68: 269–279
141. Urist MR, Hernandez A (1974) Excitation transfer in bone. Deleterious effect of cobalt 60 radiation sterilization of bone implants. Arch Surg 109: 486–493
142. von Garrell T, Knaepler H (1993) Thermal treatment of bone allografts for distinfection. Proceedings 17th Annual Meeting. American Association of Tissue Banks. Boston, Mass
143. Weintroub S, Reddi AH (1988) Influence of irradiation on the osteoinductive potential of demineralized bone matrix. Calcif Tissue Int: 255–260

144. Wells MA, Wittek AE, Epstein JS, et al (1986) Inactivation and partition of human T-cell lymphotropic virus, type III, during ethanol fractionation of plasma. Transfusion 26: 210–213

145. Yamada S, Aiba T, Endo Y, et al (1994) Creutzfeldt-Jakob disease transmitted by a cadaveric dura mater graft. Neurosurgery 34: 740–744

146. Yerly S, Chamot E, Hirschel B, Perrin LH (1992) Quantitation of human immunodeficiency provirus and circulating virus: Relationship with immunologic parameters. J Infect Dis 166: 269–276

147. Zaaiger HL, Exel-Oehlers P, Kraaijeveld T, et al (1992) Early detection of HIV-1 by third generation assay. Lancet 340: 770–772

148. Zasacki W (1991) The efficacy of application of lyophilized, radiation-sterilized bone graft in orthopedic surgery. Clin Orthop 272: 82–87

149. Zimmerman R, Bechtold J, Eastlund T, Bianco P (1992) Effect of Pasteurization on the mechanical properties of human cancellous bone. Proceedings of the 2nd North American Congress on Biomechanics. Chicago, 17

Author's address: D. Ted Eastlund, MD, American Red Cross, North Central Tissue Services, 100 South Robert Street, St. Paul, MN 55107, U.S.A.

Biomechanics of Allografts

M.G. Rock

Mayo Clinic and Mayo Foundation, Orthopaedic Department, Rochester, Minnesota, U.S.A.

The advantages of using autograft in defects less than 6 cm even in areas of high mechanical demand have been addressed elsewhere in this book (Chapter on Intercalary Reconstruction). If the defect exceeds what is possible to compensate with autograft it often becomes necessary to consider the use of allogeneic tissue. Furthermore, complications associated with autograft occur not infrequently and include blood loss and hematoma at the procurement site necessitating transfusion, infection, injury to the lateral cutaneous nerve of the thigh, fracture of the remaining iliac wing, hernia, and persistent pain and cosmetic deformity. Alternatively, allograft is associated with no morbidity with procurement, decreased operative time, allows modifying the bone graft to fit the deficiency anatomically, and theoretically unlimited supply. As such, transplant bone and soft tissue have become viable alternatives in the reconstruction of the multiply revised arthroplasty patient, after tumor resection, spinal surgery and in complex soft tissue deficiencies such as ligament reconstruction of the knee and rotator cuff repair of the shoulder. The long-term success of musculoskeletal transplantation, however, depends on the incorporation of the allograft to the host, whether it be osseous or soft tissue and avoidance of complications. Both of these factors are dependent on the biology and biomechanics of the reconstruction and are not mutually exclusive. Implications of the former to allograft success is thoroughly discussed by Dr. Hans Burchardt in a previous chapter.

Many of the complications associated with allograft reconstruction including nonunion, fracture, intra-articular collapse, and instability of the contiguous joint are not only a function of the technical aspects of the allograft reconstruction but also the status of the tissue prior to implantation which may be severely affected by a number of parameters which include the age and sex of the donor, the anatomical location of the donor bone or tendon, the metabolic condition of the donor possibly affecting the integrity of the tissue and the processing and sterilization of the tissue. These material properties of the tissue are important if it is to be used to structurally compensate for host deficiencies and contribute to the mechanical integrity of the limb, pelvis, or spine.

The donor requisites allowing procurement of large segmental allografts have become refined over the past 20 years [I, 12] excluding potential donors that may have medical or metabolic conditions affecting the integrity of the skeleton. Additionally, patients over 55 years of age are generally excluded as donors of structural grafts as there is a known 10 to 20 percent reduction in performance with tension, compression, torsion and bending in bone procured from patients over 55 years of age [10]. It has generally become accepted practice to replace the deficient anatomical area with anatomically similar allogeneic tissue. This is done recognizing the relationship between the radius of the segment and its ultimate torsional strength favoring larger diameter grafts and the limitations imposed at the recipient site with respect to approximation and closure of surrounding soft tissues and skin. The above parameters have been identified largely from the extensive use and difficulties encountered with allograft reconstructions over the past 20 years [20, 25]. The resultant emphasis on using young donors cleared of significant medical problems and whose anatomy in size and contour matches that of the proposed recipient has emerged.

Possibly the greatest effect on the biomechanical properties of the graft and which has not been nearly as effectively refined in favor of maintenance of structural integrity is that of the processing, sterilization, and maintenance of large segment allografts.

Processing

Processing involves the modification of the procured tissue for clinical application; introducing the means with which to minimize the immunologic response from the recipient and allow for safe and effective storage of the tissue prior to implantation. One of the major advances in allograft utilization was the confirmation by Wilson [38] of the marked decrease in immunogenicity of the graft if frozen to $-70°C$ and the ability to maintain this tissue in such an environment with continued anticipated clinical success. Although not totally eradicating the immunologic capabilities of the graft it markedly reduces the host response making it much less likely for the transplanted tissue to undergo extensive resorption. For ease of maintenance and dissemination, freeze drying to less than 5 percent residual moisture became quite popular due to the ability to maintain specimens at room temperature without the need for expensive refrigerating techniques. Such technology was introduced in 1951 by the United States Navy Tissue Bank and two years later by the Central Tissue Bank in Warsaw, Poland [19, 39]. With the increasing use of allograft tissue in biomechanically demanding clinical circumstances the issue of biomechanical integrity with such processing mechanisms as mentioned above became a concern. Extensive analysis of fresh frozen bone and soft tissue used for transplantation has proved that the mere act of freezing and thawing does not adversely affect the biomechanical properties of this tissue. This has included comparing fresh controls to specimens maintained at $-20°C$, $-25°C$, $-78°C$, and at $-96°C$ in the presence of liquid nitrogen and being challenged under compression, torsion, and bending (Table 1) [28].

Intrinsic in the process of the utilization of freeze dried transplant tissue is the need to rehydrate prior to implantation. This generally takes 24 hours and due to the logistics

Table 1. Effect of processing bone on mechanical properties

Technique	Control	Bone strength compression	% of control torsion
Freezing ($-20°C$)	Fresh	120	100
Freezing ($-70°C$)	Fresh	122	100
Liquid nitrogen ($-196°C$)	Fresh	117	100
Freeze dried	Fresh	120	35

From Pelker PR, Friedlader GE, Markham TC (1983) Biomechanical properties of bone allografts. Clin Orthop 174: 54–57

Table 2. Effect of processing bone on mechanical properties

Technique	Control	Ultimate strength	Ultimate strain	Modulus
Fresh frozen	Fresh	39.85	0.25	121.14
Freeze dried	Fresh	32.66	0.35	92.20

involved is very rarely performed in clinical practice. The reconstitution of the bio-mechanical properties, however, is contingent on this rehydration process as concluded by Bright, Burchardt, and Burstein [3]. The non-rehydrated freeze dried specimen were very brittle and exhibited marked reduction in all biomechanical parameters tested of human cadaveric tibia and femora. After one hour of rehydration the elastic modulus returned to normal and after four hours the yield and ultimate stresses did the same. After eight hours the ultimate strain returned to control values with the plastic modulus remaining elevated and never returning to a control value even after 24 hours of rehydration. Similarly Paulos [27] found a decrease in ultimate stress to failure in tendon grafts that were freeze dried and allowed to rehydrate before anticipated clinical use. These trends were additionally confirmed by Triantafyllou et al. who compared freeze dried specimens to $-35°C$ fresh frozen controls and found between a 10 and 45 percent reduction in bending strength and Pelker et al. comparing the properties of freeze dried tissue to fresh controls determining a 60 percent reduction in torsional properties. These effects are not entirely unexpected given the anticipated development of linear cracks in the tissue upon rehydration and the very distinct possibility of rapid freezing allowing trapped fluid to expand and propagate cracks as well (Table 1 and Table 2).

Sterilization

One of the continued concerns with transplantation of tissue is that of transmission of disease. There have been refinements in exclusionary criteria of donors introduced by The American Association of Tissue Banks [1] over the last 20 years to include the emergence of new pathogens including HIV-1 and 2, HTLV-I and HCV. This fear of transmitting disease has been heightened by the frequency with which HIV sero-conversion has occurred in the general population, the inability to control the infection, and four known cases of tissue transplantation after the era of effective HIV antibody detection [24, 33]. A recent symposium on HIV placed the world burden at 12 to 14×10^6 with 10 to 15 percent of these exhibiting symptoms of the disease. With no obvious cure in sight the anticipated population will mushroom to 110×10^6 infected and 12 million symptomatic cases by the year 2,000. Currently in the United States between .5 and 1 percent of the population is sero-positive for HIV and 1 in 800 are sero-negative HIV carriers in the window prior to conversion [4]. Unfortunately most of these patients are in the same age group as the donor pool. With the ever increasing concentration of HIV and HCV (which is currently between 1 and 2 percent of patients in the United States) the risks associated with transmission are increasing steadily. Routine assessment of the donor prior to procurement includes an extensive screening history, appropriate serologic screening, and additional testing which may include the P24 HIV antigen, reverse transcriptase, polymerase chain reaction, extensive autopsy and assessment of lymph nodes and quarantining such tissue until the results of organ recipients from the same donor are known. If screening history and serology are negative there is one chance in 10,533 of transmitting the disease from a patient who is in the process of sero-converting at the time of donation. If all the additional tests are performed that have been previously mentioned, that risk drops to 1 in 1.67 million [4]. HIV has been isolated and cultured from bone by Buck [5]. Due to the obvious concern, many banks have recommended and adopted sterilization techniques which have included gamma radiation, heat, cold, and chemical agents including ethylene oxide, hypochloride, glutaraldehyde, and cialet.

One of the more successful chemical sterilization techniques is that of incorporating ethylene oxide. Although apparently showing no significant effect on compressive strength, ethylene oxide sterilized bone as used in spinal grafting has in at least one series been found to completely resorb [14]. Contrary results have shown a 96 percent union rate in anterior cervical spine fusion and a 90 percent union rate in posterior lumbar interbody fusions using the same material [29]. Possibly the greatest concern in the use of ethylene oxide is the production of byproducts, one of which is ethylene chlorohydrin. This has recently been suggested by Jackson [15] who noticed a 6.4 percent incidence of a dramatic intraarticular reaction to bone patella bone allografts treated with ethylene oxide. The synovium from these patients showed hyperplasia, fibrosis and significant chronic inflammatory disease. Additionally, one patient who was tested revealed levels of ethylene chlorohydrin, a byproduct of ethylene oxide which is known to be toxic to biologic tissue. The toxic effects of ethylene oxide are well known and have prompted the Food and Drug Administration to propose maximum residual limits on ethylene oxide and major byproducts. Due in large part to these concerns ethylene oxide gas sterilization has not found much enthusiasm in the tissue transplant community

Although theoretically attractive and possibly simple to apply, heat inactivation may have deleterious effects on the biomechanical properties of bone and soft tissue. It has been suggested that exposure to 56°C for 30 minutes may be sufficient to inactivate most cells including HIV. When assessing the effect on biomechanical properties Knaepler [18] noted no effect at 60°C, diminution of yield point and maximum stress at 80°C, while all measured biomechanical parameters were severely affected to 60 percent of control at 100°C. The issue of heat inactivation has not yet been thoroughly determined and awaits further documentation.

By far the most commonly used means of sterilizing this tissue is that of radiation. It has been recommended by the International Anatomic Energy Commission to use 2.5 megarads. This was assumed to be enough to minimize the possibility of transmission of HIV to an acceptable bioburden of 10^{-6} TCID 50/ml. Recent studies would suggest, however, that with an assumed bioburden of an infected patient of 10^2 to 10^3 TCID 50/ml that a dose of 3.6 megarads would be necessary to inactivate to 10^{-6} [7, 11, 17, 26]. This makes the obvious assumption that one is willing to irradiate tissue from a known infected donor. However, with extensive screening and additional tests that have been outlined previously the risk of procuring from a sero-negative yet infected patient is remote and if such a case were to occur, the bioburden would likely be less than in those patients with symptomatic AIDS and/or sero-converted nonsymptomatic patients. Given all other precautionary methods in place a terminal dose of 2.5 megarads may in fact be quite appropriate. In most of these assessments, however, the virus was artificially introduced to bone assuming it would assimilate the penetration and distribution of the virus in the symptomatic patient.

It is unlikely that radiation in the prescribed dose of 2.5 megarads is going to appreciably affect the biomechanical properties of bone [2, 3, 18, 28, 36, 40] in spite of the fact that irradiation induces physical and chemical changes in the tissue which include increasing solubility of collagen and glycosaminoglycan, destroying the fibular matrix and altering collagen crosslinking. Although of concern, there has been no evidence to suggest that irradiation under these clinical circumstances produces mutagenic free radicals. For most large segment allografts the concern of interrupting osteoinductive capabilities is not an issue. Large segment allografts are osteoconductive only, and have no innate capabilities of being osteoinductive. However, the role of gamma radiation on collagenous substratum as a carrier for proteins which cause bone induction has shown no effect on its osteoinductive capability [16, 30, 32, 37]. This graft material, however, is not used in a structural environment.

As in bone the application of 2.5 megarads likely has no deleterious effect on the biomechanical properties of soft tissue allografts. In a study conducted by Gibbon, Butler and Noyes [13] in 1991 two megarads had absolutely no effect whereas 3 megarads was associated with a 27 percent reduction in maximal force and a 40 percent reduction in strain energy to maximal force suggesting that irradiation produces a dose dependent nonlinear reduction in biomechanical properties of a tendon.

Radiation by itself is rarely applied to these tissues as it is conventionally used in combination with other processing techniques. The effect of irradiation is largely precipitated by ionization, molecular excitation, and ion radical reactions. The physical state of the substrate and the temperature of application of the radiation dictate some of the effects [8]. It has been found that deep frozen tissue irradiated to 3.5 megarads induced new bone in an amount comparable to that induced by nonirradiated control whereas freeze dried tissue maintained at room temperature when irradiated was completely resorbed and did not induce any form of osteogenesis [8]. Additionally, extensive biomechanical analysis suggests marked reduction of biomechanical performance by radiation when combined with freeze drying (Tables 4 and 5) [3, 18, 19, 28, 35]. The cumulative effect of freeze drying and irradiating is very similar to what is observed to happen in aging bone which is known to experience increased cross linking of collagen thereby rendering it ineffectual in a structurally demanding environment.

Recently an extensive review of the Polish Central Tissue Bank in Warsaw has been performed with an extensive analysis of 1,014 patients who had received freeze dried radiation sterilized bone for various orthopedic reconstructive purposes [20, 39]. There was a 91.3 percent success rate. The authors identified the graft playing a significant role in mechanical support in 71 percent of the cases. Similar results have been reported elsewhere with complications including nonunion, fracture and infection equaling that

Table 3. Effect of radiation on bone strength as percent of control

Author	Control	Dose	Compression	Torsion	Bending
Komender	Fresh	3 megarads	—	90%	90%
Pelker	Fresh	6 megarads	80%	65%	70%
Bright	Frozen	3 megarads	100%	—	—
		3.5 megarads	No change		
Zhang	Frozen	2.5 megarads	No change		
Anderson	Frozen	3.1 megarads	90%		
		6.0 megarads			
Knaepler	Frozen	2.5 megarads	65%		

Table 4. Effect of irradiation and processing on mechanical properties of bone as percent of control

Author	Control	Compression	Torsion	Bending
Pelker	Fresh			
Radiation and freeze drying		—	40%	
Freeze drying and radiation		—	14%	
Triantafyllou	−35°C.			10–30%
Radiation				
Freeze drying				
Bright	Frozen	Severely diminished		
Komender	Fresh	—	70%	80%

Table 5. Effect of irradiation and processing on biomechanical properties of soft tissue

Technique	Control	Ultimate strength	Ultimate strain	Modulus
Paulos				
Fresh frozen	Fresh	39.15	0.25	121.14
Freeze dried and irradiation	Fresh	17.52	0.22	77.50

of nonirradiated tissue. It would appear that the clinical experience with irradiated tissue has not had the anticipated problems with mechanical support as would be suggested by the basic biomechanical studies.

Apart from the performance of the graft at procurement or during processing and maintenance, it is of equal significance to determine the in vivo response of the allograft tissue with time as well as the rate of incorporation of such tissue. There is a real and precipitous drop in compressive strength with all types of graft upon in vivo implantation with the bone subsequently regaining between 60 and 80 percent of its pregrafted value months after transplantation. As such if mechanically compromised tissue as would be the case with combination freeze drying irradiation is implanted, the additional significant drop in mechanical performance on in vivo introduction would potentially create a markedly compromised construct. Additionally, the time to incorporation of allogeneic tissue independent of processing and/or sterilization is markedly increased compared to autograft. Therefore, recognizing the inevitable reduction in performance of these grafts upon transplantation in vivo until incorporation occurs, the need to identify the most effective techniques to stabilize the reconstruction becomes critical. This is with the assumption that techniques to reduce the immunologic competence and to increase sterility of allografts introduce alterations in the biomechanical properties of such grafts as outlined above. Extrinsic factors that may have influence including age continues to stress the need for selecting young donors for tissue transplantation.

Fixation Concepts

The philosophy and concepts of fixation in the management of trauma patients has been well outlined principally by the AO group. Due to the unique nature of the reconstructions using large segment allografts, these concepts may not be entirely appropriate or applicable. Due to the altered mechanical properties somewhat contingent on the means of processing and/or sterilizing as well as the slow incorporation of these grafts in the host, the means with which to achieve stable fixation of allograft to host may need modification from that which has been assumed standard practice in traumatology. The use of plates and screws that has been so successful in trauma has proved problematic in large segment allografts largely due to the stress risers created by multiple screw holes in tissue that is not going to become totally revascularized and incorporated [23]. The latter has been confirmed by retrieval studies that suggest a spot weld incorporation at the allograft host juncture but no evidence of progressive and complete incorporation [9]. In an effort to minimize the possibility of peri-implant failure through allograft if plate and screws are felt to be the most appropriate form of fixation as may be true in metaepiphyseal reconstructions, the incorporation of polymethylmethacrylate into the central canal of the allograft has proved effective. This method not only removes the immunologic competent marrow cells but also allows for increased fixation of the screws, bypasses areas of stress risers, and allows the cement to be used as a vehicle for antibiotics which elute through the allograft into the surrounding soft tissues. In most other circumstances intramedullary fixation of large segment allografts either with conventional intramedullary fixation or allograft prosthetic composites with long stemmed components is the preferred means of reconstruction [23].

It has always been the desire of orthopedic surgeons to replace in whole or in part articulating segments of joints for trauma, degenerative disease, or tumor. Although theoretically possible the incorporation of articulating segments to allograft reconstructions has met nominal success [21, 31]. With some regularity articular surface collapse and degeneration occur with ultimate involvement of the contiguous joint surface. Progressive instability generally mandates conversion to allograft prosthetic composite or removal and conversion to a custom arthroplasty. Extensive work by Stevenson [34] has demonstrated that the destruction of the joint is somewhat governed by the immunologic disparity between the host and recipient and in her studies the most effective reconstruction of the articulating segments is that which is done with fresh antigen matched donor to recipient. There are many reasons why osteoarticular allografts do not work effectively. They include the inability to cryopreserve articular cartilage when subjecting the specimen to $-70°C$, size mismatch between the donor and the recipient and immunologic disparity. Various methods of identifying the most appropriate and successful cryopreservative techniques have had limited success with maximal continued viability often quoted at 20 percent. Matching the size of the donor and recipient can be theoretically accomplished by identifying the size of articulating segments by high tech imaging such as MRI [6]. The limiting factor and one that makes this impractical at this present time is the lack of sufficient numbers of articulating segments from which to make the match most precise. Until such time when there is a national or possibly international bank of osteoarticular allografts such refinement of size matching between donor and host will not be accomplished.

References

1. American Association of Tissue Banks (1987) Standard for tissue banking. Arlington, Virginia: American Association for Tissue Banks

2. Anderson MJ (1992) Compressive mechanical properties of human cancellous bone after gamma radiation. J Bone Joint Surg 74: 747

3. Bright RW, Burstein AH, Burchardt H (1983) The biomechanical properties of preserved bone grafts. In: Friedlander GE, Mankin HJ, Sell KW (eds) Osteochondral allografts. Biology, banking, and clinical applications. Boston: Little and Brown, pp 241–247

4. Buck BE, Malinin TI, Brown MD (1989) Bone transplantation in human immune deficiency virus. An estimate of risk of acquired immune deficiency syndrome (AIDS). Clin Orthop 240: 129–136

5. Buck BE, Resnick L, Shah SM, Malinin TI (1990) Human immune deficiency virus cultured from bone. Implications for transplantation. Clin Orthop 251: 249–253

6. Chao EYS, An KN, Niebur G, Westreich A, Rock M (1991) Computer aided size matching of osteochondral allograft transplantation. In: Brown KL (ed) Complications of limb salvage. Prevention, management and outcome. Sixth International Symposium of Limb Salvage, Montreal, Canada

7. Conway B, Tomford W, Mankin HJ, et al (1991) Radiosensitivity of HIV-1. Potential application to sterilization of bone allograft. AIDS 5(5): 608–609

8. Dziedzic-Goclawska A, et al (1990) Effect of radiation sterilization on the osteoinductive properties and the rate of remodeling of bone implants preserved by lyophilization and defreezing. Clin Orthop 272: 32–37

9. Enneking WF, Mindell ER (1991) Observations on massive retrieved human allograft. J Bone Joint Surg 73A: 1123

10. Evans FG (1973) Mechanical properties of bone. Springfield: Charles C. Thomas (ed), pp 43–55

11. Fideler BM, et al (1994) Effects of gamma irradiation on the human immune deficiency virus. J Bone Joint Surg 76A: 1032–1035

12. Friedlaender GE, Thomford WW (1989) Approaches to the retrieval and banking of osteochondral allografts. In: Friedlaender GE, Goldberg VM (eds) Bone and Cartilage Allografts, American Academy of Orthopedic Surgeons

13. Gibbons MJ, et al (1991) The effects of gamma radiation on the initial mechanical and material properties of goat bone patellar tendon bone allografts. J Orthop Res 9(2): 209–218

14. Herron LD, Newman MH (1989) The failure of ethylene oxide gas sterilized freeze dried bone graft for thoracic and lumbar spinal fusion. Spine 14: 496–500

15. Jackson DW, Windler GE, Simon TM (1990) Intra-articular reaction associated with the use of freeze dried ethylene oxide sterilized bone in patellar tendon and bone allograft in the reconstruction of the anterior cruciate ligament. Am J Sports Med 18: 1–10

16. Katz RW, Felthousen GC, Reddi AH (1990) Radiation sterilized insoluable collagenous bone matrix as a functional carrier of osteogenin for bone induction. Calcified Tissue Int 47: 183–185

17. Kitchen AD, Mann GF, Harrison JF, Zukermann AJ (1989) The effect of gamma radiation on the human immune deficiency virus and human coagulation proteins. Vox Sang 56: 223–229

18. Knaepler H, Haas H, Puschel HU (1990) Biomechanical properties of heat and radiation application to bone. Unfall Chirurgie 17: 194–199

19. Komender J, et al (1976) Radiation sterilized bone grafts evaluated by electron spin resonance technique in mechanical tests. Transplantation Proceedings 8 [2 Suppl]: 25–32

20. Komender J, et al (1990) Therapeutic effects of transplantation of lyophilized and radiation sterilized allogenic bone. Clin Orthop 272: 38–49

21. MacDonald DJ, McQuire MH (1991) Complications with large fragment allografts. In: Brown KL (ed) Complications of limb salvage. Prevention, management and outcome, Sixth International Symposium of Limb Salvage, Montreal, Canada

22. Mankin HJ, et al (1992) Current status of allografting for bone tumors. Orthopedics 15(10): 1147–1154

23. Markel M, Rock MG, et al (1992) Mechanical characteristics of proximal femoral reconstruction after fifty percent resection. J Bone Joint Surg (in press)

24. MNWR (1988) Transmission of HIV through bone transplantation. A case report and public health recommendation. MNWR 37: 597–599

25. Musculo DL, et al (1992) Massive femoral allografts. Follow-up for 22 to 36 years. Report of six cases. J Bone Joint Surg 74B: 887–892

26. Oakeshott R, et al (1994) Radiation sterilization of bone for transplantation. Presented at the European Association of Tissue Bank Meeting, Vienna

27. Paulos L, et al (1987) Comparative material properties of allograft tissues for ligament replacement: effects of type, age, sterilization, and preservation. Trans Orthop Res Soc 12: 129

28. Pelker RR, et al (1983) Biomechanical properties of bone allografts. Clin Orthop 174: 54–57

29. Prollo DJ, et al (1980) Ethylene oxide sterilization of bone, duramater, and fascia-lata for human transplantation. Neurosurgery 6: 529–539

30. Pruett AB, et al (1990) Investigation of the effect of low dose gamma radiation on the collagenous and noncollagenous proteins of bone matrix. Presented at the American Society for Bone and Mineral Research, Atlanta, GA

31. Rock MG, Chao EYS, et al (1991) Osteoarticular allografts for reconstruction after tumor excision about the knee. In: Brown KL (ed) Complications of limb salvage. Prevention, management and outcome, Sixth International Symposium of Limb Salvage, Montreal, Canada

32. Schwartz N (1988) Irradiation and sterilization of rat bone matrix gelatin. Acta Orthop Scand 59: 165–167

33. Simonds RJ, et al (1992) Transmission of human immune deficiency virus Type 1 from a sero-negative organ in a tissue donor. N Engl J Med 326(11): 726–732

34. Stevenson S, et al (1991) The fate of cancellous and cortical bone after transplantation of fresh and frozen tissue antigen matched and mismatched osteochondral allografts in dogs. J Bone Joint Surg 73A: 1143–1156

35. Triantafyllou N, et al (1975) The mechanical properties of lyophilized and irradiated bone grafts. Acta Orthop Belg 41: 35–44

36. Whittenberg RH, et al (1990) Compressive strength of autologous and allogenous bone graft for a thoracolumbar and cervical spinal fusion. Spine 15(10): 1073–1078

37. Wientroub S, Reddi AH (1988) Influence of irradiation on the osteoinductive potential of demineralized bone matrix. Calcified Tissue Int 42: 255–260

38. Wilson PD (1947) Experiences with a bone bank. Ann Surg 126: 932–946

39. Zasacki W (1991) The efficacy of application of lyophilized radiation sterilized bone graft in orthopedic surgery. Clin Orthop 272: 82–87

40. Zhang Y, et al (1993) A comprehensive study of physical parameters. Biomechanical properties and statistical correlation of iliac crest bone graft wedges used in spinal surgery. The effect of gamma radiation on mechanical material properties. Spine 19: 304–308

Authors' address: Michael G. Rock, M.D., Orthopedic Department, Mayo Clinic, 200 First Street SW, Rochester, MN 55905, U.S.A.

Preserved, Allogeneic Bone Grafts in Orthopaedic Reconstructions

J. Komender[1], H. Malczewska[2], and A. Komender[1]

[1] Central Tissue Bank in Warsaw, Department of Transplantology, Poland
[2] Department of Histology and Embriology, Medical School in Warsaw, Poland

Preserved allogeneic bone grafts have been used in orthopaedic reconstructions for many years [1, 2, 4, 10, 12]. Therapeutic effects of such transplantations have been reported in numerous papers [3, 5–7, 11, 13, 15]. General opinions about the effect of such transplantations are favorable. Literature reports have dealt mainly with the use of grafts in particular clinical situations and that do not permit the direct evaluation of the role of grafts. This study has been undertaken in our tissue bank to elucidate the role of preserved bone grafts based on a significant number of patients undergoing bone transplantation [9]. Having cooperation with nearly 200 hospitals throughout the country, we have selected patients from three units in which over 100 transplantations were performed in one year. The analysis covered approximately 45% of the patients operated in those units during that time. Data concerning 1014 patients have been collected. The mean age of patients was 14.3 years, with a very high standard deviation (S.D.) of 15.8 years. The prevailing diagnoses included congenital lesions (37.7%), benign tumors (18.3%) and scolioses (10.8%). Pathologic malformations requiring surgery were localized mainly in the hips (37.9%), vertebral column (25.6%) and femur (15.4%). The patients were examined 24 to 63 months after surgery. The effect of treatment and patient condition was determined by the same team that had performed the surgery. In this manner data on 1014 patients were collected. Some biological and clinical variables were coded and their correlations with the results of treatment were analysed. The following conclusions are based on this material.

General Results of Treatment

Table 1 presents the results of treatment in various diagnostic groups. Over 91% of transplantations in orthopaedic operations were completed with full restoration of form and function (37.1%—very good) or satisfactory (54.2%—satisfactory) as a result of treatment. Thus, the general conclusion seemed to confirm the clinical analysis published earlier. However, 5.1% of patients did not demonstrate any positive effects of treatment. We should also note that the largest group consists of children and very young patients.

Numerous sources have confirmed that the regeneration of bone and the rebuilding of bone grafts is better in younger patients. It is worth to note that in our material we found no correlation between the results of treatment and the age of patients in the Ch^2 test ($p = 0.2$).

Table 1. Results of treatment in various diagnoses

Diagnoses	Result of treatment									
	Very good number	%	Satisfactory number	%	Difficult to estimate number	%	Unsatisfactory number	%	Total number	%
Traumas	11	1.1	19	1.9	2	0.2	6	0.6	38	3.8
Benign tumors	107	10.6	68	6.7	6	0.6	5	0.5	186	18.4
Malignant tumors	0	0	2	0.2	0	0	0	0	2	0.2
Unspecific inflammations	6	0.6	30	3.0	1	0.1	4	0.4	41	4.1
Specific inflammations	42	4.2	86	8.5	5	0.5	7	0.7	140	13.9
Degenerative changes	34	3.4	38	3.8	3	0.3	7	0.7	82	8.1
Congenital changes	141	14.0	213	21.1	11	1.1	17	1.7	382	37.8
Scolioses	25	2.5	73	7.2	7	0.7	4	0.4	109	10.8
Others	9	0.9	18	1.8	1	0.1	2	0.2	30	3.0
Total	375	37.1	547	54.2	36	3.6	52	5.1	1010	100

$Chi^2 = 75.479$; degrees of freedom, 24; $p < 0.01$

Dispersion of successful results of treatment was found to depend on diagnosis, localization of pathology, and post-surgery observation period.

It maybe of significance to find out the sequence of various biological and clinical variables influencing the result of treatment. Some statistical trials based on Chi^2 permit to arrange some variables of non-parametric analysis according to the values of coincidence indices (c.i.). Analysis of this index (14) reveals that the strong correlation with the final results of treatment concerns mainly rebuilding of the graft (0.633), early estimated result (0.596), reoperation (0.519), complicated wound healing (0.364) and diagnosis (0.304). Further, some biologic or clinical traits of the analysis, such as the duration of illness before surgery (0.209), level of disability before surgery (0.157), age (0.127) and general complaints (0.112) were found not to correlate with the final result of treatment.

The whole analyzed group included 166 patients (11.4%) with concomitant diseases. The incidence of unsatisfactory results was higher (approx. 11%) in this group ($p < 0.001$). It is, however, difficult to asses the influence of various diseases on the result of bone transplantation, as the group was not homogeneous (circulatory illnesses, infectious diseases, neuropathology, tumors and others).

This gives an idea of the importance of various factors affecting the results of bone transplantation in the group under analysis.

Fitness for Work after Bone Transplantation

Fitness for work after bone transplantation, especially in the case of manual workers seems to be a good indication of successful treatment. We have been interested in this topic for many years [8]. In the group of patients analyzed recently, 73% of transplanted patients were found to be capable of physical effort and they did not have to change their

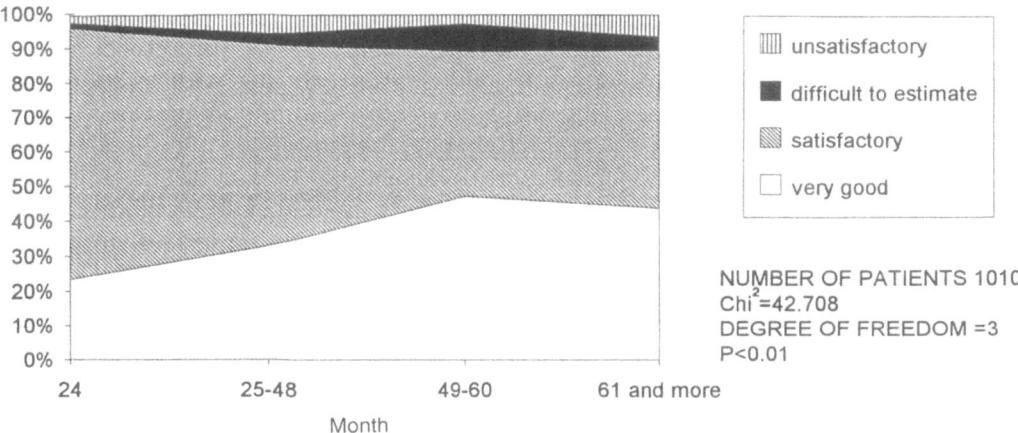

Fig. 1. Results of bone transplantation estimated at various times after surgery

occupation. This means that most patients after treatment may be regarded as fully fit. Among them 20.4% were able to work but had to change the occupation, due to some physical limitations, while 6.6% of the patients were not fit for any manual work.

Comparison of the coincidence indices of various traits of analysis reveals that the main factors affecting the capacity for work after bone transplantation were age (0.557), diagnosis (0.556), physical disability (0.517), rebuilding of the graft (0.448), and reoperation (0.292). Such variables as intra and postsurgery complications (0.179), handicap level (0.209) and general state before surgery (0.218) are of less importance.

Fitness for work after preserved bone transplantation seems to be closely related to age. The number of the patients unable to work increased with age and reached 47.7% in the group over 50 years of age. Between the ages of 11 and 25 years, the necessity for patients to change their occupation or occupational training appeared more often than in other groups ($p < 0.01$).

Evaluation of Results of Treatment During Different Post-Surgery Times

Analysis of the coincidence of positive results of treatment in relation to the post-surgery observation time (Fig. 1) reveals the increasing number of "very good" results until 60 months of observation followed by a certain decrease, with accompanying reduction in the number of satisfactory results and a higher incidence of unsatisfactory results. This correlation seems to be significant ($p < 0.01$) in the Ch^2 test. However, when we calculate the c.i. for "observation time after surgery" with the "final result of treatment" its value is very low (0.223), suggesting that the coincidence is of limited importance.

Rebuilding of the Bone Graft as Prognosis for Result of Treatment

Rebuilding of the bone graft after transplantation is strongly correlated with good result of treatment (value of c.i. = 0.633) and with fitness for work (value of c.i. = 0.448). Other traits of analysis seem to confirm this phenomenon. Unrebuilt grafts were infrequent i.e. in 30 patients (approx. 3%), while among the unsatisfactory results the absence of graft rebuilding was observed in 56.6%. Graft rebuilding also correlated with "reoperation" (when the graft is often removed), "diagnosis" (less advanced rebuilding was found in posttraumatic malformations and congenital changes than in benign tumors and specific inflammations), "complaints after treatment" (frequent with delayed graft rebuilding), "localization" (better in the arm, hips and femur and not as good in the vertebral column and lower legs). Proper bone graft rebuilding seems to be an important prognostic factor.

Allogeneic Bone Enriched by Autogenous Bone for Transplantation

In 46 patients in the course of surgery the allogeneic bone from the tissue bank was enriched with the patient's own bone. However, this did not improve the result of treatment. The number of unsatisfactory results of treatment among these patients was higher (10.9%), while the proportion of positive results was diminished. The difference in dispersion of evaluated results of treatment between the patients who received their own bone together with preserved bone and those who received only bank bone was significant ($p < 0.05$). It might be possible that the addition of the patients' own bone during reconstruction was performed in specially difficult clinical situations.

The Problem of Deep-Frozen and Lyophilized Bone Grafts

The problem of optimal bone preservation has been discussed for many years, and the arguments in this matter become very emotional. Since our analysis has been based mostly on the observation of patients who received lyophilized and radiation-sterilized bone, we would like to compare our results with those obtained by transplantation of deep-frozen and radiation-sterilized bone (Table 2). In the tissue banks in Poland both techniques of preservation have been equally used for ten years. In 1993 W. Marczyński published the results of orthopaedic reconstructions when only deep-frozen bone grafts were used [11]. Table 2 presents a comparison of the results of our earlier analysis

Table 2. Results of treatment after preserved bone transplantation. Comparison of the results of treatment with lyophilized and deep-frozen bone grafts

Result	Bone preserved by				p Value
	Lyophilization*		Deep freezing*		
	Number	%	Number	%	
Very good	375	37.1	261	57.7	~ 0.001
Satisfactory	547	54.2	147	32.6	~ 0.001
Difficult to estimate	36	3.6	35	7.9	~ 0.001
Unsatisfactory	52	5.1	8	1.8	= 0.01
Total	1010	100	452	100	

*Radiation-sterilized — 33 kGy

with those of Marczyński. The observation of patients operated with the use of deep-frozen bone was carried out by Dr. Marczyński who also evaluated clinical effects. The only element in common in those studies was the tissue banking performed in the same unit.

It is clear that the number of very good results is much higher in the group transplanted with the use of deep-frozen grafts than that with lyophilized grafts, with the difference being highly significant. The opposite may be observed in the group of unsatisfactory results. The number of unsatisfactory results in the group with lyophilized grafts is nearly three times as high as that with deep-frozen grafts. This is a very strong argument for the use of frozen bone grafts in orthopaedic reconstructions.

Conclusion

Allogeneic bone grafts prepared by the tissue banks are useful for skeletal reconstruction. The methods of grafts preservation seem to be of significance in surgical applications. The result of treatment after bone transplantation was found to depend on numerous biological and clinical variables.

References

1. Burchardt H, Enneking WP (1978) Transplantation of bone. Surg Clin North Am 58: 403
2. Burwell RG (1969) The fate of bone grafts. In: Apley AG (ed) Recent advances in orthopaedics. London: Churchill, p 115
3. Czitrom AA (1992) Indications and use of morsellized and small-segment allograft bone in general orthopaedics. In: Czitrom AA, Gross AE (eds) Allografts in orthopaedic practice. Baltimore: Williams & Wilkins, p 47
4. Dodd CA, Fergusson CM, Freedman L, Houghton GR, Thomas D (1988) Allograft versus autograft bone in scoliosis surgery. J Bone Joint Surg 70: 431
5. Friedlaender GE (1987) Bone banking: In support of reconstructive surgery of the hip. Clin Orthop 225: 17
6. Head WC, Malinin TI, Berklacich F(1987) Freeze-dried proximal femur allografts in revision total hip arthroplasty. Clin Orthop 215: 109
7. Komender J, Komender A (1977) Evaluation of radiation-sterilized tissues in clinical use. In: Gaughram ERL, Goudie AJ (eds) Sterilization of medical products by ionizing radiation. Montreal: Multiscience, p 188
8. Komender J, Malczewska H (1981) Fitness for work after preseved bone transplantation. Arch Immunol Ther Exper 29: 535
9. Komender J, Malczewska H, Komender A (1991) Therapeutic effects of transplantation of lyophylized and radiation-sterilized allogeneic bone. Clin Orthop 272: 38
10. Kowalenko PP (1975) Kliniczeskaja Transplantologia. Rostowskie Kniznoje Izdat, p 188
11. Marczyński W, Tylman D, Komender J (1993) Frozen and radiation-steriled allogenic biostatic bone grafts in the clinical use. In: Ricciardi L (ed) Recent advances in oral and orthopaedic prostheses: Bone implant interface. Milano: Pubblideale S.r.L., p 197
12. Melloning JT, Bowers GM, Cotton WR (1981) Comparison of bone graft materials. Part II. New bone formation with autografts and allografts: A histological evaluation. J Peridontol 52: 297
13. Miller F, Sussman M, Stamp W (1984) The use of bone allograft: A survey of current practice. In: Jacobs RR (ed) Pathogenesis of idiopathic scoliosis. Proc Internatl Conference, p 174
14. Pearson K (1904) On the theory of contingency. (Memoirs, Biometric series, No 1) London: Drapers, p 119
15. Zasadzki W (1991) The efficacy of application of lyophilized, radiation-sterilized bone graft in orthopaedic surgery. Clin Orthop 272: 82

Authors' addresses: Prof. Dr. med. Janusz Komender and Dr. med. Andrzej Komender, Central Tissue Bank in Warsaw, Department of Transplantology, Medical School in Warsaw, PL-02-004 Warszawa, ul. Chałubińskiego 5, Poland. Dr. biol. Hanna Malczewska, Department of Histology and Embriology, Medical School in Warsaw, PL-02-004 Warszawa, ul. Chałubińskiego 5, Poland.

Allogeneic Bone Grafts: Study of Radiation Sterilized Bone Tissue by Electron Paramagnetic Resonance Spectrometry and a New Model of Periosteal Induction of Osteogenesis

K. Ostrowski[1], K. Wlodarski[1], A. Dziedzic-Goclawska[2], J. Michalik[3], and W. Stachowicz[3]

[1] Department of Histology, Medical Academy, Warsaw, Poland
[2] Department of Transplantology, Institute of Biostructure, Medical Academy, Warsaw, Poland
[3] Institute of Nuclear Chemistry and Technology, Warsaw, Poland

Summary

The positive clinical result of bone grafting depends on rebuilding of the graft i.e. its resorption and induction of new bone formation by the host. In our research on induction of bone formation a new experimental system was described based on induction of periosteal bone formation in mice by Moloney virus. No direct clinical application is proposed.

The fate of radiation sterilized bone grafts can be controlled by a new type of biological marker. This marker is induced by ionizing radiation in the form of stable paramagnetic centers in the crystalline lattice of bone hydroxyapatite. These can be measured by electron paramagnetic resonance (EPR) spectrometry and can serve as biological markers for the evaluation of crystallinity of bone mineral, quantitation of the rebuilding process of radiation sterilized bone grafts and estimation of doses of absorbed ionizing radiation.

Introduction

The positive clinical result of bone grafting is based, after a period when the bone graft serves as a mechanical prosthesis, on the rebuilding process of the graft. Rebuilding of grafted bone means its resorption and creeping substitution by the host's own newly formed bone tissue. New bone formation is induced by many, nowadays well defined factors, contained in grafted bone matrix. The process of bone preservation performed in the Tissue Banks can lower or even destroy the inductive potency of bone grafts.

In this short review paper we will discuss two results which were achieved by our group in the field of research: 1. on bone induction and 2. on control of the fate of radiation sterilized bone grafts.

A new experimental system of induction of periosteal bone formation was described and the use of a new biological marker in the form of radiation induced paramagnetic centers in the grafts' mineral is proposed.

Induction of Periosteal Bone Formation

It was demonstrated that in rodents, the murine Moloney sarcoma oncogenic RNA virus (Mu-MSV) induces upon muscular inoculation a rapidly growing tumor, which regresses spontaneously due to the host immune reaction within 3–4 weeks. The growing sarcoma induces proliferation and osteoblastic differentiation of cells in the adjacent periosteal membranes. Within 5–6 days post virus inoculation the periosteum becomes a thick membrane, composed of 7–20 layers of osteoblasts and fibroblasts. Deposition of osteoid within this hyperplastic periosteum begins. In some cases chondrogenesis in this activated membrane is observed. After 2–3 weeks the newly formed cancellous bone covering the old original cortex of long bones is 3–5 times thicker than the original bone. This orthotopic induced bone formation sometimes affects the whole periphery of bone, sometimes is asymmetric but always affects the site adjacent to the tumor. The regression of Moloney sarcoma is accompanied by cessation of periosteal growth and the start of rebuilding and maturation of cancellous bone which lasts for 6 months. Although this model has no direct clinical application, it serves as a research tool in the quickly developing field of induction of bone formation.

Radiation-induced Paramagnetic Centers Used as Markers in the Research of Bone Tissue

Deproteinized bone, as well as synthetic HA, irradiated at room temperature, both in vacuo and in the presence of atmospheric oxygen shows an asymmetric ESR singlet with spectral width (ΔH) of 8, 56 G and a spectroscopic splitting factor $g\perp = 2.036$ and $g\| = 1.9978$. This stable ESR singlet (Fig. 1) is attributed to the paramagnetic centers generated by ionizing radiation in the crystalline lattice of bone HA. Although a lot of experiments have been done, there are still controversial opinions concerning the structure of these centers. According to one opinion, these centers are holes trapped in the Ca^{2+} vacancies of the Ca column of the crystalline lattice of HA. The alternative view is that this signal is connected with carboxyl radicals contained in bone mineral [1, 6]. The two possibilities do not exclude each other.

Whatever the nature of these centers, the radiation-induced ESR singlet possesses three important features: 1) it originates from crystals of tissue mineral, 2) it is stable at room temperature for years and 3) its intensity is dose dependent in a wide range.

All these features have been examined and explored for their usefulness in biomedical research.

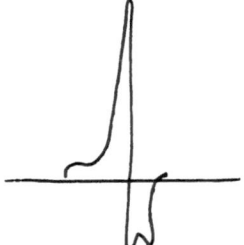

Fig. 1. The asymmetric ESR singlet with spectra width (ΔH) of 8, 56 G and spectroscopic splitting factor $g\perp = 2.036$ and $g\| = 1.9978$. This stable ESR singlet is attributed to the paramagnetic centers generated by ionizing radiation in the crystalline lattice of bone HA

Crystallinity of Bone Mineral

In the course of the synthesis of HA in vitro as well as during the process of mineralization in vivo, the primary HA crystals differ from the mature ones. They are small, they exhibit distortions in crystalline lattice, and they have a low calcium-to-phosphorus molar ratio. In the course of synthesis in vitro as well as in vivo the perfection and the size of crystals increase, as expressed by increased crystallinity. This process is described as a process of maturation of the mineral and it plays an important role in biology. As a rule, the higher the crystallinity of the mineral the better are the mechnical properties of bone tissue.

The definition of crystallinity of tissue mineral is a purely operational one, because the measured values depend on the resolution of the applied method. X-ray diffraction and infrared spectrometry have been used mainly for this purpose [11]. Generally crystallinity is defined as the ratio of the measurable fraction of HA crystals to the total amount of mineral in the tissue. Comparison of the intensity of the stable ESR singlet in different kinds of skeletal tissues such as cartilage, compact bone, tooth enamel and synthetic HA allowed the observation that in tissues characterized by a higher degree of crystallinity, as determined by X-ray diffractometry [8], the yield of radiation-induced stable paramagnetic centers is markedly higher (Fig. 2).

Experiments performed on synthetic HA of different average crystal sizes (c-axis) support the observations described above and show that the yield of radiation-induced stable paramagnetic centers is proportional to the average crystal size (in the range of 7–50 nm), as determined by X-ray diffraction (Fig. 3). This phenomenon can be explained in terms of surface effect. In smaller crystals the contribution of surface atoms to the overall number of atoms within the crystal is greater than in larger ones. This factor increases considerably the possibility of annealing of the discussed paramagnetic centers localized on or near the surface, which is in direct contact with the surrounding medium. This interpretation is supported by the time-dependent decay of paramagnetic centers in samples of HA differing in their crystal sizes (Fig. 4). The smaller the average crystal size, the more advanced is the decay of the intensity of the ESR singlet measured at various time intervals after irradiation. In crystals of average size of 7 nm the spin concentration decreases by approximately 40% and reaches a plateau value after 8 days of storage. In the case of bigger crystals (48 nm) the decrease is by 10% and the plateau is reached within 2 days. If the average crystal size is below a certain value, i.e., less than 3 nm,

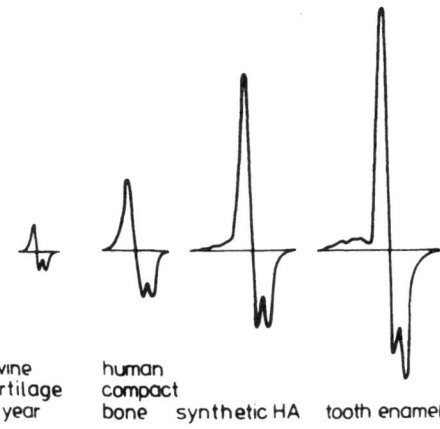

bovine
cartilage
1.5 year

human
compact
bone   synthetic HA   tooth enamel

Fig. 2. In tissues characterized by a higher degree of crystallinity, as determined by X-ray diffractometry, the yield of radiation induced stable paramagnetic centers is markedly higher

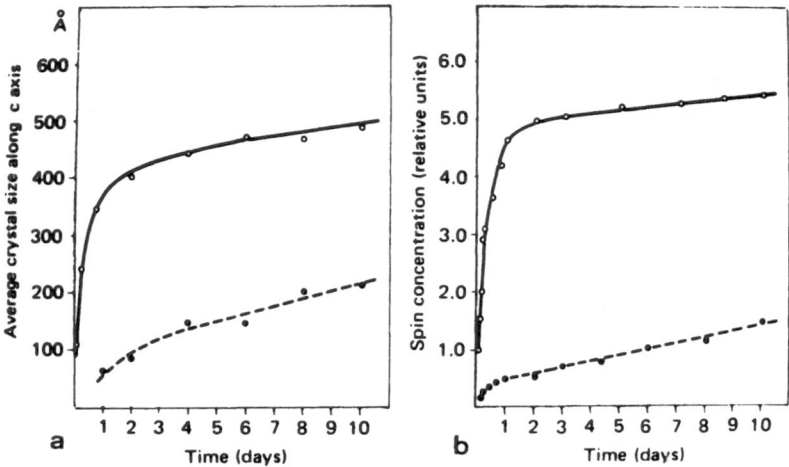

Fig. 3. The yield of radiation-induced stable paramagnetic centers is proportional to the average crystal size (in the range of 7–50 nm), as determined by X-ray diffraction

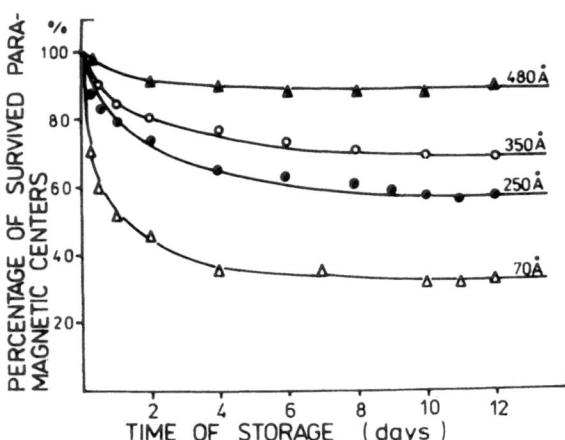

Fig. 4. The time-dependent decay of paramagnetic centers in samples of HA differing in their crystal sizes

complete decay of the described paramagnetic centers is observed. This fraction of mineral is called by operational definition— noncrystalline or "amorphous" [8].

On the basis of the described model experiments the "crystallinity coefficient" has been defined as the ratio of the amount of the described radiation-induced, stable, paramagnetic centers to the total mineral content in the tissue sample. In practice, to evaluate this parameter the lyophilized, powdered bone samples are irradiated at room temperature with a saturation dose of 100 kGy (10 Mrads). After annealing all other unstable paramagnetic entities (usually 5 weeks after irradiation) the concentration of the described stable paramagnetic centers is measured at the X band in the ESR spectrometer and related to the total mineral content after ashing of tissue samples. The value of the crystallinity coefficient is expressed in arbitrary units.

The example of maturation of bone mineral is provided by comparison of mineral content and crystallinity of bone mineral in growing and adult rats (Table 1). In the femoral diaphysis the amount of mineral in young rats was lower by about 13% in comparison to the adult ones. One the other hand, the crystallinity coefficient of mineral

Table 1. Age-dependent changes in mineral content and its crystallinity coefficient in femur diaphyses in rats

Age, wk	n	Mineral content, g/g dried mass	Crystallinity Coefficient, arbitrary units
5	7	0.66 ± 0.012	23.72 ± 4.08
15	7	0.76 ± 0.023*	37.16 ± 0.93*

Values are means ± SD. *Statistically significant differences evaluated by Wilcoxon test (α = 0.01).

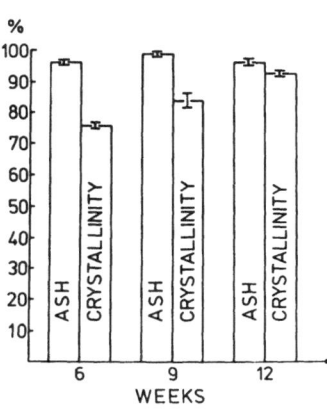

Fig. 5. The experiment was performed on 45 adult rabbits. Standard defects near the tibial tuberosity were performed with the use of rotating knife. The amount of mineral and its crystallinity were measured in the newly formed callus at various time intervals after fracturing and compared with the values characteristic for normal, healthy bone in the same individuals. Six weeks after fracture the amount of mineral deposited in the newly formed callus reached 95% of the value of control bone, while at the same time the crystallinity of mineral was low, less than 80% of control value

in the young animals was lower by about 36% when compared with the adult rats. This signifies the immaturity of bone mineral in growing animals [2].

Bone healing is another example of maturation of mineral (Fig. 5). The experiment was performed on 45 adult rabbits. Standard defects near the tibial tuberosity were performed with the use of a rotating knife. The amount of mineral and its crystallinity were measured in the newly formed callus at various time intervals after fracturing and compared with the values characteristic for normal, healthy bone in the same individuals. Six weeks after fracture the amount of mineral deposited in the newly formed callus reached 95% of the value of control bone, while at the same time the crystallinity of mineral was low, less than 80% of control value. The crystallinity of mineral deposited in the callus increased with time, reaching nearly 95% of control value only 12 weeks after fracture [4].

Changes in the crystallinity of bone mineral were found in some systemic bone diseases, such as in congenital osteopetrosis, which occurs in many mammalian species, humans included. There are many different types of this disease, but the common features of all kinds of osteopetrosis are increased skeletal mass, disturbance in development of bone marrow cavities in long bones, pathological fractures of bones and disturbance in development and eruption of teeth. Generally speaking, the process of bone remodelling is inhibited due to the decrease of bone resorption. In many types of osteopetrosis, changes in the ultrastructure of osteoclasts demonstrated by underdevelopment of the ruffled border, the structure responsible for resorptive properties, were described. Some types of osteopetrosis in mammalian species can be cured by transplantation of normal syngeneic bone marrow.

Table 2. Mineral content and its crystallinity coefficient in femur diaphyses in normal, osteopetrotic, and osteopetrotic-cured rats

Rat group	n	Age, wk	Mineral content, g/g of dried mass	Crystallinity coefficient, arbitrary units
Control	5	14	0.71 ± 0.01	30.6 ± 2.8
op/op	5	14	0.74 ± 0.01*	24.8 ± 0.9*
op/op cur	3	19	0.72 ± 0.01	28.2 ± 2.5

Values are means ± SD. op/op, osteopetrotic rats; op/op cur, osteopetrotic-cured rats.
*Statistically significant differences in comparison to control evaluated by Student's t test ($\alpha = 0.01$).

In osteopetrotic rats (op/op) a significant increase of the amount of mineral accompanied by the marked decrease of its crystallinity was observed in femoral diaphyses (Table 2), which might be one of the reasons for pathological fractures occurring in this disease. After syngeneic bone marrow transplantation the normalization of both values was observed. These results demonstrate that evaluation of crystallinity of mineral, based on ESR spectrometry, may be useful for diagnosis and monitoring of therapeutic effects in the treatment of osteopetrosis [5].

ESR spectrometry was also used to evaluate the crystallinity of mineral deposited in pathological calcification in heterotopic places, namely in arterial walls in the course of arteriosclerosis. In advanced arteriosclerotic lesions the crystallinity of deposited mineral is as high as in compact bone tissue [3].

Quantitative Evaluation of the Rebuilding Process of Radiation-Sterilized Bone Grafts

The stability of radiation-induced paramagnetic centers in bone mineral (over 10 years of observation) allowed their use as a new marker for the evaluation of the rate of resorption as well as substitution of radiation-sterilized bone grafts by the host's own, newly formed bone tissue. The rate of resorption is calculated by measuring the decrease of the total amount of radiation-induced paramagnetic centers introduced with the graft into the recipient at different time intervals after transplantation. The radiation-sterilized bone graft loses its paramagnetic markers only through the process of dissolution of HA crystals. This happens in the course of graft resorption. This marker is never reutilized, in contrast to radioisotopical markers. The rate of substitution is calculated by a comparison of the concentration of spins in the grafted bone before implantation and the concentration of spins at definite times after grafting. The ingrowing, newly formed bone "dilutes" the radiation-induced paramagnetic centers present in the graft. The rate of this "dilution" describes quantitatively the rate of the "creeping substitution" of the graft [7].

Dosimetry of Absorbed Dose of Ionizing Radiation Based on ESR Spectrometry

Although the exact nature and origin of ESR signals induced in bone tissue by ionizing radiation are not clearly defined, the suggestion to use them for dosimetry of absorbed dose of ionizing radiation was proposed. A linear relationship between the yield, at room temperature, of stable paramagnetic centers and the applied dose of ionizing radiation has been found in the wide range of doses, up to 20 ky (2 Mrads). Various kinds of ionizing radiation differing in nature and energies give different yields of stable paramagnetic centers in bone HA crystals. This depends on different linear energy transfer (LET) values. Therefore the dose-dependence curves for gamma radiation, and X-rays (250 kV) differ in their slopes. These curves can be used as nomograms for estimation of the dose of ionizing radiation absorbed by bone tissue in the living organism. With the use of ESR spectrometry the dose absorbed in bone tissue in the range of 1 Gy (100 rads) can be measured, but with the use of enamel as the dosimeter, absorbed doses as low as 0.5 Gy can be detected. This is due to the fact that in tooth enamel the crystallinity of mineral is much higher than in bone and therefore the yield of generation of stable paramagnetic centers is higher [8].

Skeletal tissues might serve as a biological dosimeter in the case of accidental exposure even when the applied dose and the geometry of irradiation are unknown. Small samples of bone or teeth, weighing a few milligrams, could serve for estimation not only of the absorbed dose but also for scanning of those parts of the skeleton that escaped irradiation. This idea was substantiated in model experiments performed on the human pelvis embedded in paraffin wax and irradiated according to the scheme used by radiation therapists for the treatment of ovarian cancer [10].

References

1. Doi Y, Aoba T, Moriwaki Y, Takahashi I (1980) Orientation of carbonate ions in human tooth enamel studied with use of $^{13}CO_3$ radical ions probes. J Dent Res 59: 1473–1477
2. Dziedzic-Goclawska A (1984) Crystallinity of Mineral and Spatial Distribution of Collagen Fibers in Normal and Pathologically Changed Bone Tissue. PhD thesis J. Warsaw; Medical Academy of Warsaw
3. Dziedzic-Goclawska A, Fuchs U, Ostrowski K, Stachowicz W, Michalik J (1984) Crystallinity of mineral deposited in arterial walls in the course of arteriosclerosis in diabetics and in patients with normal carbohydrate metabolism. Basic Appl Histochem 28: 21–28
4. Dziedzic-Goclawska A, Michalik J, Stachowicz W, Zasacki W, Ostrowski K (1976) Theoretical basis for evaluation of the kinetics of mineralization of newly formed bone and the process of ageing of calcified tissues by electron spin resonance spectroscopy. Nova Acta Leopold. 44: 217–224
5. Dziedzic-Goclawska A, Ostrowski K, Stachowicz W, Moutier, R (1979) Decrease of crystallinity of bone mineral in osteopetrotic rats. Metab Bone Dis Relat Dis 2: 33–37
6. Geoffroy M, Tochon-Danguy HJ (1985) Long lived radicals in irradiated apatites of biological interest: an ESR study of apatite samples treated with $^{13}CO_2$. Int J Radiat Biol Relat Stud Phys Chem Med 48: 621–633
7. Ostrowski K, Dziedzic-Goclawska A (1976) Electron spin resonance spectrometry in investigations on mineralized tissues. In: Bourne GH (ed) Biochemistry and physiology of bone, 2nd edn. New York: Academic, Vol IV, p 303
8. Ostrowski K, Dziedzic-Goclawska A, Stachowicz W (1980) Radiation-induced paramagnetic entities in tissue mineral and their use in calcified tissue research. In: Pryor W (ed) Free radicals in biology. New York: Academic, vol IV, p 321
9. Ostrowski K, Dziedzic-Goclawska A, Stachowicz W, Michalik J (1974) Accuracy, sensitivity and specificity of electron spin resonance analysis of mineral constituents of irradiated tissues. Ann NY Acad Sci 238: 186
10. Ostrowski K, Komender A, Liniecki J, Cisowska B, Stachowicz A, Michalik J (1975) Distribution of absorbed dose of ionizing radiation in bone in simulated therapeutic irradiation measured by means of ESR technique. Nukleonika 20: 877–880

11. Posner AS, Betts, F, Blumenthal N (1979) Bone mineral composition and structure. In: Simmons D (ed) Skeletal research. New York: Academic, pp 167–187

Authors' addresses: Prof. Kazimierz Ostrowski, M.D., Ph.D. and Prof. K. Wlodarski, M.D., Ph.D., Department of Histology, Institute of Biostructure, Medical Academy, Chalubinskiego 5, PL-02-004 Warsaw, Poland; Prof. Anna Dziedzic-Goclawska, M.D., Ph.D. Department of Transplantology, Institute of Biostructure, Medical Academy, Chalubinskiego 5, PL-02-004 Warsaw; Ass. Prof. Jacek Michalik and Dr. Sci. W. Stachowicz, Institute of Nuclear Chemistry and Technology, Dorodna 16, Warsaw, Poland.

Bone Replacement Studies Using Titanium Chamber Models in Small Animals

P. Aspenberg

Department of Orthopaedics, Lund University Hospital, Lund, Sweden

Summary

When Kiel bone was introduced clinically, animal experiments seemed to demonstrate its efficiency. It later became obvious that the utilized experimental models were insufficiently sensitive. This presentation discusses the demands on a model for evaluating materials with claimed "osteoconductive" properties, and describes some attempts to meet these demands by using titanium bone chamber techniques. A new type of chamber allows studies of the osteoconductive performance of cancellous bone grafts in rats. This model makes it possible to carry out large series of experiments. It was shown that defatting increased bone graft incorporation, and that defatted bone grafts performed even better if they were pretreated with basic Fibroblast Growth Factor (bFGF). Ethylene oxide sterilization had a dramatic negative effect even though residuals were below levels recommended by the FDA. Radiation had no effect. As fibrous tissue ingrowth into porous materials was usually affected in the same way as bone ingrowth, it appears that the term "osteoconduction" has to be further defined.

Introduction

Kiel bone was introduced clinically after having passed the "spongiosa test" [25], which means that the material was found to be incorporated in 5 mm diameter burr holes in cancellous bone of dogs. In 1961 Maatz and Bauermeister [24] reported 316 patients with mostly excellent results. During the 1960-ies Kiel bone was widely used for various indications including fresh fractures, delayed unions and osteomyelitis. While good clinical results were reported by several authors, a failure rate of 42% in 142 cases has been recorded [21]. Hallén reproduced the result of the "spongiosa test" in dogs, and also performed the same test in 4 patients comparing fresh autografts, frozen allografts and Kiel grafts. No differences could be recorded between these very different types of grafts [19]. It appears that the healing capacity of these small holes was good, regardless of the grafting material used.

Schweiberer [30] increased the sensitivity of the "spongiosa test" by increasing the diameter of the burr hole. Now the method could distinguish between different types of grafts. In a large experimental study in dogs, Schweiberer reported negative effects of Kiel bone. Autologus bone, prepared as Kiel-bone, was not better. He also implanted Kiel bone into healing fractures of dogs, and in almost all cases the Kiel bone was shown to rather inhibit than facilitate bone healing. Cortical bone was regularly seen sequestered by fibrous tissue. Schweiberer's thesis in 1970 [30], and increasing negative clinical experience caused Kiel-bone to disappear from orthopaedic practice almost totally.

In neurosurgery, however, Kiel bone has proven useful for vertebral fusion due to the fact that it is not incorporated. A Kiel bone dowel remains unchanged, therefore giving better immobilization than an autograft which might remodel and soften, and thus allow intervertebral mobility [28].

The Kiel-bone experience raises many questions, two of which will be discussed: 1) How can we evaluate bone replacement materials in animal models? 2) In what situations is incorporation and remodelling desirable?

Osteoconduction

Regarding the evaluation of bone replacement materials, I will concentrate on bone ingrowth, but then we must ask ourselves by which mechanisms the material affects ingrowth. The answer to that question is usually "by osteoconduction". However, there is no good definition of osteoconduction: usually words like "trellis' or "scaffold" are used. These descriptive metaphors would mean a rather simple mechanical function by which a porous material could protect a preosteoblastic tissue from deformation which would disturb its differentiation into bone [5, 17]. This "mechanical function" also includes the effects of pore size, elasticity and the ability to isolate a bone defect from soft tissue. However, bone conduction is sometimes thought of as a surface phenomenone, which should indicate that the surfaces of an osteoconductive material selectively favour the anchorage of bone forming cells. Cell adhesion is dependent on the protein film which forms on any implanted material, which in turn may be dependent on the surface characteristics of the material. A selective affinity for osteoblasts is theoretically possible, for example if an implant is artificially covered with a protein with affinity for cell surface attachment molecules (integrins) on osteoblastic cells. Bone Sialoprotein (BSP) may have selective affinity to osteoblasts (even though the receptor seems nonspecific), but experiments in our laboratory have failed to show increased "osteoconduction" of BSP-coated hydroxyapatite (unpublished data). If an implant has not been manipulated for selective osteoblast affinity, it is probably wise to expect "mesenchymal tissue conduction" or "callus conduction" rather than bone conduction. When comparing empty defects and porous hydroxyapatite, the most striking effect of the porous hydroxyapatite in our experiments has been that on fibrous tissue ingrowth [6]. The extent to which this tissue was metaplastically ossified seemed to depend more on other factors, e.g. mechanical load, or distance from loaded bone, although the osteoblasts tended to lay down their matrix on hydroxypatite surfaces.

Bank bone is a bone replacement material which contains large quantities of a variety of potent growth factors, such as BMP and TGF-ß, believed to play a role in fracture repair and bone remodelling. However, the biological significance of these factors in a non-demineralized bone graft is unknown. Certainly, if these growth factors are not activated in the bone grafting situation, a bone allograft would have no biological advantage over a synthetic bone replacement material. Although the significance of the naturally occurring endogenous growth factors in a bone graft is uncertain, it is clear that an addition of exogenous growth factors has stimulatory effects [29, 33, 36, 37]. Thus, osteoconduction (viz material effects) and osteoinduction (viz BMP-effects) are not the only mechanisms by which a bone replacement material may act. Between these two extremes, there is room for other hypothetical bone stimulatory mechanisms, of which growth factors are only one.

Chamber Models

It is clear from the above that we do not know what determines tissue ingrowth into a porous material, and to what extent the ingrowth tissue forms bone. In order to find the best material, we can only compare ingrowth distances under as standardized conditions as possible. The complexity of the factors which make up osteoconductive properties indicates that we may need an assay model which is simple and allows a large number of experiments, i.e. a model in small animals. Usually this means rabbits. In smaller animals it is practically difficult to create large enough defects, at least in cancellous bone. In the rabbit, large burr holes in the distal femur have been able to discriminate between various degrees of bone ingrowth [22], but the variation in this model is great and may necessitate the use of larger animals like the swine [29].

In order to standardize a defect in the rabbit for studies in the osteoconduction by bank bone, our group applied the Bone Harvest Chamber (BHC; Fig. 1). This a cylinder made of pure titanium, with a 1 mm wide transverse canal for tissue ingrowth. The canal acts as a standardized bone defect. Ingrown tissue can be harvested from the canal in the interior of the device via a subcutaneous opening. Bone formation in this model has been shown to be quite sensitive to various forms of disturbance. Small amounts of particulate

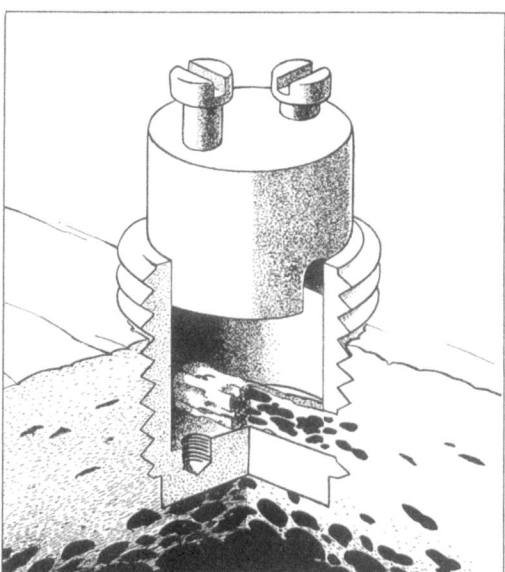

Fig. 1. The Bone Harvest Chamber (BHC) is a 7 mm high and 6 mm wide titanium cylinder which is threaded so that it can be screwed into the proximal tibial methaphysis of adult rabbits. The cylinder contains a piston-like core with a $1 \times 1 \times 5$ mm groove facing the bottom of the cylinder. This groove is co-axial with holes in the outer cylinder, providing a continous canal through the entire device for tissue ingrowth. The cylinder will osseointegrate, but one end sticks out of the bone. From this end, the core can be pulled out, thus exposing the tissue inside the ingrowth canal, which can be harvested without disturbing the surrounding bone. The chamber can be used for repeated harvesting, and bone formation in the chamber has been shown to be quite sensitive to various forms of disturbance

biomaterials (bone cement, high density polythylene, titanium alloy and crome-cobalt, but not hydroxyapatite) diminished bone ingrowth, as did demineralized bone matrix [2, 16, 18]. This chamber has been modified for continuous drug application to the bone ingrowth canal [1, 3], and for micromotion [5, 16].

The BHC has the advantage that one animal can be used for several consecutive experiments. The bone production is reproducible over a considerable time [23]. In fact, we have harvested rabbits more than 20 times over a time period of one and a half years. An analysis of 340 paired specimens, from the second to the 20th operation of the animal, showed no decay with time in 99mTcMDP scintimetric activity [34]. The harvested bone can be used as a graft, which is formed under standardized conditions with a predetermined shape. When grafted into another chamber, it fits the site to be grafted.

Using the BHC, our group has shown that frozen allogeneic bone grafts are better incorporated if they are defatted [4]. This effect is due to both a removal of debris and a lessened immune reaction to alloantigens [32, 34]. However, the differences were small, probably because the conditions were favorable for healing of the defect, regardless of treatment. The favorable conditions for bone formation in this model caused a seemingly paradoxical finding: osteoinductive demineralized bone matrix had a negative effect [2]. The disturbance from the foreign material was greater than the benefit from the osteoinductive factors, which were unnecessary.

When evaluating osteoconductive properties, the defect should be big, so as to challenge the adjacent bone with a space that it can hardly fill spontaneously. However, if one uses a large segmental defect in a long bone, surrounding soft tissues will compete with the bone resection ends to fill the defect. In the middle of the defect, all ingrown cells will be derived from soft tissues, and thus we are in reality studying an extraskeletal site. If the surrounding soft tissues are shielded off, we arrive at what is called "guided tissue regeneration", which has proven a highly useful principle in the treatment of periodontal bone defects. Only if soft tissues are shielded off and the defect still does not heal, do we have the appropriate conditions to evaluate osteoconduction.

In order to fulfill these criteria, our group designed the Bone Conduction Chamber (BCC). In this device, the bone enters one end of a cylindrical space at the cortical level. This space extends far out into the subcutaneous region, and the ingrown bone-derived tissue has the possibility to fill the chamber without competition with other tissues. Without an osteoconductive material in the space, new tissue will fill a small portion of the chamber within 6 weeks, most of it bone. With an osteoconductive implant, the entire chamber is filled with ingrown fibrous tissue, but ingrown bone will still not reach more than a third of the distance from the ingrowth openings to the other end of the cylinder. Different osteoconductive materials have shown different bone ingrowth distances. Although the interior space in the BCC is 5 times larger than in the BHC, it can be used in 300g rats, which allows much greater numbers of animals than the previous rabbit chamber models and thus more experiments per time period. Further, ingrowth distances can be measured in the BCC at 6 and 10 weeks after grafting, a time by which the bone in the BHC is completely remodelled, so that such measurements would be meaningless. The BCC has also been modified to allow adaptation of a minipump for drug application, and a device for mechanical loading of an implant in the chamber.

Our group tried to demonstrate increased bone healing using several growth factors in the old BHC model, without success [33]. The best result was a slight increase in osteoid area, when adding bFGF to bone allografts. When the same experiments was repeated in the BCC, the stimulatory effect of bFGF was striking [36].

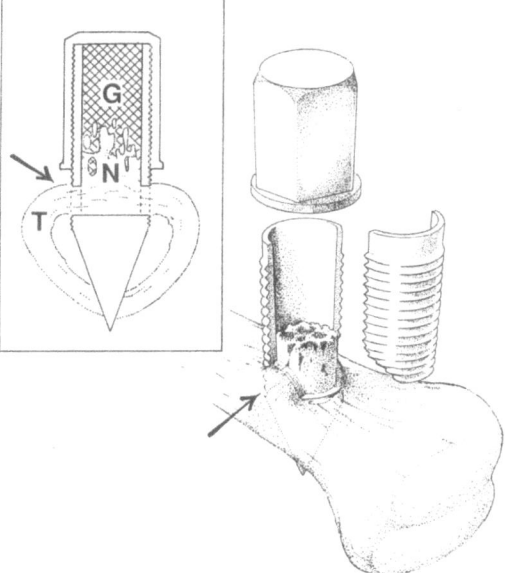

Fig. 2. The BCC consists of a threaded titanium cylinder formed from two half cylinders, which are held together by a hexagonal closed screw cap. There are two bone ingrowth openings, 1 mm in diameters, at the bottom of the chamber (arrows). The ingrown bone-derived tissue has the possibility to fill the chamber without competition with other tissues. If implanted empty, only the lower part will be filled with new tissue. With an osteoconductive implant in the chamber (inset schema), ingrown fibrous tissue will reach the top of the chamber, but bone will still only form in the lower part, The amount of new bone can be increased by various pretreatments of the osteoconductive material. The overall length is 13 mm. The bone ingrowth chamber has an inside diameter of 2 mm, and an inside length of 7 mm. (Reproduced with permission from Europ J Exp Musculoskel Res)

Bone Graft Preparation

Defatting by various solvents is a common procedure when producing lyophilized grafts for clinical use. We compared frozen bone grafts with grafts that had also been defatted in chlorophorm-methanol, using the BCC model. At 6 weeks, there was a 58% increase in bone ingrowth distance [35]. This difference was also seen when syngeneic rats were used as donors and recipients. In previous BHC experiments we made similar findings, but only with short implantation times.

When defatted grafts were sterilized with ethylene oxide, the bone ingrowth distance at 6 weeks in the BCC was diminished by 68% ($p < 0.001$). This finding is surprizing considering that the concentration of remaining ethylene oxide and its metabolites were well below the limits recommended by the American Food and Drug Administration. Radiation at 2.5 Mrad had no deleterious effect.

When defatted grafts were pretreated with bFGF, the effect was apparent as an increased scintimetric activity after 2 weeks, and as increased ingrowth distances after 4–6 weeks [9]. The difference in bone ingrowth persisted for at least 10 weeks and possibly increased until then. A dose response study showed a biphasic curve, with a positive effect within a dose range of 8 to 200 ng of bFGF per implant (9). When applying bFGF to porous hydroxyapatite instead of bone allografts, the findings were similar, with a 70% increase of the bone ingrowth distance [8]. Both with bone allografts and hydroxyapatite, the soft tissue invasion reached about twice as long into the material as did the bone, and the soft tissue invasion was increased to a similar degree with bFGF [8, 9]. Systemic growth hormone treatment, which caused constantly elevated IGF 1 levels in serum, had no effect on bone ingrowth [7].

In another type of experiment, we have studied the effects of morselized cortical bone after deproteinization with a gentle ceramic process (low temperature, high pressure), which leaves the bone minerals unchanged. Deproteinization caused a slight decrease in bone ingrowth, but a larger negative effect on fibrous tissue ingrowth. To our knowledge, this is the first study to demonstrate the long hypothesized stimulatory effect of the organic components of undemineralized bone grafts.

Remodelling

The above discussion is based on the presumption that bone ingrowth into a bone replacement material is desirable. However, this may be disputable. The reason to aim at maximal bone ingrowth is to reinforce the replacement material in order to avoid fatigue fractures. If fatigue fractures can be avoided by other means, the amount of ingrowth is sufficient when the implant is "mechanically united" with the host. In resorbable materials like bone graft, ingrowth may lead to bone resorption, which can jeopardize the mechanical function. This is a serious problem which has led to frequent late failures when structural auto- or allografts were used in total hip revisions [20, 26]. In retrospect, these failures should have been easy to predict: the structural grafts consist of devascularized femoral heads, and the behavior of mechanically loaded devascularized femoral heads is known from spontaneous osteonecrosis. It is clearly established that osteoneocrotic bone collapses as a result of osteoclastic resorption, which is a part of the repair process that follows the ingrowth of new blood vessels [12, 13, 14, 15].

In normal bone remodelling, there is a close coupling between osteoclasts and osteoblasts. Osteoblasts prepare a site for an osteoclasts to start resorbing the bone, and the resorption "pit" is subsequently filled by osteoblasts. Several bone matrix proteins are involved in controlling this process; among them the TGFß, which is released from the bone matrix during resorption. TGFß might serve in a local self-regulatory system, since it can inhibit further osteoclastic activity and initiate the local replacement of the resorbed volume [19, 27]. In bone allografts and osteonecrosis, the osteoblast-osteoclast coupling is disturbed, perhaps because important bone matrix proteins are destroyed. The disturbed spatial organisation of osteoclastic and osteoblastic activity during revascularisation of osteonecrosis leads to stress concentration at interfaces between resorbed and sclerotic areas, causing microfractures and collapse.

At least one calcium-phosphate material has been claimed to undergo osteoclastic resorption followed by bone formation in a "normal" remodelling cycle [11]. This is quite remarkable, since there is evidence that osteoclasts utilize a specific bone protein (osteopontin) for their attachment to bone. Further, the subsequent remodelling seems to be dependent on the release of other bone matrix proteins. A possible explanation for the remodelling of a calcium-phosphate material would be that necessary proteins are absorbed to its surface. However, it seems unlikely that a sound balance between resorption of the material and formation of bone could be maintained that way. Thus, a risk of collapse must be anticipated. Other calcium-phosphates resorb or dissolve spontaneously, without osteoclasts. In that case, new bone formation is of course not a result of a coupling between resorption and formation. Rather, new bone formation would be due to a prolonged healing response to the insertion trauma, and the persistance of this response with time would be uncertain: formation may not keep up with resorption.

The above discussion suggests that the term "osteoconduction" is unclear and that there are other considerations besides conduction when choosing a bone replacement material.

References

1. Aspenberg P, Albrektsson T, Lohmander LS, Thorngren K-G (1988) Drug test chamber: a titanuim implant for adminstration of biochemical agents to a standardized bone callus in situ. J Biomed Eng 10: 70–73

2. Aspenberg P, Kälebo P, Albrektsson T (1988) Rapid bone healing delayed by bone matrix implantation. Int J Oral Maxillofac Implants 3: 123–127

3. Aspenberg P, Albrektsson T, Thorngren K-G (1989) Local application of growth-factor IGF-1 to healing bone. Experiments with a titanium chamber in rabbits. Acta Orthop Scand 60: 607–610

4. Aspenberg P, Thoren K (1990) Lipid extraction enhances bank bone incorporation. An experiment in rabbits. Acta Orthop Scand 61: 546–548

5. Aspenberg P, Goodman S, Toksvig-Larsen S, Ryd L, Albrektsson T (1992) Intermitent micromotion inhibits bone ingrowth. Experiment using titanium implants in rabbits. Acta Orthop Scand 63: 141–145

6. Aspenberg P, Wang JS (1993) A new bone chamber used for measuring osteoconduction in rats. Eur J Exp Musculoskel Res 2: 69–74

7. Aspenberg P, Choon P, Wang JS, Thorngren K-G (1994) No effect of growth hormone on bone graft incorporation in the normal rat. Acta Orthop Scand 65 (4): 456–461

8. Aspenberg P, Wang J-S (1996) Porous hydroxyapatite loaded with bFGF. Titanium chamber study in rats. In: Buchhorn W HG (ed) Ceramic implant materials in orthopedic surgery. Accepted for publication

9. Aspenberg P, Wang JS (1994) Basic fibroblast growth factor. Dose and time-dependence in rats. Trans Orthop Res Soc 19: 181

10. Bonewald LF, Mundy GR (1990) Role of transforming growth factor beta in bone remodelling. Clin Orthop 250: 261–276

11. Constantz BR, Young SW, Kienapfel H, Dahlen BL, Summer DR, Turner TM, Urban RM, Galante JO, Goodman SB, Gunasekaran S (1994) Calcium phosphate cement in a rabbit femoral canal and a canine humeral plug model: A pilot investigation. Materials Research Society symposium proceedings, Vol 252. Tissue-inducing biomaterials (ed: Cima LG, Ron ES)

12. Gardeniers JWM (1988) Behaviour of normal, avascular and revascularizing cancellous bone in the femoral head of an African pygmy goat. ISBN 90-9002151-5 Thesis, Nijmegen

13. Glimcher MJ, Kenzora JE (1979a) The biology of osteonecrosis of the human femoral head and its clinical implications: I Tissue biology. Clin Orthop 38: 284–309

14. Glimcher MJ, Kenzora JE (1979b) The biology of osteonecrosis of the human femoral head and its clinical implications: II. The pathological changes in the femoral head as an organ in the hip joint. Clin Orthop 139: 283–312

15. Glimcher MJ, Kenzora JE (1979c) The biology of osteonecrosis of the human femoral head and its clinical implications: III. Discussion of the etiology and genesis of the pathological sequelae; comments on treatment. Clin Orthop 140: 273–312

16. Goodman SB (1994) The effects of micromotion and particulate materials on tissue differentiation. Bone chamber studies in rabbits: Thesis Acta Orthop Scand [Suppl 258] 65: 1–43

17. Goodman S, Aspenberg P (1993) Mechanical stimulation and the differentiation of hard tissues. Biomaterials 14: 563–569

18. Goodman SB, Aspenberg P, Wang JS, Doshi A, Regula D, Emmanual J, Lidgren L (1993) Cement particles inhibit bone ingrowth into titanuim chambers implanted in the rabbit. Acta Orthop Scand 64: 627–633

19. Hallen LG (1996) Heterologous transplantation of Kiel bone. An experimental and clinical study. Acta Orthop Scand 37: 1–19
20. Hooten Jr JP, Engh Jr CA, Engh CA (1994) Failure of structural acetabular allograft in cementless revision hip arthroplasty. J Bone Joint Surg (Br) 76: 419–422
21. Hopf A (1963) Citation from Haasch K. Klinische Erfahrungen mit dem Kieler Span. Der Chirurg 34: 21
22. Katthagen B-D (1986) Knochenregeneration mit Knochenersatzmaterialien. Eine tierexperimentelle Studie In: Hefte zur Unfallheilkunde. Berlin: Springer
23. Kalebo P, Jacobsson M (1988) Recurrent bone generation in titanium implants. Biomaterials 9: 295–301
24. Maatz R, Bauermeister AB (1961) Klinische Erfahrungen mit dem Kieler Span. Langenbeck Arch Chir 208: 239
25. Maatz R, Lent W, Graff R (1954) Spongiosa test on bone graft. J Bone Joint Surg (Am) 36: 721
26. Mulroy RD, Harris WH (1990) Failure of acebular autogenous grafts in total hip arthroplasty. Increasing incidence: a follow-up note. J Bone Joint Surg Am 72: 1536–1540
27. Oursler MJ (1992) Osteoclast synthesis and secretion and activation of latent transforming growth factor beta. J Bone Mineral Res 9: 443
28. Ramani PS, Kalbag RM, Sengupta RP (1975) Cervical spinal interbody fusion with Kiel bone. Br J Surg 62: 147–150
29. Schnettler R, Dingeldein E, Wahlig H, Tausch W (1992) Potential of porous HA and bFGF loaded porous HA on bone repair in cancellous bone in mini pigs. Trans World Biomat Congr 4: 260
30. Schweiberer L (1970) Experimentelle Untersuchungen von Knochentransplantaten mit Unveränderter und mit Denaturierter Knochengrundsubstanz. Ein Beitrag zur kausalen Osteogenese. In: Hefte zur Unfallheilkunde. Berlin: Springer
31. Sweet DE, Madewell DJE (1988) Pathogenesis of osteonecrosis. In: Resnick D, Niwayama G (eds) Diagnosis of bone an joint disorders. London: Saunders WB
32. Thoren K, Aspenberg P, Thorngren K-G (1993) Lipid extraction decreases the specific immunologic response to bone allograft in rabbits. Acta Orthop Scand 64: 44–46
33. Thoren K, Aspenberg P (1993) Effects of basic fibroblast growth factor on bone allografts. A study using bone harvest chambers in rabbits. Ann Surg Gyn 82: 129–135
34. Thoren K, Aspenberg P, Thorngren K-G (1995) Lipid-extracted bank bone. Bone conductive and mechanical properties. Clin Orthop 311: 232–246
35. Thoren K, Aspenberg P (1995) Increased bone ingrowth distance into lipid extracted bank bone at 6 weeks. A titanuim chamber study in allogenic and syngenic rats. Arch Orthop Trauma Surg 114: 167–171
36. Wang JS, Aspenberg P (1994) Basic fibroblast growth factor increases allograft incorporation. Bone chamber study in rats. Acta Orthop Scand 65: 27–31
37. Wipperman BW, Zwipp H, Junge P, Saeman T, Tischerne H (1994) Healing of a segmental defect in the sheep tibia filled with a hydroxyapatite ceramic augmented by basic fibroblast growth factor and autologous bone marrow. Trans Orthop Res Soc 19: 545

Author's address: Per Aspenberg, Department of Orthopaedics, Lund University Hospital, S-221 85 Lund, Sweden.

Histological Observations on Retrieved Human Allografts

R. M. Bloem[1], W. W. Tomford[2], and H. J. Mankin[2]

[1] University Hospital Leiden, Department of Orthopaedic Surgery, Leiden, The Netherlands
[2] Massachusetts General Hospital, Department of Orthopaedic Surgery, Orthopaedic Research Laboratories, Boston, Massachusetts, U.S.A.

Introduction

Massive human allografts are frequently being used in reconstructive surgery of the skeleton especially after resection of a malignant bone tumor. Despite their frequent use little is known about the incorporation of massive allografts in humans. The present study reports on the histological findings in eight retrieved massive allografts all of which had been implanted in the course of surgery for malignant bone tumors at the Massachusetts General Hospital in Boston.

Material and Methods

The retrieved grafts have been implanted in four males and four females with a mean age of 39 years (range 20–65). The grafts had been in situ for various periods of time ranging from four to ninety months. Five grafts were recovered because of a fracture, two because of a nonunion and one graft was recovered because of a local recurrence of a chondrosarcoma, this particular graft functioned well at the time of retrieval.

After recovery the grafts were stored at temperatures of minus 80° Celsius. For analysis the dimensions of the specimens were recorded and photographs and radiographs were obtained. The grafts were initially cut transversely at three to four centimeter intervals to form blocks. These blocks were embedded in polymethylmethacrylate and cut into sections approximately two millimeters thick which were ground using a machine grinder to a thickness of approximately 350 microns and stained with Toluidine Blue on the polished surface according to a technique described by Schenk [8]. The distance between the sections studied depended on the original thickness of the sections and the number of sections lost during the grinding process. The final distance between the sections studied varied from five to fifteen millimeters. Bone remodeling was evaluated on these transvers sections by macroscopic and microscopic examination of three different envelopes: an outer periosteal envelope, a cortical or Haversian envelope and an endosteal envelope. Resorption was evaluated by examination of periosteal and endosteal surfaces for irregular borders and cavities. New bone

Work supported by the Gisela Thier foundation of the medical faculty of the University of Leiden Holland and by US Public Health Services Grant AR #21896.

formation was judged by the presence of osteocytes, the architecture of the bone and the color. Using Toluidine Blue, young not fully mineralized bone stains darker blue when compared to mature fully mineralized bone.

Results

In six grafts remodeling was unimpressive. Three of these grafts were distal femoral osteoarticular allografts, two humeral intercalary allografts and one osteochondral allograft of a proximal humerus. These specimens revealed little biological activity, almost all of which was confined to the periosteal envelope and the outer layers of the Haversian envelope. Small patches of new bone formation were present at random locations and never seemed to extend more than two or three millimeters into the bone. Haversian remodeling was relatively rare and usually occurred in the vicinity of areas of periosteal bone formation. Bone resorption seemed more prominent but was also limited to the outer layers of the graft leaving the necrotic inner layers undisturbed. The duration of time the graft had been in situ (range 4–90 months) did not appear to influence the extent of remodeling.

Two proximal femoral allografts revealed locally far more active patterns of remodeling. One graft was implanted as an osteoarticular allograft. This particular graft did not unite and fourteen months after implantation the AO plate failed. A new plate was applied and an autologous cancellous bone graft was performed at the junction site. The junction site subsequently healed uneventfully. Forty six months after implantation a subtrochanteric fracture occurred which was treated with a dynamic hip screw and an autologous bone graft. This fracture did not heal and the graft had to be removed nine months later.

The second graft to be discussed was a proximal femur which was implanted in combination with a Moore prosthesis. Twenty-one months after implantation a diaphyseal fracture of the allograft occurred which was treated with cerclage wiring and autologous bone grafting. This fracture healed but was followed by a second fracture eighteen months later after which the graft was recovered.

Both macroscopic and microscopic examination of the sections through the region of the allograft which had previously been treated with autologous bone grafting (for nonunion in the first case and for fracture in the second case) revealed areas of extensive remodeling involving all three envelopes of the allograft. Figure 1 illustrates the retrieved specimen described in the first case history. Section one (Fig. 2) is the bottom section (closed arrow). Since the junction site between allograft and host bone had healed, it is hard to tell whether or not this section is through the proximal part of the host bone or the distal part of the allograft. It is however clear that there is a highly porous structure of the bone and the histology showed areas of living bone next to areas of necrotic bone. Figure 3 represents the macroscopic view of a section located six millimeters more proximal. The original cortex of the allograft can be clearly distinguished. Also one can appreciate the bubble like appearance of the callus which overlaps part of the allograft. The structure of the allograft underneath this highly porous woven bone has a moth eaten appearance indicating resorption of allograft bone. A micro-photograph of a part of the cortical envelope represented by the little square on the bottom of Fig. 3 shows that remodeling of allograft bone has taken place in a rather random fashion (Fig. 4). Bands of dark staining newly formed bone have filled in resorption cavities like those still present in the upper part of the photograph. The original structure of the necrotic allograft bone can be seen as the light staining tissue in the right hand corner. Similar

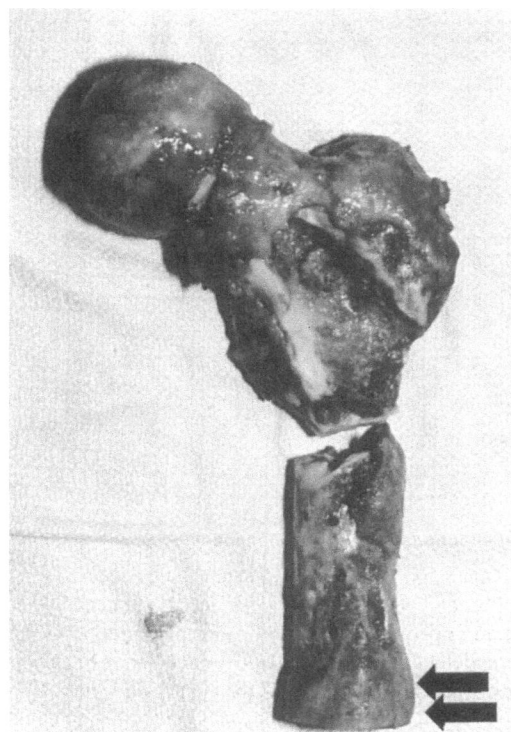

Fig. 1. Proximal femoral allograft retrieved for a fracture in the subtrochanteric region. The arrows indicate the two sections illustrated in the region close to the junction site. Note the fusiform appearance of the enveloping callus in this region

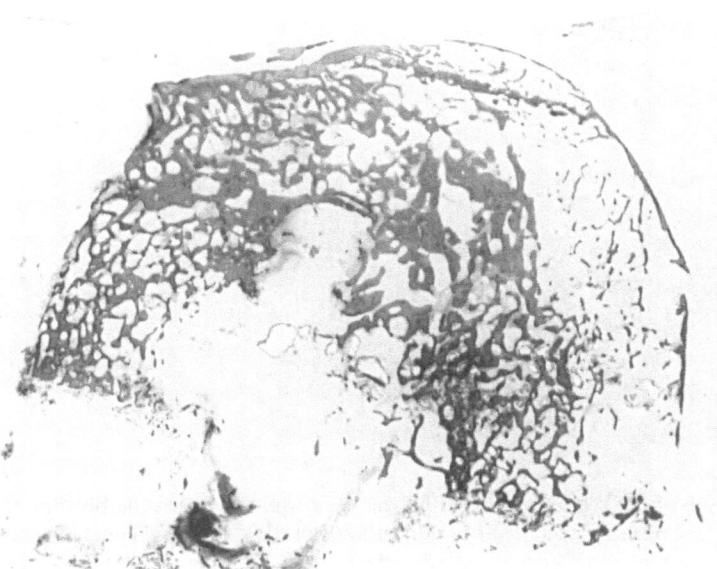

Fig. 2. Macroscopic view of the most distal transverse section (Fig. 1). Note the extreme porosity of the cortex

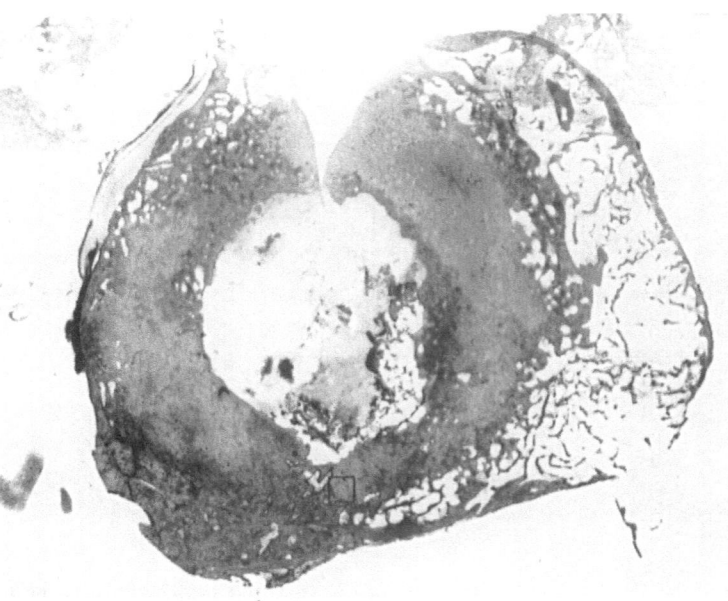

Fig. 3. Macroscopic view of a transverse section taken approximately 6 mm more proximal (Fig. 1) than the section illustrated in Fig. 2. The wedge shape defect at the top is an artefact. Note the high porosity of the callus on the right hand side and the moth eaten appearance of the cortex underneath it

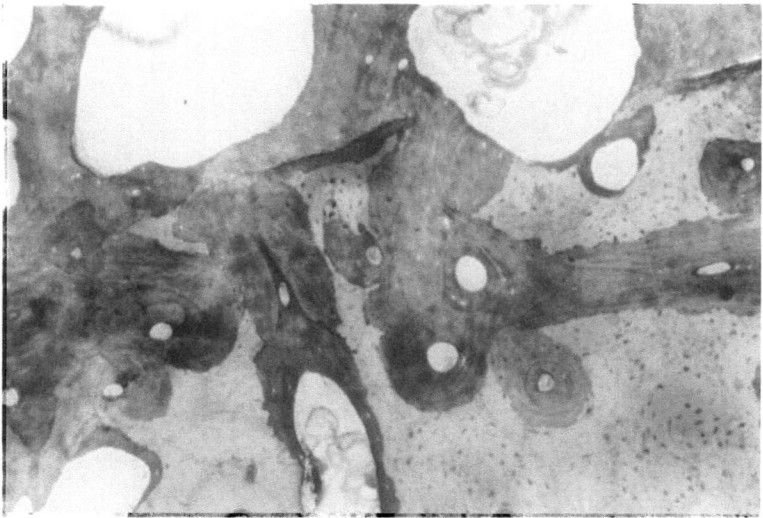

Fig. 4. Microscopic view ($\times$ 100) of the region presented by the little square box on the bottom of Fig. 3. Mark the large resorption cavities especially at the top. Bands of dark staining newly formed bone cross the original light staining necrotic allograft bone

findings were observed in the second allograft in the region of the first healed fracture. Extensive remodeling was also observed in this particular area sometimes affecting the entire thickness of the cortex but never the entire circumference. In both grafts this extensive type of remodeling was only observed in areas which were treated with an autologous bone graft for a nonunion or a fracture. Further away from these "healed problem sites" the pattern of remodeling resembled that of the other six allografts discussed before.

Discussion

The biological sequence of events in the incorporation of small cancellous or osteochondral allografts has been well described [1, 3, 4, 6] but few papers have reported on the remodeling of massive bone grafts in humans [2, 5, 7]. The excellent paper by Enneking and Mindell published in 1991 presented the most complete study so far. In our study two patterns of cortical remodeling were observed. These two types differed in extent and organization. The periosteal type was confined to the outer layers of the allograft. Remodeling occurred randomly along the periosteal surface of the cortex, and was usually modest. Bone resorption appeared more extensive than bone formation, and osteonal remodeling was a rare phenomenon. These findings are in agreement with the observations made by Enneking and Mindell [7].

A different and more extensive type of remodeling was observed in two grafts: one which had been successfully treated with an autologous bone graft for a nonunion and one graft which was successfully treated for a fracture with osteosynthesis and an autologous bone graft. Allograft bone close to callus showed extensive cortical remodeling, including large resorption cavities and bands of newly formed bone traversing the original cortex. The structure of the remodeled bone was completely different from the well organized osteonal structure of the necrotic allograft bone. This type of remodeling did not correspond to the well organized type of osteonal remodeling described by Burchardt and Enneking in an animal model [3]. It is likely that the process of bone induction in a very active area of callus formation enhances the remodeling of adjacent allograft bone. One of the most striking findings was the disorganized fashion in which this seemed to occur. The remodeling often seemed to be disorganized and in some areas the original cortex must have weakened significantly due to the increase in porosity and the thinning of the cortex which was observed.

In summary our observations showed that in the majority of the allografts studied, cortical remodeling was limited to the superficial layers of small areas of the allograft. Under certain conditions however, an extensive type of remodeling occurred affecting relatively large areas of the allograft and at times the entire thickness of the cortex but never the entire circumference. This extensive type of remodeling was only observed in areas with callus formation after a fracture or a nonunion suggesting that the allograft merely participated in the bone formation process of that particular area. It is important to realize that the allograft bone may be weakened during this process because resorption of bone is often more extensive than the formation of new bone. Because of this, remodeling of allograft bone does not necessarily have to beneficial for the patient but is on the other hand essential for the long term survival of the graft. The real question is how to control the remodeling process to make patients benefit from a truly biological implant.

References

1. Barth A (1893) Über Histologische Befunde nach Knochen Implantationen. Arch Klin Chir 46: 409–417
2. Broström LA, Nilsonne U, Nilsson OS (1988) Survival of frozen bone allograft. Ann Chir Gyn 77: 85–89

3. Burchardt H (1983) Biology of cortical bone graft incorporation. In: Friedlaender GE et al (eds) Osteochondral allografts; Biology, banking and clinical applications. Little Brown and Co, pp 51–57
4. Burchardt H (1987) Biology of bone transplantation. Orthop Clin N Am 18: 187–196
5. Coutelier L, Delloye Ch, de Nayer P, Vincent A (1984) Aspects microradiographiques des allogreffes osseuses massives chez l'homme. Rev Chir Orthop 70: 581–588
6. Enneking WF, Burchardt H, Puhl JJ, Piotrowsky G (1975) Physical and biological aspects of repair in dog cortical bone transplants. J Bone Joint Surg 57-A: 237–252
7. Enneking WF, Mindell ER (1991) Observations on massive retrieved human allografts. J Bone Joint Surg 73–A: 1123–1142
8. Schenk RK, Olah AJ, Hezmann W (1984) Preparation of calcified tissue for light microscopy. In: Glenn R Dickson (ed) Methods of calcified tissue preparation. Elsevier, pp 1–56

Author's addresses: Rolf M. Bloem, University Hospital Leiden, Department of Orthopaedic Surgery, P.O. Box 9600, NL-2300 RC Leiden, The Netherlands; W. W. Tomford and H. J. Mankin, Massachusetts General Hospital, Department of Orthopaedic Surgery, Orthopaedic Research Laboratories, Boston, Massachusetts, U.S.A.

Repair of Massive Allografts: Histological, Nuclear Medicine and CT-Studies

A. J. Aho[1], T. Ekfors[2], J. Knuuti[3], K. Mattila[4], and J. Heikkilä[1]

[1] Department of Surgery, Orthopaedic Unit,
[2] Department of Pathology,
[3] Department of Nuclear Medicine, and
[4] Department of Diagnostic Radiology, University of Turku, Turku, Finland

Summary

The repair of massive osteoarticular allografts was evaluated by invasive and non-invasive techniques utilizing histological biopsies, isotopes, particularly the SPECT method, and computed tomography (CT) techniques.

With regard to osteogenesis four different morphological anatomic areas were found. New bone formation began first at the host-graft junction induced by the host's periosteum and the autogenous bone grafts. In the cortex postresorptional osteogenesis occurred as a thin appositional layer of lamellar bone. In the subchondral bone cyst-like small cavities resulting from resorption of Haversian canals revealed new lamellar bone of varying degree lining the cavity walls. However, large areas of the grafts remained necrotic and the new bone formation event (creeping substitution) was a long drawn-out process lasting years. The proportion of new bone formation averaged 36% (range 5–75%). Bone scans and SPECT (Single Photon Emission Computed Tomography) studies with ^{99m}TcDPD indicated slight activity only at the outer layer of the cortex corresponding to histological observations. Computed tomography (CT) studies revealed first thinning and irregular defects of the cortex and small subcortical cysts. Later these resorptive changes repaired by gradual thickening of the cortex. On CT a neocortex, a circumferential bony structure inside the normal cortex was found to develop over several years.

Introduction

For clinical purposes, there is a pressing need for an improved understanding of the metabolic biological events occurring during the incorporation of massive allografts in orthotopic surgical allograft procedures. In the treatment of bone defects, large bone allografts may be used as osteoarticular, cylindrical, intercalary or various types of bloc replacements (e.g. flat bones for the pelvis, or strut type for hip repair). The concept of massive allograft characteristically implies the use of a bloc consisting of an intact corticocancellous bone structure. The incorporation of allografts into the host comprises several distinct phases: (1) haematoma, (2) inflammation, (3) resorption, (4) regeneration of new bone or other tissues (creeping substitution), (5) mature bone formation, and (6) remodeling. Characteristic for the allograft metabolism are the morphological and time-dependent changes of these phases in different parts of the graft. In this study, the repair process was studied by using histological biopsies, nuclear medicine techniques, and computed tomography (CT) methods.

Material and Methods

The findings reported here are based on a total of sixty patients treated with massive allografts during the period 1973–1994 in the Department of Surgery, Turku University Central Hospital. Twelve dogs with metaphyseal osteoarticular allografts of the distal femur have also been utilized for the histological studies. After resection of the half or hemi-joint, the allograft was fixed with AO-plates and screws. In the patients, autogenous chips were transplanted to the osteosynthesis site at the host-graft junction (Fig. 1). The storage temperature for the human grafts was −70–80°C, and for the canine grafts −50–70°. The follow-up time varied between 1 month and 8 years for the human patients; for the dogs it was 2 weeks −3 years. Details of the other techniques used are presented in the relevant sections below.

Histology

Biopsies for histological evaluation (obtained during re-operations, plate removals, and post-mortem) were taken from thirteen human massive allografts and from twelve dogs. Inflammatory round cells were found located around the graft and at the host-graft junction for a period of some weeks after transplantation. There are four different morphological structural anatomic areas to be distinguished with regard to osteogenesis and the creeping substitution phenomenon in osteoarticular grafts: 1) the host-graft junction, 2) the cortex, 3) the cancellous metaphyseal area, 4) the subchondral cancellous bone, and 5) the cartilage as a distinct biological entity (Fig. 1).

The Host-Graft Junction

New bone appeared first as woven bone growing from the host periosteum, and then as new lamellar bone forming a Haversian lamellar structure with a variety of orientations.

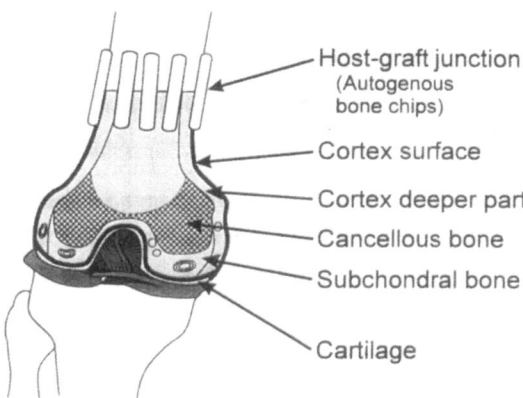

Host-graft junction
(Autogenous
bone chips)

Cortex surface

Cortex deeper part

Cancellous bone

Subchondral bone

Cartilage

Fig. 1. Schematic drawing of an osteoarticular allograft of the distal femur illustrating different histological areas relevant to the incorporation process of the osteoarticular allograft

This was seen relatively early, beginning at one month after operation. However, bone union was a slow process, lasting several years, as seen by the appositional bone formation found around the host-graft junction in repeated radiographs. Autograft bone chips transplanted to this site showed both active new bone formation, and resorption, influencing the initiation of osteogenesis.

The Cortex

Cortical remodeling appeared in two distinct morphological modes. At the outer layer of the cortex, signs of resorption (erosion pits) were evident during the first month after transplantation. These resorption areas were later replaced, first by woven bone, and later, at about 6–12 months, by appositional lamellar bone (Fig. 2). One distinct feature of this appositional new bone was its variation in thickness, ranging between 0–5 mm. This new bone was most likely derived from tissues consisting of both adjacent periosteal and/or muscle insertion tissues of the host bed. At deeper endosteal parts of the cortex, on the other hand, the graft remained dead. Osteoclastic resorption occurred in many old Haversian canals, widening them into cavities rounded or oval in shape. This kind of changes was seen most often near the metaphyseal areas consisting of cancellous bone and resembled those in the subchondral area.

The Cancellous Metaphyseal Area and the Subchondral Bone

The histology of the metaphyseal cancellous and the subchondral areas of the osteoarticular frozen allografts was characterized by large areas with necrotic bone trabeculae.

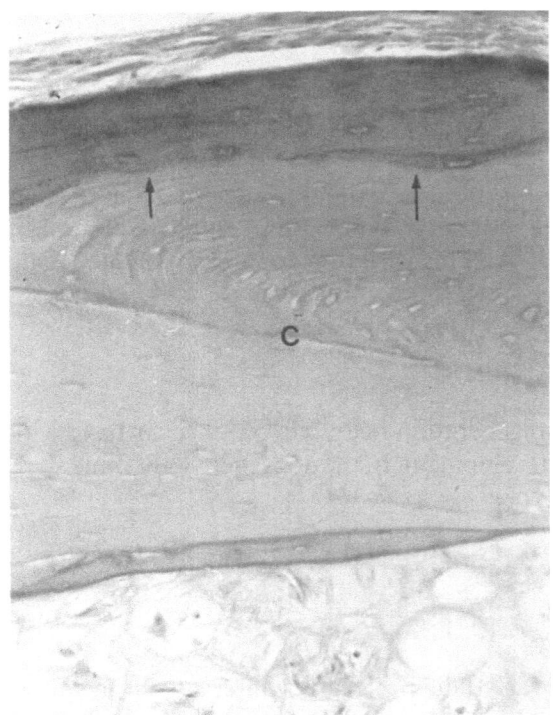

Fig. 2. Appositional lamellar new bone formation of the outer superficial layer of the human cortex (arrows). The deeper part (C) of the cortex is old, necrotic donor bone. The biopsy is from a retrieved human allograft at one year after transplantation. H-E staining, × 60

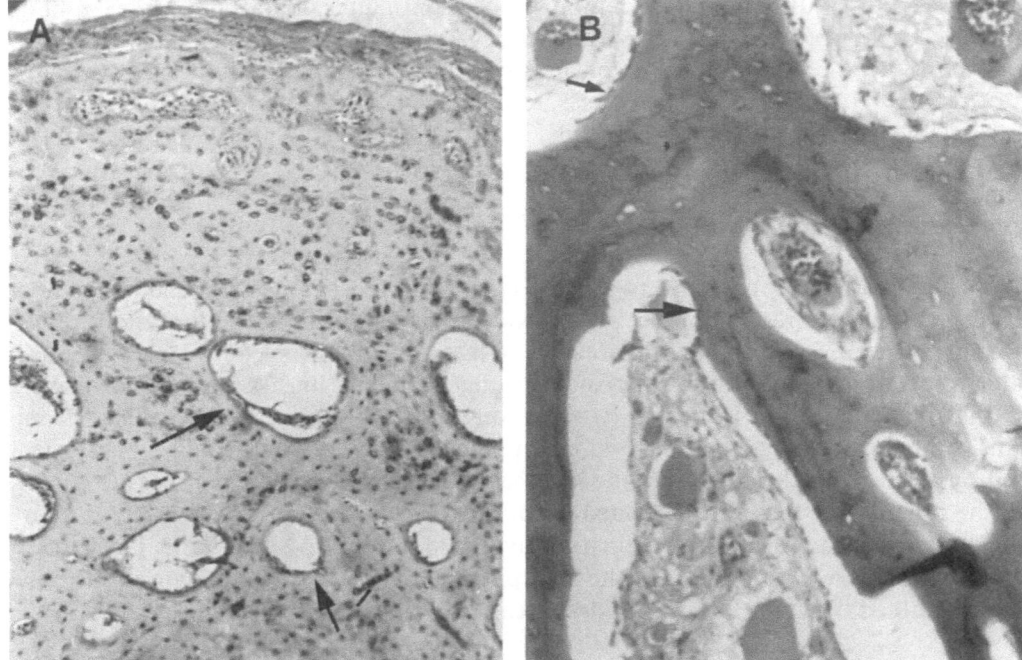

Fig. 3. A. Histological picture of subchondral bone of an osteoarticular allograft in a dog. A fibrous cartilage layer is seen on the top towards the joint space. Rounded cyst-like aversion resorption cavities (arrows) are seen at seven months after transplantation (Alcian Blue staining, × 95). **B.** Histological specimen of a proximal humeral allograft 7 years after transplantation. Widened Haversian canals are seen with new lamellar viable bone (arrows) an old necrotic lamellae. H-E, × 100

In addition, cyst-like small cavities resulting from resorption of the walls of the Haversian canals were evident (Fig. 3A). The cavities displayed a visual pattern of porosity, and often revealed osteoid and new bone lining the walls in a lamellar osteon-like orientation (Fig. 3B). The proportion by volume of new-bone formation calculated from the human biopsies varied greatly, with initial subjective histologic evaluations ranging from 5–75% (mean 36%). This variation apparently resulted from the use of two different biopsy techniques, either hollow drill or bloc.

The Cartilage

In general, in the humans, joint surface regeneration occurred via fibrocartilage with some focal tendency to "better" cartilage development. In the dogs there were some signs of persistence of cartilage of the hyaline type.

Nuclear Medicine Studies

The incorporation of human allografts was studied at regular intervals by means of isotopes, using 3-phase radionuclide scintigraphy and single-photon emission computer tomography (SPECT) with ^{99m}Tc DPD. In the early post-operative period, phase 1 (blood flow) and phase 2 (blood volume and soft tissue) images indicated increased perfusion, which subsequently decreased. Phase 3 planar images indicating total uptake of graft and surrounding tissues showed an uptake area continuing for many years at the united host-graft junction and at the cortex. However, more reliable spatial information was obtained from thin tomographic SPECT slices (3–4 mm in thickness) at the graft uptake site. The radioactivity was high at the united host-graft junction, but slight and limited in the more outer layers of the cortex (Fig. 4), and this pattern was maintained for several years.

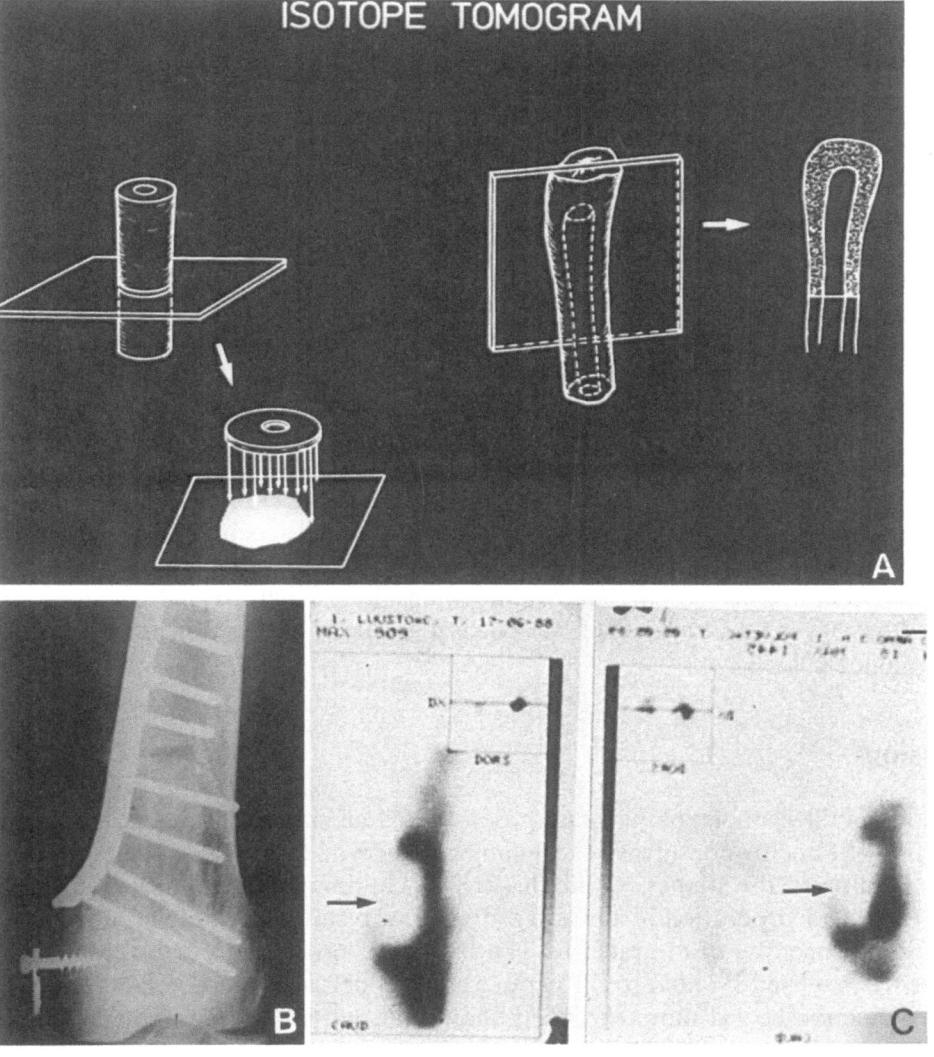

Fig. 4. A. A schematic drawing illustrating the distribution of the isotope activity in a three dimensional format as thin slices. **B.** Radiograph of an osteoarticular allograft of the distal femur at one year after transplantation. **C.** A SPECT frontal slice illustrates very slight uptake in the cortical layer (arrow) both at one year (on the left) and at two years (on the right) after transplantation

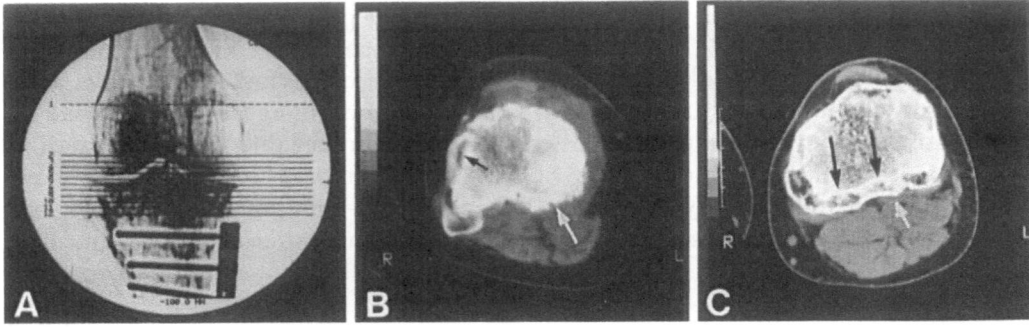

Fig. 5. A. A computed tomogram showing the subchondral area of the knee used for CT-studies. **B.** Irregular resorptive defects (arrow) developing in the cortex during the first six months to one yea1. A simultaneous cyst (short arrow) is also seen. **C.** Reorganization of the cortex at two years and onwards as a thickened continuous layer (short arrow). Neocortex is seen as a new circumferential bone structure (arrow)

CT-Studies

Osteoarticular knee allografts were studied by repeat CT examinations 0–101 months postoperatively. Transaxial sections through the subchondral bone were used to avoid artifacts caused by the osteosynthesis devices (Fig. 5). The thickness of the sections varied between 3 and 5 mm (GE 9800 and Siemens Somatom CR). Resorptive thinning, and defects in the circumferential continuity of the cortex were observed during the first six months. Simultaneously, the formation of subcortical cyst-like resorption cavities, some exceeding 1 cm in diameter, was seen with an increase in the structural irregularity of the cortex and subcortical bone. Later on, the cortex became more continuous again and thickened gradually. A new finding was the identification of a circumferential sclerotic bony structure inside the subcortical cystic layer. It was named neocortex. The neocortex developed over several years postoperatively. The CT studies revealed fatigue fractures in the subchondral bone earlier than routine plain films. When treated adequatively these fractures healed by formation of sclerotic bridges along the fracture lines deep into the cancellous bone.

Discussion

The findings in these studies of the repair process of frozen massive allografts, examined both by invasive and by non-invasive techniques confirm and complete earlier observations. According to the studies by Burchardt [3], Goldberg and Stevenson [8], and Delloye [5] the incorporation of a massive allograft is a slow, long drawn-out process appearing in a necrotic dead graft [4]. The biological process in our osteoarticular allografts was in general similar to the various graft models used by other authors. The host-graft junction healed more effectively than other parts of the graft, as has been observed earlier in experimental grafts [1]. The use of autogenous bone grafts transplanted to the host-graft junction is of fundamental significance for primary union of the osteosynthesis site [2]. At this site, the massive allografts serve as a scaffold for the ingrowth of new host bone allowing union. All three methods used here for assessing the repair of allografts showed parallel results, indicating slow and only partial remodeling of the graft. However, the use of the techniques employed here made it possible to obtain a more comprehensive picture of the repair process in different parts of the osteoarticular allograft. Resorption, for example, was morphologically different at the cortical surface from that seen in the Haversian canals. They widened to cyst-like holes in the cancellous subcortical bone, resembling a porotic bone pattern. The resorption is preceded by the invasion of vascular buds through pre-existing Haversian-Volkmann canals [7]. Remodeling, by osteo-conduction or osteo-induction (stimuli from the matrix in the form of BMP and related proteins), was not active enough to restore normal bone architecture and bone content. The proportion of new-bone formation in allografts has been reported as varying between 43% in a dog's fibula [5] and 20% in retrieved human grafts [6]. The slight perfusion of the allograft cortex illustrated by the SPECT studies corresponds closely with the slight appositional new-bone growth demonstrated in the cortex by histology. Interestingly, the CT studies indicated continuous bone formation. During the follow-up over several years, in addition to some empty hole-like cysts, reorganization of the cortex and an entirely new structure, termed neocortex, was found [9]. This observation suggests that the cortex reorganizes in response to stimuli derived from long-term weight bearing loads in accordance to Wolff's law.

Overall, the repair of massive osteoarticular allografts is a lengthy process. The repair continues for several years, and displays variable patterns in different anatomical parts of the graft, even though in principle it conforms to the classical model of direct, intramembranous osteogenesis. The clinical massive allografts with significant structural changes as described, resist weight bearing loads. However, they are mechanically vulnerable and the described findings can explain the occurrence of clinical complications such as fatigue fractures.

References

1. Aho AJ, Penttinen R, Niinikoski J, Aho HJ (1992) Incorporation of massive half-joint allografts in dogs. In: Lindholm ST (ed) New trends in bone grafting. Tampere, Finland: University of Tampere, pp 176–185
2. Aho AJ, Ekfors T, Dean PB, Aro HT, Ahonen A, Nikkanen V (1994) Incorporation and clinical results of large allografts of the extremities and pelvis. Clin Orthop 307: 200–213
3. Burchardt H (1987) Biology of bone transplantation. Orthop Clinics North Am 18: 187–196
4. Chase SN, Herndon CH (1955) The fate of autogenous and homogenous bone grafts: A historical review. J Bone Joint Surg 37-A: 809
5. Delloye C (1990) The bridging capacity of a cortical bone defect by different bone grafting materials and diaphyseal distraction lengthening. An experimental study. Thesis. Louvain
6. Enneking WF, Mindell ER (1991) Observations on massive retrieved human allografts. J Bone Joint Surg 73-A: 1123–1142
7. Friedlaender GE (1982) Current concepts review: Bone banking. J Bone Joint Surg 64-A: 307
8. Goldberg VM, Stevenson S (1987) Natural history of autografts and allografts. Clin Orthop Rel Res 225: 7–16
9. Mattila KT, Heikkilä JT, Aho AJ, Manner I, Dean PB (1995) Structural changes in large human osteoarticular knee allografts studied with CT. Radiology 196: 657–660

Author's addresses: Allan J. Aho, M.D., Ph.D. and J. Heikkilä, M.D., Department of Surgery, Orthopoedic Unit; T. Ekfors, M.D., Ph.D., Department of Pathology; J. Knuuti, M.D., Ph.D., Department of Nuclear Medicine; K. Mattila, M.D., Department of Diagnostic Radiology, University of Turku, Turku, Finland.

Revision Joint Replacement

Bone Allograft Reconstruction in Revision Hip Replacement

B. Loty

Orthopaedic Department Hospital Cochin, Paris, France

Introduction

Major bone defects are frequently encountered in revision total hip arthroplasties. We use bone allografts to reconstruct both acetabular and femoral sides to allow successful implantation of a new prosthesis.

Our Bone Bank provides two types of allografts to support this activity. Frozen femoral heads are used for all kinds of acetabular defects and for small femoral defects. Irradiated massive cortical bones are used for major deficiencies of the femur.

Acetabular Reconstructions

Femoral Head Allografts

Femoral head bone banking began in our hospital in 1975. Their use in revision prostheses increased rapidly, as revisions became more and more frequent, and 200 of them are implanted each year in our department.

Procurement is performed by living donors undergoing hip arthroplasty for arthrosis. Complete preoperative examination and routine biology testing is performed when the bone is retrieved, including use of the polymerase chain reaction for HIV and Hepatitis C, allowing strict and efficient selection [2, 5]. Procurement sterility conditions are ideal, because of the operating environment and are verified with bacteriological samples cultured for a month. A computerized data-base allows graft validation and traceability.

Acetabulum Reconstruction Technique

Acetabuli are reconstructed with one or several bone blocks. The grafts are shaped to fit the defect, cartilage is removed and the grafts are impacted and fixed with screws to obtain primary stability. The screws are directed parallel to the mechanical forces, and we protect the reconstruction with a cruciate plate each time we need a large graft or when the acetabulum is fractured. We consider secure fixation to be mandatory for good graft healing and for preventing collapse during the remodelling period. A Charnley cemented cup is finally implanted.

Results

We reviewed our first ten years experience from 1975 to 1984 [3] with 122 large acetabulum grafts excluding the small grafts. All but 3 had very good results at follow-up ranging from 1 to 11 years. There were two infections unrelated to the grafts (negative preoperative graft cultures). One graft collapse occurred at 6 months in a large acetabular defect reconstruction without a cruciate plate (such a plate would have been used in later years). This case was revised with a new allograft and plate with a good final result. In all other cases, the radiological gap between graft and host acetabulum disappeared between the sixth and twelfth month, but healing still progressed during the following two or three years. From the third year all grafts showed union and consolidation, and no further change was observed.

In another study [8], we reviewed the results of 90 one step septic revision arthroplasties, performed between 1980 and 1988, with a two to ten year follow-up. Half of these cases needed femoral head allografts for reconstruction. The use of allografts did not influence the final results (46 cases with allograft: 3 septic recurrences; 44 cases without allograft: 5 septic recurrences). The infection failures were only correlated with the type of bacteria and not with the use of allografts.

Femoral Reconstructions

Small femoral defects were reconstructed with banked femoral heads. The small grafts used for repairing cortical holes or calcar deficiencies healed and, despite frequent superficial areas of resorption, all showed good cortical repair. Major femoral bone loss is not easily reconstructed with femoral heads: primary stability is hard to obtain and requires the use of long stem prostheses. Even with these long stem reconstructions, we observed resorption of grafts. Since 1985 we have therefore used massive cortical allografts in large femoral defect reconstructions.

Irradiated Massive Cortical Allografts

The higher risk of graft contamination due to cadaver procurement, led us to sterilize bones by gamma irradiation [4, 6, 7]. There is no risk of induced tissue radioactivity, owing to the low energy of Cobalt Sixty gamma rays, and tissue penetration is excellent. The efficiency of irradiation depends on the dose, the nature of treated tissue, the type and amount of initial contamination, and the temperature at which irradiation is performed (low temperature stops the sterilizing effect of free radicals). Radiation sterilization increases safety but is no substitution for donor screening. The irradiation dose cannot be increased without deleterious effects on bone strength. A previous experimental study, following the preparation procedure used in our bone bank [4] showed that bending strength decrease on femoral cortical samples was less than 20% after 27000 Gray and 35% after 35000 Gray. The bacteriological safety of this procedure (clean retrieval, graft washing, freezing, and room-temperature gamma irradiation), has been determined [5] using an experimental and statistical method [1]: a 10^6 Stability Assurance level for bacteriological contamination and achieved after 18500 Gray.

The bone banking procedure follows strict guidelines: after checking the removal authorizations, donor selection includes the same criteria as with unsterilized allografts (medical history, routine serology including (PCR), and autopsy whenever possible). Harvesting is performed in the mortuary operating room, avoiding any massive contamination. Grafts are cleaned, washed, packed, X-rayed, and stored at minus eighty degrees Celsius. The grafts are irradiated at room temperature, with accurate dosimetry. Computerized record keeping is very important for safety, efficiency, and traceability.

Large Femoral Defect Reconstruction Techniques

We used different surgical procedures with circular or strut allografts combined with prosthesis, according to the type of bone deficiency encountered, the goal being to preserve as much host bone as possible for implantation of the new prosthesis.

1) Segmental reconstructions consisted in massive circular allografts replacing the proximal femur or impacted into it.

   When we had to replace complete bone loss, as in replacement of a failed massive femoral prosthesis, we used an allograft and a long stem prostheses. Caution was paid to obtain the anatomical femoral length, alignment and rotation. A long stem prosthesis was cemented in the allograft, and the composite implant finally cemented into the host shaft. The junction was cleaned from cement, and spongious autograft was added.

   When the proximal femur was weak and fragmented, it was replaced by a segmental allograft and a long stem prosthesis with the same technique, but the remnant host femoral cortex was carefully preserved with its soft tissues attachments, and wired around the massive allograft. When a thin, enlarged, but continuous femoral metaphysis remained (egg shell looking metaphysis), the remnant host bone was preserved entirely, and a massive allograft was shaped and introduced into it. In a few cases, a long stem prosthesis was cemented both into the host femur and the allograft. In the other cases the allograft appeared strongly secured after impaction, and a standard short stem prosthesis was used, cemented only into the allograft.

2) When the loss of bone concerned only one side of the femoral shaft, we replaced it by a semi-circular allograft strut.

   Cortical defects were replaced by struts shaped to fit the defect, wired with the remnant cortex before cementing the prosthesis. Attention was paid to remove cement from the graft-femur junctions.

   A weak or fractured cortex was reinforced with long onlay struts, laid on the host femur and secured with cerclage wiring.

3) The approach was always trans-trochanteric, greater trochanters being strongly wired or fixed by a trochanteric plate. Standard or long stem Charnley prostheses were cemented with gentamicin loaded bone cement. All patients received systemic cephamandole and gentamicin during the operation and postoperativly for 4 days, followed by oral cephalosporin treatment for 5 days. Patients with a past history of infection had adapted oral antibiotic treatment for at least 6 months. Weight bearing was immediate, protected with two crutches for 1 to 3 months.

Results

We reviewed the results of upper-femur reconstructions in revision arthroplasties performed at Chochin from 1985 to December 1991. 102 revision procedures were performed in 99 patients.

   The average age of patients was 64 years (23 to 88 years, average 64 ± 13). Most had already had more than three previous hip surgery procedures.

Table 1. Massive allograft femur reconstruction procedures

---

102 Femoral massive allograft reconstructions in revision total hip arthroplasties (Cochin
1985–December 1991)
51 Segmental allografts: 6–28 cm (average 14 ± 6 cm)
   —16 replacing complete bone loss (loosened custom massive prosthetic replacement)
     Long stem prostheses
   —15 covered with remnant fragmented cortex
     Long stem prostheses
     20 shaped, impacted in enlarged deficient femur
   —15 short stem prostheses
     5 Long stem prostheses
51 Semi-circular strut allografts: 7–20 cm (average 14 ± 3 cm)
   —15 Cortical Replacements
     Longitudinal cortical bone loss
   —36 Cortical Reinforcements
     Weak or fractured femurs

The indications were: loosened prostheses in 88 cases (including twelve massively loosened femoral components) and femoral fractures around femoral prosthetic stems in 14 cases. Previous infection was present in 23 hips.

We used circumferential segmental allografts, or longitudinal struts in an equal number of cases, the different procedures being described in Table 1. The average length of the grafts was 14 cm.

Clinical and radiological examinations were performed at one, three and six months after surgery, and then each year.

1. *Complications*

Medical complications occurred twice in the series: one 87 year old patient with a fractured and loosened femur, died soon after operation, and one hemiplegia occurred in another patient.

No infection was observed among the aseptic revisions. Among the 23 previously infected hips, one infection recurred after a two step septic exchange arthroplasty, requiring removal of the graft and prosthesis. Two allograft struts were used as reinforcement in case of persistent aseptic loosening. In both the prostheses were revised secondarily and the allograft struts had united and were conserved.

Three technical errors were corrected by reoperation early with final good results (1 insufficient femoral lengthening, 1 acetabulum misorientation, and 1 screw replacement).

Trochanteric nonunion occurred in 14 cases among the 67 greater trochanter fixations to allografts. Three had no displacement and no clinical consequences, two were responsible for claudication in old patients and were not reoperated. Nine were revised because of recurrent dislocation or claudication: one was wired without success and 8 were plated with 7 good functional results although bony union was not observed in 4 cases. It is to be noted that one graft fractured when applying the plate.

There were no nonunions, but we observed 3 partial resorptions after massive prosthetic replacement. One strut, badly applied to the femur using a single wire resorbed distally, without any consequences.

Subsidence of implants was observed in 5 cases.

Some millimeters subsidence of an impacted allograft occurred early, but appears to be stabilized at 4 years follow-up.

In two cases subsidence of the prostheses occurred through the segmental allograft without damage to the graft. One of them had to be revised by cementing a new stem in the allograft, the other soon needs the same procedure.

Two other loosenings were associated with fragmentation of inlay allograft struts and will necessitate complete revision.

One fracture occurred 4 years after segmental grafting around a very small diameter long stem. It was revised by stem replacement, keeping the allograft in place.

2. *Final Results*

Six patients were lost from follow-up within the first year (1 post-operative and 1 unrelated death, 2 foreigners returned home, 2 old patients over 80 years). The maximum follow-up was 7 years, with a 3.5 years average (41 ± 18 months). Final results were evaluated in ninety six reconstructions: 90% of them had good or excellent functional results (Merle d'Aubigne-Posted score); 9 hips had poor results related to complications (1 infection, 4 instable hips, 4 loosenings).

The radiological evolution differed according to the type of reconstruction performed. Replacement segmental allografts were easy to assess: they showed union occurring during the first year, clearly promoted by the large spongy autograft adjunct. Union was quick and extensive when host remnant cortex was wired around the allograft. Fusion was harder to evaluate when allografts were included into the host femur, but always appeared to be taking place with progressive union between the allograft and the thin remaining metaphysis. Onlay struts always showed obvious and early union, even when located on the lateral side of the femur.

Conclusions

Frozen femoral heads proved to be reliable in reconstructing the acetabulum after more than fifteen years experience.

Massive irradiated allografts appear to be an effective method in major femoral reconstructions. Onlay struts had excellent results, always united, and had rare complications. Segmental allografts had a higher complication rate. The frequency of trochanteric complications (20%) indicates the need for strong initial fixation, better accomplished with plates, even at the risk of placing screws through the graft with resulting damage as it occurred once. Graft or prosthesis failures were rare, and occurred mainly with large segmental allografts used in custom massive prosthetic replacements, the conditions being then exactly comparable to reconstruction surgery after the resection of malignant tumors. When complications occurred, the benefit of initial bone stock repair was preserved in most cases, allowing easy further revision.

These results rely on safe bone banking procedures, which require predefined and strictly controlled methods, as defined by the GESTO in France [2]. Good results also depend on special surgical techniques, good graft stability, secure muscle reattachment, and reliable prostheses. The aim of the different surgical techniques used in revision arthroplasties is to obtain anatomical alignment and length with maximum preservation of remnant host bone.

References

1. Darbord JC, Laizier J (1987) A theoretical basis for choosing the dose in radiation sterilization of medical supplies. Int J Pharmaceutics 37: 1–10
2. GESTO (Association pour l'étude des Greffes Et Substituts Osseux en Orthopédie) (1993) Guide pour le prélévement, la sélection et la conservation des allogreffes osseuses. Monographie éditée par le GESTO, sous l'égide de la SOFCOT, Paris, Novembre 1993
3. Hedde C, Postel M, Kerboul M, Courpied JP (1986) La réparation du cotyle par homogreffe osseuse conservée au cours des révisions de prothése totale de hanche. Rev Chir Orthop 72: 267–276
4. Loty B (1988) Irradiation des allogreffes osseuses. Rev Chir Orthop 74: 109–159
5. Loty B (1992) Greffes osseuses: aspects fondamentaux et techniques de conservation en 1992. Cahiers d'enseignement de la SOFCOT, Conférences d'enseignement 1992: 211–237, Expansion Scientifique, Paris
6. Loty B, Courpied JP, Tomeno B, Kerboull M, Postel M, Forest M (1991) Allogreffes osseuses massives stérilisées par irradiation: bilan aprés 5 ans d'utilisation. Acta Orthopaedica Belgica 57 [Suppl II]: 35–43
7. Loty B, Courpied JP, Tomeno B, Postel M, Forest M, Abelanent R (1990) Radiation sterilized bone allografts. Intern Orthop 14: 237–242
8. Loty B, Postel M, Evrard J, Matron Ph, Courpied JP, Kerboull M, Tomeno B (1992) Remplacements en un temps des prothéses totales de hanches infectées et reconstructions osseuses par allogreffes: Etude de 90 reprises dont 46 avec allogreffes osseuses. Intern Orthop 16: 330–338

Author's address: B. Loty, Orthopaedic Department, Hospital Cochin, 27 rue du Faubourg Saint Jacques, F-75014 Paris, France.

The Use of Allografts in Revision Hip Alloarthroplasty

D. Bettin

Klinik und Poliklinik für Allgemeine Orthopädie, Westfälische Wilhelms Universität Münster, Federal Republic of Germany

Introduction

Many publications described the progressive bone destruction in endoprosthetic surgery [4, 9, 11, 18, 22]. After removal of the cement or curretage of an infection the quality of the bone bed is impaired [13]. Often a new prosthesis cannot be fixed firmly. Increasingly these bone defects cannot be reconstructed with autogenous bone transplants alone [5, 16]. Allografts offer structural stability and osteoconductive properties [3]. However, large parts of the bone transplants remain avital. If the osteointegration at the junction sites has taken place, the allograft offers an improved biomechanical situation [9, 15].

The basis for a successful revision operation is precise planning and early recognition of the bone stock deficiency [4]. It is important to avoid waiting for special implants or transplants during the operation. The clinical examination of the patient, classification of the defect and the intra-operative reconstruction are all of the same importance [4]. Because of the three dimensional distribution of acetabular and femoral defects alone classification by preoperative radiographs is insufficient and has to be always completed by an intraoperative description [8, 18, 19]. Diseases of the patient, which might influence osteointegration (e.g. chemotherapy or radiation) have to be considered in advance. All infections have to be diagnosed by hip joint aspiration, leukocyte cell counting and cultures [4, 12].

Material and Methods

Classification

Since 1991 the German Society of Orthopedics and Traumatology (DGOT) started a nation wide Multi Center Study in 20 different clinical centers concerning the indications and results of bone transplantation in revision total hip arthroplasty [14]. The new classification was designed taking into account former classifications by Morscher, Paprowski and Chandler [4, 18, 19]. The new classification was done in relation to the question, whether a certain segment of the acetabulum or femur is able to withstand the mechanical load of the body weight. This correlates with the distinction of minor ($<50\%$) or major segmental defects ($>50\%$) [9]. We also classified constrained defects and non-constrained defects. In type 1 we see only little irregularities at the acetabular

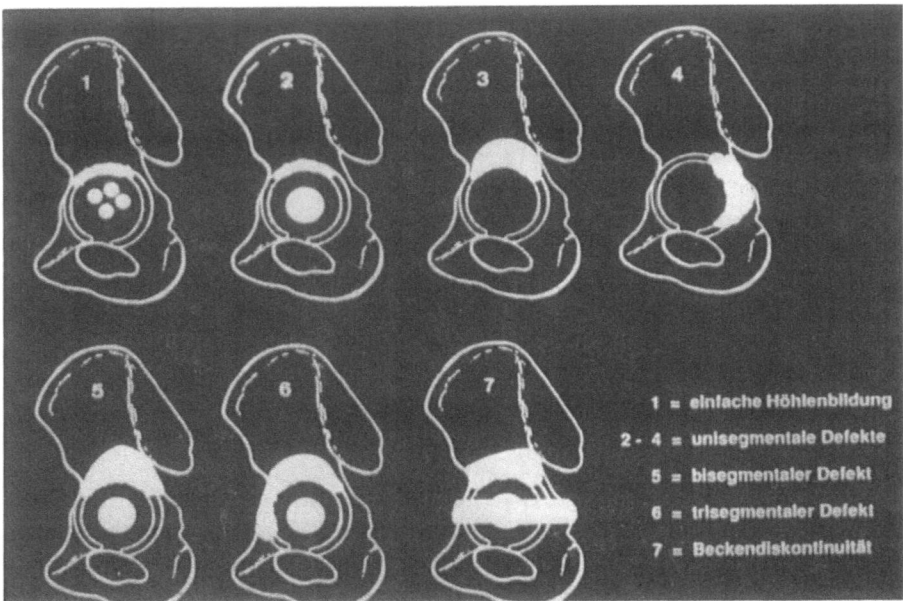

Fig. 1. Acetabulum defects, classification of the German Society of Orthopedics and Traumatology (DGOT)

floor with an intact acetabular hemisphere. In the segmental defects type 2–4 only one segment is destroyed. Type 5 and 6 present two or three segmental defects of the acetabular ring and floor. In type 7 a total pelvic instability can be seen after perforation of the acetabular floor (Fig. 1).

On the femoral side we distinguish 6 different types of deficiency. Type 1 demonstrates only an intramedullary cancellous deficiency. In type 2 the trochanter major is deficient. Type 3 represents a large calcar resorption down to the trochanter minor region. In type 4 and 5 a medial and lateral cortical shaft defect is present due to varus or valgus movement of the former prosthetic stem. In type 6 a complete circular loss of the femoral bone is present (Fig. 2).

At the Orthopedic Department at the University of Münster we analyzed the results of acetabular reconstruction in 19 patients, who demonstrated severe acetabular destruction with complete pelvic instability after multiple revision operations. The mean age at operation was 65.1 years (48–79) and the mean follow-up time was 27.1 months (1–55). Most of the patients were treated with a structural tibial allograft (11 cases). Sometimes we used a femur (6 cases) or combinations of femoral heads (6 cases) or patellas (2 cases). In a few cases we used a reconstruction ring for additional fixation to improve the load distribution in the acetabulum: Münster ring (5 cases), Schneider ring (2 cases), Müller ring (1 case). In 7 patients the polyethylene cup was directly cemented into the allograft.

Reconstruction Technique

After exposure of the acetabulum it is important to do a precise intraoperative measurement of the real defects (Fig. 3) with a special device (Fig. 4). We intended to have

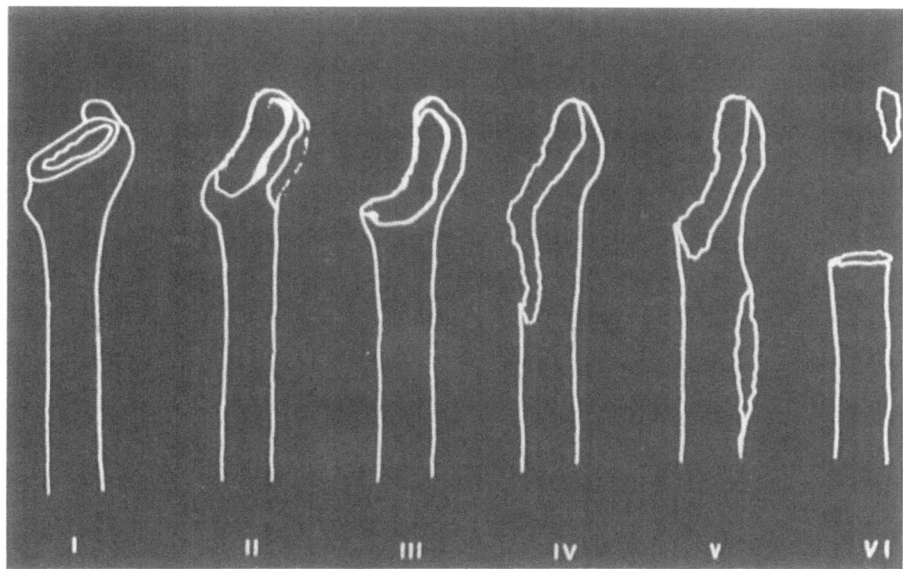

Fig. 2. Femur defects, classification of the German Society of Orthopedics and Traumatology (DGOT)

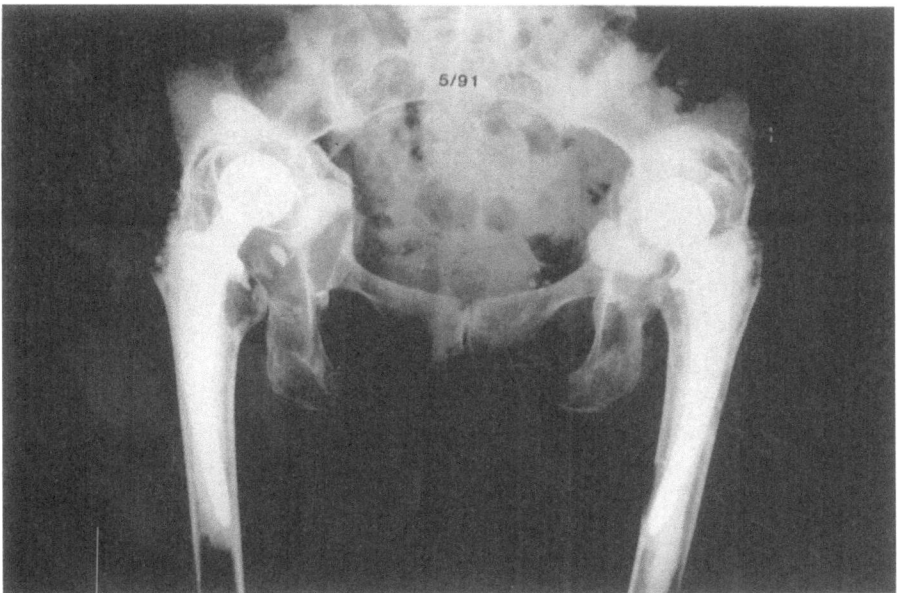

Fig. 3. 48 year old women with rheumatoid arthritis, bilateral central dislocation of both prostheses, fracture in the right ilium due to the soft bone structure, immobilization in a wheel-chair because of the severe pain

a "press fit implantation" of the allograft into the defect. We can do exact measurements also at the inside of the pelvis. On a separate working bench the chosen allograft is prepared. The allograft is reamed under the posterior part of the plateau to make a new acetabulum. Depending on the size of the tibia cup diameters up to 50 mm can be covered circumferentially. After preparation the whole tibia, which should be at least

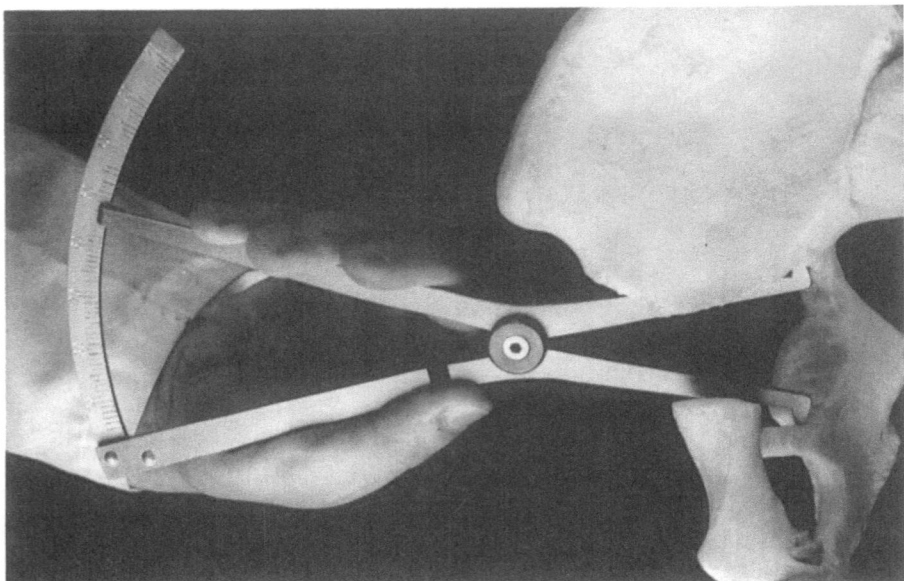

Fig. 4. Intraoperative defect measuring device for press-fit implantation

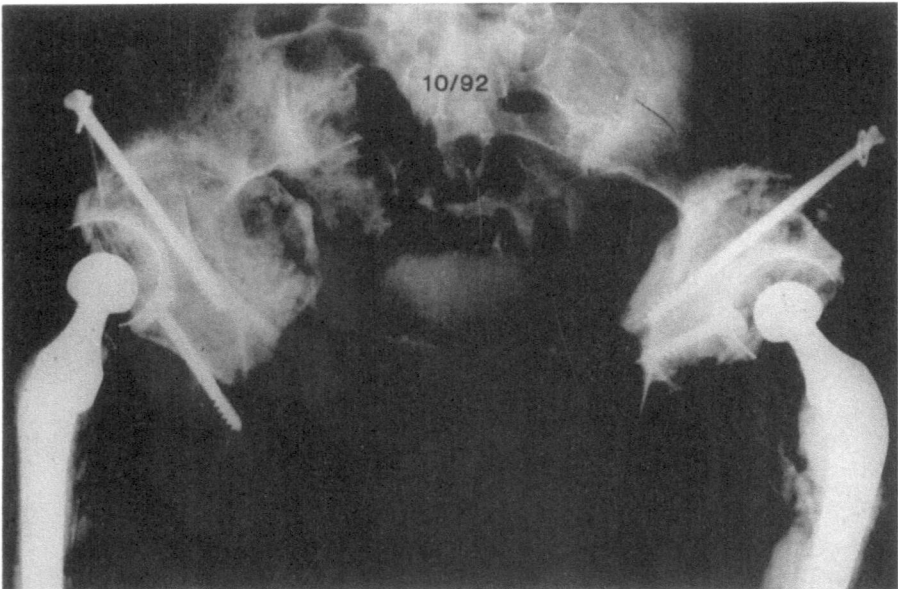

Fig. 5. Radiographic follow-up at 2.5 years after structural allograft, unchanged position of the allograft, good bone incorporation in the upper acetabulum area, no pain and good hip function, no lytic lines in the cement anchorage of the Charnley cup

5 mm greater than the defect, is impacted into the defect. For additional anchorage pelvic reconstruction plates can be applied from the outside or two screws can be inserted from the ilium to the pubis or the ischium (Fig. 5). In some cases reaming of the acetabulum can be done in situ after implantation of the tibia. In these cases the calculation of the definite cup inclination and position is easier.

Results

Our clinical follow-up according to the criteria of Enneking [7] (1 = excellent, 4 = poor) demonstrated improvements from preoperative to postoperative mean values concerning the pain from 3.3 to 1.6, leg length from 2.5 to 2.1 and general activity from 3.7 to 2.3. Changes in gluteal force from 2.9 to 2.9, Trendelenburg sign from 3.3 to 2.8 and contractures from 1.4 to 1.4 were not significant.

Complications

In 17 patients normal wound healing occurred while in 2 patients prolonged drainage was seen. As late complications (> 4 weeks) we noticed one loosening of screw anchorage after 7 months. After 4 months we saw one fracture of the allograft, which could be related to a technical failure of the osteosynthesis. Lytic lines between the acetabular cup and the allograft bone were not seen. Two patients required reoperation because of allograft fracture and dislocation of the prosthesis. One infected allograft was treated with a Girdlestone procedure.

Discussion

Both auto and allografts can incorporate reliably into the recipient bone and are able to restore bone stock [3, 13, 16]. However, large defects cannot be treated only by autografts. Allografts can be used as cancellous, cortico-cancellous or structural bone. In revision operations we normally found a poorly remodelling atrophic and sclerotic bone bed, which had to be first prepared by removal of all granulomatous tissue and drilling of the sclerotic bone to increase vascularization [4, 21]. The primary strength of the allograft is depended on the age and sex of the donor and can also be influenced by different processing methods [9]. The best strength can be expected from femoral heads, distal femurs or proximal tibias of young male donors [9]. Those solid structural allografts should be used in areas of high biomechanical stress loads e.g. in the upper acetabulum [11, 13]. Cortico-cancellous transplants or crushed bone are weaker but offer a greater surface area for revascularisation and quicker osteointegration [3]. Cortico-cancellous allografts should be protected against high stress loading until their final osteointegration [1, 5]. Sometimes this process needs several months [1]. Therefore cortico-cancellous allografts are more often used as filling material in cavities in combination with other reconstruction devices [1, 8]. Large defects of the acetabulum can be bridged with metallic supporting rings [1, 4, 8]. These are able to transmit the weight load to the remaining intact areas of the acetabular bone [8]. At least a three point fixation of the acetabular ring is required to avoid swinging or rotation of the whole construct. The long term anchorage of an alloimplant to the recipient bone is often compromised by osteogenic bone and can result in early failure [1]. Often the supporting ring is lined with bone grafts. However, if a cancellous bone graft is used alone, the primary stability of this construct is mainly dependent on screw anchorage [8]. Additional support can only be expected, if the transplant unites and integrates with the recipient bone. During this time the bone transplant has to be protected against full weight bearing [3]. Therefore only young patients, which are able to do partial weight bearing, are suitable for this treatment. Otherwise implant failure at the screw anchorage site has to be expected.

Defects with pelvic instability can also be bridged by large structural allografts [4, 10, 19]. With the use of large structural bone grafts, e.g. femur or tibia the pelvic continuity can be restored. In our experience these allografts can be implanted with a "press fit technique" or stabilized with plates or screws to the recipient bone to gain good primary stability [15, 17]. The contact area between the donor and recipient bone should be plane [3]. This way micro or macrofactures in the transplant during compression in the implantation procedure can be avoided. Additional impaction of the transplant improves the contact areas to the vital osteoblasts of the recipient. Rigid fixation of graft to host bone should always be done. The fixation to living host bone improves osteointegration [4]. Osteosynthetic fixation and acetabular ring devices are essential to maintain stability under load bearing [1, 8]. Cementing is only indicated if the stability can not be achieved with any other technique. In every allograft reconstruction good primary stability is essential [11, 22]. This allow early partial weight bearing, which is important for further bone incorporation [3]. Mankin described progressive bone resorption especially in the non-weight bearing parts of structural allografts [15]. In our early experience with large allografts we always gained a good primary stability with the "press fit implantation technique". All patients could be mobilized immediately with partial weight bearing and progressed to full weight bearing after 15 weeks.

To date the influence of biomechanical stability of different bone transplants on the long-term surviour ship rates of allo-implants remains uncertain. Long-term results can be influenced by fractures due to the remodelling process or lack of allograft integration at the recipient interface [2, 4]. It can be expected that structural bone allografts will loose their primary biomechanical stability during the process of revascularization after a few years [2].

This may be the reason for an increased failure rate in allograft transplantation-reported Mankin after 1–3 years [15]. We emphasize, in accordance to the studies of Pauwels, that early postoperative partial and dynamic biomechanical loading is very important for bone remodelling [20]. Resorption has to be expected in not stress bearing areas of the acetabulum as we can impressingly see in resorption of the iliac ring in hemipelvic allografts [10, 17].

References

1. Aebi M, Richner L, Ganz R (1989) Langzeitergebnisse der primären Hüfttotalprothese mit Acetabulumstützring. Orthopäde 18: 504–510
2. Bloem R (1989) A study on cortical remodelling and cartilage in a series of retrieved tumor allograft. International Symposium on Allografts. Leuven, Belgium
3. Burchardt H (1983) The biology of bone graft repair. Clin Orthop Rel Res 174: 28–42
4. Chandler HP, Penneberg BL (eds) (1989) Bone stock deficiency. In: Chandler HP (ed) Total hip replacement classification and management. Thorofare: SLACK
5. Convery, R, Minteer-Convery M, Devine S, Meyers M (1990) Acetabular augmentation in primary and revision total hip arthroplasty with cementless prosthesis. Clin Orthop Rel Res 252: 167–175
6. Delloye Ch, Vincent A, Nayer P (1989) Contribution of Allografts in prosthetic surgery. In: Abstract book, 5th International Symposium on Limb Salvage, Saint Marlo
7. Enneking WF (1983) Musculoskeletal tumor surgery. Philadelphia: Saunders
8. Ganz R (1993) Pfannenprobleme bei Hüftprothesenwechsel. 42. Jahrestagung der Vereinigung Norddeutscher Orthopäden, Hannover
9. Gross A, Lavoie M, McDermott P, Marks P (1985) The use of allograft bone in revision of total hip arthroplasty. Clin Orthop Rel Res 197: 115–122
10. Harrington K (1992) The use of hemipelvic allografts or autoclaved grafts for reconstruction after wide resection of malignant tumors of the pelvis. J Bone Joint Surg 74 A (3): 331–341

11. Harris W, Crothers O, Indong O (1977) Total hip replacement and femoral head bone grafting for severe acetabular deficiency in adults. J Bone Joint Surg 59 A (6): 752–759

12. Härle A (1981) Die postoperative Wund-Saug-Drainage and ihr Einfluss auf die Wundheilung. Habilitationsschrift Münster.

13. Jasty M, Harris W (1987) Total hip reconstruction using frozen femoral head allografts in patients with acetabular bone loss. Orthop Clin North Amer 18 (2): 291–299

14. Katthagen B-D (1993) Knochentransplantation beim Prothesenwechsel. 42. Jahrestagung der Vereinigung Norddeutscher Orthopäden, Hannover

15. Mankin H, Gebhardt M, Tomford W (1987) The use of frozen cadaveric allografts in the management of patients with bone tumors of the extremities. Orthop Clin North Amer 18 (2): 275–289

16. McCollum D, Nunley J, Harrelson J (1980) Bone grafting in total hip replacement for acetabular reconstruction protrusion. J Bone Joint Surg 62 A (7): 1065: 1073

17. Mnaymneh W, Malinin T, Mnaymneh L, Robinson D (1990) Pelvic allograft, a case report with a follow-up evaluation of 5.5 years. Clin Orthop Rel Res 255: 128–132

18. Morscher E, Jick W, Seeling W (1989) Klassifikation der Knochendefekte bei Hüftpfannenrekonstruktion. Orthopädie 18: 428

19. Paprowsky W, Lawrence J, Schwarzt C, Cameron H (1989) Methods of allografting in deficient acetabulum—an eight year clinical experiment. 57th annual meeting of the American Academy of Orthopaedic Surgeons New Orleans LA

20. Pauwels F (1965) Gesammelte Abhandlungen zur funktionellen Anatomie des Bewegungsapparates. Berlin, Heidelberg, New York: Springer

21. Trancik T, Toledo B, Stulberg B, Wilde A, Feiglin D (1989) Allograft reconstruction of the acetabulum during revision total hip arthroplasty. J Bone Joint Surg 68 A (4): 527–533

22. Wagner H (1987) Revisionsprothese für das Hüftgelenk bei schwerem Knochenverlust. Orthopäde 16: 295–300

Author's address: Priv. Doz. Dr. D. Bettin, Klinik und Poliklinik für Allgemeine Orthopädie, Westfälische Wilhelms Universität Münster, Albert-Schweizer-Strasse 33, D-48149 Münster, Federal Republic of Germany.

Revision Joint Replacement: Proximal Femoral Replacement

M. G. Rock

Mayo Clinic and Mayo Foundation, Orthopedic Department, Rochester, Minnesota, U.S.A.

Introduction

One of the more difficult problems encountered by orthopedic surgeons today is periarticular loss of bone as a result of aseptic loosening in the multi-revised arthroplasty patient, massive osteolysis in response to debris accumulation from the articulating components, stress shielding, fracture, infection or even iatrogenic damage. Such bone loss precludes the use of conventional arthroplasty components due to the lack of mechanical support. Femoral revisions relying on extensive cementation have failed prematurely [5, 22, 28]. It has become apparent that revision hip arthroplasty performed in the presence of poor quality bone will fail with further aseptic loosening, stem breakage, femoral fracture, or femoral subsidence. The importance of reconstituting quality bone to the revision arthroplasty patient is assuming greater significance in light of the lack of clinical success when performing such operations in patients with compromised or deficient bone.

The advantages of biologic reconstruction include ultimate incorporation with the host, tailoring the graft to fit the anatomic deficiencies and in the case of allogeneic tissue potential unlimited supply and lack of morbidity. The magnitude and shape of most proximal femoral deficiencies preclude the use of autogenous tissue and therefore greater reliance on a safe source of allograft tissue has become apparent. In spite of increasing difficulties in maintaining viable tissue banks at tertiary centers across the United States the use of large segment allografts has risen exponentially particularly among adult reconstructive surgeons. The technical nuances associated with allograft reconstruction of proximal femoral deficiencies have evolved over the past several years with a noticeable reduction in the complications [1, 13, 14, 20, 26].

Preoperative Planning

Prior to the reconstruction appropriate radiographs are taken to determine the extent of bone loss and/or deficiency on both sides of the articulation. Segmental loss of bone in the proximal femur is generally easy to identify on plane radiographs. Lesions with significant endosteal bone loss are somewhat more difficult to quantitate. Using the cortical index of Barnett and Nordin [3] as applied to the hip by Gruen [15] is an effective way of quantitating bone quality in such circumstances. Most of these endosteal erosions will be due to osteolysis and may be present in otherwise stable implants as

Table 1. AAOS classification of femoral defects

1. Segmental
      Proximal
      Partial
      Complete
      Intercalary
      Greater trochanter
2. Cavitary
      Cancellous
      Cortical
      Ectasia
3. Combined segmentary and cavitary
4. Malalignment
      Rotational
      Angular
5. Stenosis
6. Discontinuity

confirmed by aspiration arthrography. Anticipating the use of large metallic components in combination with allogeneic tissue it becomes imperative to rule out the possibility of concomitant infection.

It has become apparent that classifying bone deficiencies provides for a framework to develop and evaluate treatment outcomes internationally and it aids in preoperative planning of the surgical reconstruction. There are numerous classifications of proximal femoral deficiency in total hip arthroplasty [2, 14, 16, 27]. In 1990 The American Academy of Orthopaedic Surgeons through task force recommendations proposed the femoral deficiency classification noted in Table 1 [2]. Allograft utilization will principally apply to segmental proximal and 'intercalary' deficits as well as cavitary cancellous and cortical deficiencies. The latter will be discussed in cancellous impaction grafting by Professor Sloof in a subsequent section. As such we will concentrate on the use of large bulk allografts to reconstruct segmental deficiencies of the proximal femur and cortical cancellous strut grafts to address the former and intercalary deficiencies created by osteolysis, implant penetration of the proximal femoral cortex or iatrogenic created access to facilitate cement removal.

Anticipating segmental cortical deficiencies and/or the possible penetration of cortex in the process of removing cemented components, it will become necessary to expose or skeletonize the proximal femur for adequate exposure. In circumstances that do not mandate an extensive reconstruction of the acetabulum, a vastus slide as recommended by Head et al. [19] allows for mobilization of the anterior abductors along with an intact vastus lateralis as a solid anterior sleeve exposing the lateral and anterior aspect of the femur. If extensive acetabular exposure is necessary a modification of this has been recommended by the same authors utilizing an extended trochanteric osteotomy which is continued 3–10 cm distal to the vastus tubercle allowing for unprecedented exposure of the acetabulum but also access to the proximal femur for removal of cement and implant [29]. The extended nature of the trochanteric osteotomy allows for repositioning of the trochanteric segment, increases exposure of the trochanteric segment of the proximal femur, and allows for more effective and rigid fixation.

Reconstruction of the Deficient Femur with Cortical Strut Allografts

The principal indications for cortical strut allografts include the loss of cortical bone through osteolysis, fracture, penetration by implant, iatrogenic access to the cement and component, or even in primary total hip arthroplasties with patients who otherwise have significant compromised bone quality. Much of the anticipated and subsequent realized success of allograft struts was based on the experience of treating fractures of the adult dog radii with freeze dried cortical strut allografts [12]. It became evident from that study that within two months of application the struts had uniformly attached to the underlying host bone and had reconstituted 80 percent of the mechanical strength of the underlying radius. Within an additional four weeks complete bridging of the allograft to the host had occurred and the biomechanical performance of the grafted radius was similar to that of the control contralateral side. The graft radiographically and microscopically underwent a progressive healing course which included rounding off of the proximal and distal ends of the strut graft, scalloping which reflects soft tissue invasion, bridging to the host cortex and then progressive cancellization. Areas not in direct contact with the underlying host bone resorb but in areas in which there is intimate contact, vascularized tissue and new bone formation is seen extending into the strut. This observation underscores the need for absolute approximation of the strut to the underlying host femur and to contour the strut to facilitate this. As such, it may be necessary to choose a proximal femoral or tibial metadiaphyseal segment of allograft that is slightly larger than the host to allow for contouring of the strut to the surface of the native bone. Most allograft struts will be applied to either the lateral, anterior or medial aspect of the proximal femur.

With the rather successful application of this technique in the canine model, the use of allograft struts has increased significantly and replaced large segment bulk allografts of the proximal femur when the indications allow. Surgical nuances of the application have become apparent and have been well documented by several authors [1, 7, 9–12, 20, 31, 33]. Generally the struts should buttress one-half the diameter of the host allowing for preservation of blood supply through soft tissue attachments to the native femur. Given that hoop stresses do not normalize for two diameters of the bone away from cortical deficiencies the strut lengths should extend 8 cm proximal and distal to the defect and be approximately 1.5 to 2 cm wide. Prior to application the strut should be contoured to allow maximal contact between the allograft and the host (Fig. 1). This is often best accomplished with a high speed burr. The struts are applied to the native bone and maintained in position with 2 mm Dall-Miles cables that are separated at 2 1/2 cm intervals. Prior to formally tightening the cables, autogenous cancellous bone is applied at sites of allograft host juncture where there is not absolute contact. With cable application, the autogenous graft is compressed between the allograft and the host (Fig. 2). Ideally the femoral component should bypass any areas of cortical transgression by at least two diameters of the native femoral shaft and should rest on native bone proximally. Relying solely on allograft reconstitution of the calcar has not been successful with many of these patients experiencing migration of the component [9–11, 14]. It may, therefore, be necessary as is routinely done by Emerson, Head and associates [9–12], to use a calcar replacement long-stemmed femoral component.

The short and mid-term results of cortical strut utilization are now becoming available. Possibly the greatest experience has been that of Emerson, Head and associates who have recently reported on 106 patients followed up for a minimum of two years with a range of 24 to 69 months [12, 20]. The average time to radiographic union was 8.4 months and the incidence of graft union which was assumed to occur if 50 percent

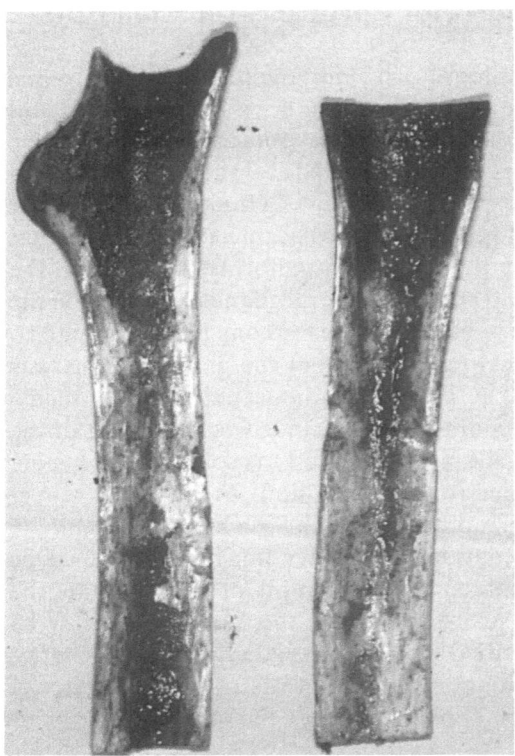

Fig. 1. Proximal femoral strut allografts fashioned with a high-speed burr to fit the contour of a deficient proximal femur

of the allograft and host had evidence of union was 98 percent. The average preoperative Harris hip score for this patient population was 48.1 and the average postoperative Harris hip score at final follow-up was 79.6. Twenty of the 106 patients were judged to be clinical failures, 10 of which were attributed to the femoral side. Eight of the 10 femoral failures were due to subsidence. Many of these patients [5] were early in the series where reliance was placed on calcar allograft replacement which has been abandoned in favor of calcar replacement prosthesis.

In an extensive review of proximal femoral allografts and revision hip arthroplasty, Allan [1] reviewed seven cortical strut allografts with a mean length of 5.8 cm. They uniformly united and remodeled indicating revascularization. The success in this patient population in their hands was 86 percent with preoperative hip scores of 36.6 proceeding to a postoperative score of 78.8. There were no structural failures and no subsidence of the components. In an additional review, Chandler assessed 22 cortical struts for similar indications as mentioned [6, 7]. Union was achieved in 100 percent radiographically with one fracture of the graft and femur that ultimately went on to heal with conservative measures. In 19 of the 22 patients conventional short-stemmed femoral components were used with the tip being proximal to the cortical deficiency. It is now recommended that a long-stemmed femoral component or dual struts at right angles to each other be applied in circumstances where there is a sizable (greater than 2 cm) deficit of the lateral femoral cortex.

The use of allograft struts has increased significantly at our institution. The use of allograft prosthetic composites has in large part stabilized but the use of struts has increased almost two-fold every year since 1991 suggesting that in situations in which the native femur can be maintained the use of strut allografts are associated with successful

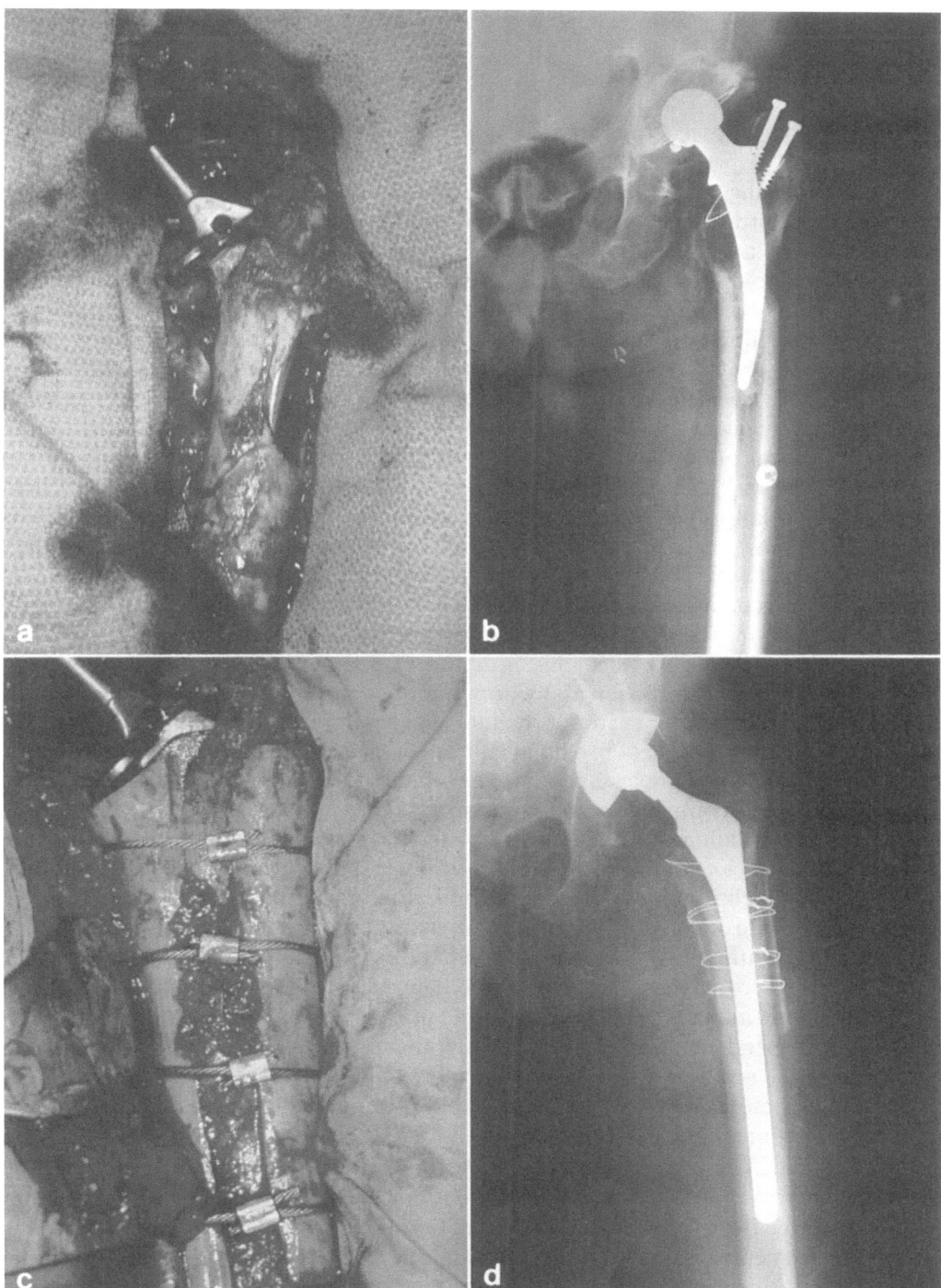

Fig. 2. **a** Large intercalary deficiency of the proximal femur in a multiply revised total hip arthroplasty patient exhibiting marked deficiency in the proximal medial aspect of the femur and proximal lateral cortex; **b** A trial prosthesis in place revealing the deficient medial and lateral proximal femoral cortex; **c** Trial prosthesis in place after the allograft cortical struts have been applied and maintained with circumferential Dahl-Miles 2 mm cable separated by 2 cm. Note the extensive autogenous grafting applied between the allograft and the native femur; **d** Reconstructed proximal femur showing the strut allografts in place prior to formal union

reconstitution of bone without some of the inherent problems that large bulk allograft introduce.

Allograft Prosthetic Composite

When encountering complete loss of the proximal femur several options exist including conversion to girdlestone arthroplasty, the use of custom tumor proximal femoral replacement implants or the use of allograft prosthetic composites. The latter has all the advantages of biologic reconstruction discussed previously. Girdlestone arthroplasty is not a serious consideration in this patient population given that the extensive loss of proximal femur allows pistoning, shortening and inevitably results in a flail uncontrolled lower limb. The proximal femoral replacement prosthesis for non-tumor conditions has recently been reviewed at our institution [32]. Most of the patients had numerous failed previous total hip arthroplasties with a smaller contribution from patients experiencing proximal femoral nonunions with underlying severe hip arthrosis. Preoperative hip scores were 44 and at last follow-up 68. There was improvement in pain as well as 'severity of the limp' that were statistically significant but the need for external aids persisted. There was a 12 percent femoral component revision due to aseptic loosening with an acetabular revision rate of 21 percent. The femoral component survivorship was a predicted 72 percent at 12 years. There was, however, a high dislocation rate of 22 percent. With no means of advancing the abductor mechanism to the implant, attempts are generally made to advance this into the IT band or the vastus lateralis and reconstitute soft tissue tension in abduction. It is often necessary to lengthen the limb to increase the stability of the custom proximal femoral implant. It was the conclusion of the authors to limit the use of proximal femoral custom implants for reconstruction to older and inactive patients who otherwise could not undergo the more extensive allograft prosthetic composite reconstruction [8, 21, 30].

Selection of the allograft to be used prior to surgery should match the diaphyseal and metaphyseal diameters of the host to minimize a step-off deformity at the allograft host juncture site as well to minimize excessive bulk proximally that may preclude effective soft tissue coverage or closure of skin. The surgical approach should minimize soft tissue injury while maintaining blood supply to whatever proximal native femur exists [1]. Trochanteric osteotomy may be necessary to gain access to the acetabulum if extensive reconstruction is anticipated [29]. Due to the magnitude of the operation it is best to have two independent teams working simultaneously. The first team can work on exteriorizing the proximal femur, removing all remaining cemented components, identify proximal femoral segments with native blood supply and tagging these for future application around the allograft and attending to any surgical necessities on the acetabular side. The other team can be working on the back table fashioning the proximal femoral allograft to receive a long-stemmed femoral component. The amount of bone removed from the endosteal surface of the allograft should be minimized and the component cemented in place utilizing antibiotic impregnated cemented preventing cement from appearing at the step-cut osteotomy site. A mirror image step-cut is performed on the host femur distally to allow for increase in overall contact between the allograft and host as well as to afford some additional rotational stability to the construct which is often compromised due to the expanded intramedullary portion of the native distal femur (Fig. 3). The allograft prosthetic composite is then advanced into the host. A cortical strut can be applied at the allograft host juncture site along with considerable autogenous grafting to expedite healing. Generally it is best to avoid side

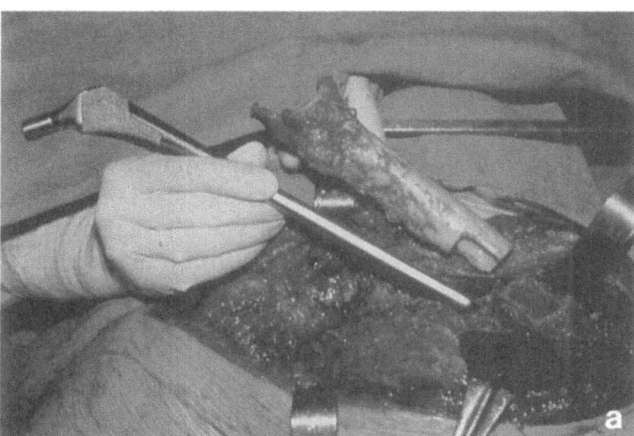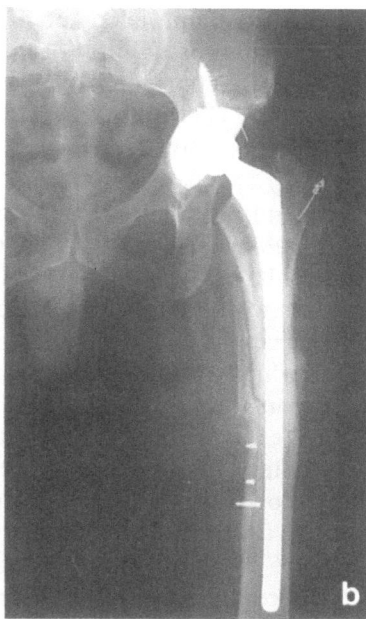

Fig. 3. **a** Large segmental loss of the proximal femur for which allograft prosthetic composite was felt to be the most appropriate reconstruction. The long stem femoral component is shown prior to cementation into the allograft and advancement into the host. Note the step-cut orientation of the allograft/host juncture site; **b** Reconstructed proximal femur with allograft cortical strut being applied at the juncture sites and after union has occurred to the host

plates as screws applied into the allograft act as stress risers through which fractures can occur. Studies performed at our laboratory show the very distinct advantage of using an intramedullary stem as fixation at the allograft host juncture site and the added rotational stability of the step-cut [23]. Plate and screw application at the juncture site under rotational stresses create fractures emanating from the most proximal screw site directed up into the allograft to the lesser trochanteric region. Given the lack of blood supply and lack of total incorporation of the allograft, these fractures often will not unite demanding revision of the allograft prosthetic composite. The strut application affords not only the possibility of increasing overall bone quality with incorporation but also contributes to torsional stability. Proximally the native greater trochanter is reapplied to the proximal allograft maintaining it in position with the Dahl-Miles grip and cable system introducing the cables just underneath the lesser trochanter and through the bulk of the lesser trochanter through a small 2 mm drill hole made to accommodate the 2 mm cable.

With segmental loss proximal to the lesser trochanter the calcar replacement prosthesis is preferred over any attempts at grafting the calcar region as this is often associated with resorption and migration of the components [10, 11, 14, 18]. Gross [1, 14, 26] reviewed 40 large bulk proximal femoral allograft implant composites with an average length of these grafts being 10.4 cm. The overall success rate was 85 percent with radiographic union occurring in 81 percent. Unstable nonunions necessitating additional grafting and fixation occurred in 8 percent. The preoperative Harris hip score was 30.5 and the average postoperative score, 65.8 with an average improvement of 35.3. Trochanteric union occurred radiographically in 38 percent with a stable fibrous union without trochanteric escape in an additional 42 percent. Subsidence occurred in four hips and no gross failures of the construct occurred. Similarly, Head and Emerson [17, 18, 20] have reported their experience of large segment allografts with success rates of 73 percent and Harris hip scores that are not dissimilar from the experience of Gross et al. [14]. Preoperative Harris hip scores were 26 and postoperatively 65. They did notice, however, a 4.5 percent infection rate, a 25 percent dislocation rate, a nonunion rate of 25 percent and a fracture rate of 2 percent. These complications exceed those in which only strut grafts were used. As such, these authors have recommended minimizing the use of large bulk proximal femoral allografts in revision surgery. Gitelis [13] presented 26 patients with allograft prosthetic composites for failed total hip arthroplasty in 1988. The success rate was 88 percent with 90 percent achieving radiographic evidence of union which took 5.8 months on an average to occur. The authors suggest repairing the abductors into the allograft greater trochanter utilizing drill holes and nonabsorbable tape. We have, in our series, noticed several cases of extensive resorption of the greater trochanter when drill holes are made and soft tissue is advanced into the allograft. This may be on the basis of trochanteric fragmentation because of the stress riser associated with the drill holes or by possibly introducing immunologically competent cells from the host into the allograft marrow compartment. Regardless, we are now either advancing the native greater trochanter onto the allograft trochanter with the Dahl-Miles cable grip system or advancing the abductor tendon (if the trochanter is missing) to the preserved gluteal tendon on the allograft utilizing nonabsorbable sutures in a modified Krakow type suture. This affords good soft tissue tensioning, minimizes dislocation of the component, serves to return some of the abductor power and preserves the allograft greater trochanter as we have not witnessed bone loss or absorption. A similar smaller series of allograft prosthetic composites for hip arthroplasty have been reported by Borja [4] and McGann [24] and Roberson [31] who report, as larger series do, 80 percent success rate and postoperative hip scores of approximately 70. A recent review at our institution of 41 total hip arthroplasties utilizing allograft prosthetic composite for massive femoral bone loss were reviewed [25]. The mean follow-up was 2.8 years with a mean allograft length of 15 cm. The host allograft juncture site was augmented with cortical strut grafts in 29 patients. The average preoperative Harris hip score improved from 54 points to 76 points at one year and subsequently to 79 at two years. Survivorship at three years using reoperation as the endpoint was predicted at 76 percent. The infection rate was 7.3 percent, the dislocation rate was 7.3 percent, intraoperative fractures of the native bone occurred in 17 percent. Progressive radiolucent lines were evident in 14 percent of the femoral components in zone 1 and in 19 percent in zone 7.

One of the more devastating complications associated with this form of reconstruction is that of infection. Our infection rate of 7 percent is in keeping with that of Gitelis 6 percent [13], Allan 8 percent [1], Gross 6 percent [14]. It has become apparent that effective soft tissue coverage over the reconstruction is necessary and given the multiple revision nature of most of these-cases, it may be necessary to consider transposition or even free flaps to cover the reconstruction area. The infection rate is the same, however, if a large segment custom proximal femoral replacement was to be used.

Summary

There is no doubt that extensive revision arthroplasty will become more of the practice pattern of most arthroplasty surgeons. Although technically demanding, allograft reconstruction of the proximal femur has had gratifying results. The indications for large segment allograft prosthetic composites and allograft struts are different and therefore effective comparisons between the two reconstructive options is not appropriate. However, current tendency is to minimize the use of large bulk allografts whenever possible and to utilize host vascularized tissue augmented with struts. The complication rate of this form of reconstruction is no different than the other alternatives addressing such clinical problems and deficiencies. The operative nuances that have increased the success are becoming apparent as are consistent processing techniques of large segment allografts for safer and more reliable application by the orthopedic surgeon. These forms of reconstructions are not to be compared with primary arthroplasty and the limitations associated with this type of surgery and the ultimate functional result so achieved has to be thoroughly discussed with the patient before proceeding with operations of this magnitude.

References

1. Allan DG, Lavoie GJ, Gross A (1991) Proximal femoral allografts in revision hip arthroplasty. J Bone Joint Surg 73B: 235–240
2. American Academy of Orthopedic Surgeons Committee on the Hip (1990) Classification and management of bone deficiencies of the acetabulum and femur. Presented as a Scientific Exhibit at the Annual American Academy of Orthopedic Surgeons Scientific Meeting, New Orleans, LA
3. Barnett E, Nordin BEC (1960) The radiographic diagnosis of osteoporosis. A new approach. Clin Radiol 11: 166–174
4. Borja F, Mnayneh W (1985) Bone allograft in salvage of difficult hip arthroplasties. Clin Orthop Rel Res 197: 123–130
5. Callaghan JJ, Salvati EA, Pellicci PM, et al (1985) Results of revision for mechanical failure after cemented total hip replacement. J Bone Joint Surg 67A: 1074–1095
6. Chandler H, McCarthy J, et al (1993) Reconstruction of major segmental loss of the proximal femur. Read at the Annual Meeting of the American Academy of Orthopedic Surgeons Knee and Hip Society, San Francisco, CA
7. Chandler HP (1992) The use of strut allograft in the reconstruction of failed total hip replacements. Orthopedics 15(10): 1207–1218
8. Chao EYS, Sim FH (1990) Composite fixation of salvage prosthesis for the hip and knee. Clin Orthop Rel Res 276: 91–101
9. Emerson RH, Cuellar AD, Head WC, Peters PC (1993) Reconstruction of the deficient femur with cortical strut allografts. Tech Orthop 7(4): 27–32
10. Emerson RH, Head WC, Malinin TI, Matlin JA (1990) Allograft femoral reconstruction in revision hip arthroplasty. Part I. Surg Rounds Orthop 4: 15–22
11. Emerson RH, Head WC, Malinin TI, Matlin JA (1990) Allograft femoral reconstruction in revision hip arthroplasty. Part 11. Surg Rounds Orthop 4: 31–39
12. Emerson RH, Malinin TI, Head WC, et al (1992) Cortical strut allografts in the reconstruction of the femur in revision total hip arthroplasty. Basic designs and clinical study. Clin Orthop Rel Res 285: 35–44
13. Gitelis S, Heligman D, Quill G, Piasecki P (1988) The use of large allografts for tumor reconstruction and salvage for failed total hip arthroplasty. Clin Orthop Rel Res 231: 62–70
14. Gross AE, Lavoie JV, et al (1985) The use of allograft bone in revision of total hip arthroplasty. Clin Orthop Rel Res 197: 115–122
15. Gruen TA, Hedley AK, Borden LS, Hungerford DS (1991) Adaptive bone remodeling associated with cementless porous coated femoral total hip replacement components. Five year minimum follow-up radiographic analysis. Scientific Exhibit at the Annual Meeting of the American Academy of Orthopedic Surgeons, Anaheim, CA
16. Gustillo RB, Pasternak HS (1988) Revision total hip arthroplasty with titanium ingrowth prosthesis and bone grafting for a failed cemented component loosening. Clin Orthop 235: 111
17. Head WC, Berklacich F, Malinin TI, Emerson RH (1987) Proximal femoral allografts in revision total hip arthroplasty. Clin Orthop Rel Res 225: 22–36

18. Head WC, Malinin TI, Berklacich F (1987) Freeze dried proximal femur allografts in revision total hip arthroplasty. A preliminary report. Clin Orthop Rel Res 215: 109–121

19. Head WC, Mallory TH, Emerson RH, et al (1987) Extensile exposure of the hip for revision arthroplasty. J Arthroplasty 2(4): 265–273

20. Head WC, Wagner RA, Emerson RH, Malinin TI (1993) Restoration of femoral bone stock in revision total hip arthroplasty. Read at the Annual Meeting of the American Academy of Orthopedic Surgeons Hip Society, San Francisco, CA

21. Inglis AE, Carter SR, Walker PS (1991) Long term radiographic evaluation of massive proximal femoral replacement. In: Langlais F, Tomeno B (eds) Limb salvage major reconstructions in oncologic and non-tumoral conditions. Berlin, Heidelberg: Springer

22. Kavanagh BF, Ilstrup DM, Fitzgerald RH (1985) Revision total hip arthroplasty. J Bone Joint Surg 67A: 517–526

23. Markel MD, Rock MG, et al (1994) Mechanical characteristics of proximal femoral reconstruction after fifty percent resection. J Bone Joint Surg (in press)

24. McGann W, Mankin HJ, Harris WH (1986) Massive allografting for severe failed total hip replacement. J Bone Joint Surg 68A: 4–12

25. Nelson T, Rock MG (1995) Revision hip arthroplasty with proximal femoral allograft. Mayo Clinic experience. (Submitted to the American Academy of Orthopedic Surgeons for podium presentation)

26. Oakeshott RD, Morgan DAF, Gross A, et al (1987) Revision total hip arthroplasty with osseous allograft reconstruction. Clin Orthop Rel Res 225: 37–60

27. Paprosky WG, Lawrence J, Cameron H (1990) Femoral defect classification. Clinical application. Orthop Rev 19: 9–15

28. Pellicci PM, Wilson PD, et al (1985) Long term results of revision total hip replacement. J Bone Joint Surg 67A: 513–516

29. Peters PC, Head WC, Emerson RH (1992) An extended trochanteric osteotomy for-revision total hip arthroplasty. J Bone Joint Surg 75B: 158–160

30. Postel M, et al (1991) Segmental total hip and knee replacement: A long term review. In: Langlais F, Tomeno B (eds) Limb salvage major reconstructions in oncologic and non-tumoral conditions. Berlin, Heidelberg: Springer

31. Roberson JR (1992) Proximal femoral bone loss after total hip arthroplasty. Orthop Clin N Amer 23(2): 291–302

32. Seteceri J, Sim FH, et al (1994) Proximal femoral replacement for non-tumor conditions. Mayo Clinic experience. J Bone Joint Surg (submitted)

33. Stiehl JB (1992) Femoral allograft reconstruction in revision total hip arthroplasty. Orthop Rev 21: 1057–1063

Author's address: Michael G. Rock, M.D., Orthopaedic Department, Mayo Clinic, 200 First Street SW, Rochester, MN 55905, U.S.A.

Revision Arthroplasty of the Acetabulum with Restoration of Bone Stock

A. E. Gross[1], D. Garbuz[2], and E. S. Morsi[3]

[1]Division of Orthopaedic Surgery, University of Toronto, Toronto, Ontario, Canada
[2]Clinical Fellow, Mount Sinai Hospital, Toronto, Ontario, Canada
[3]Mount Sinai Hospital, Department of Orthopaedic Surgery, University of Menoufyia, U.S.A.

Introduction

The goal of revision arthroplasty of the hip is to achieve a stable implant with restoration of anatomy. This may be achieved relatively easily or with great difficulty depending on the available bone stock.

The primary goal is to implant new components against host bone with restoration of anatomy and leg lengths. This can be done with or without the use of cement depending on the characteristics of the patient and the preferences of the surgeon [22, 11, 18, 2, 4, 9, 10, 12, 23, 24, 26, 29, 30, 33, 31, 32].

If the primary goal cannot be achieved, the secondary goal would be to achieve stable components and restore anatomy and leg lengths but with help from bone grafts or prosthetic design. If bone graft is used it is either morsellized or noncircumferential (cortical strut) so that the implant is supported primarily by host bone. Some implants are designed to compensate for minimal to moderate loss of bone stock. Femoral components with calcar replacing stems and several neck lengths, and oblong asymmetric cups are examples of this [32, 3].

When the bone loss is more severe and the implants cannot be stabilized primarily against host bone, then a decision has to be made whether to sacrifice or to restore anatomy and leg length.

If the components can be stabilized primarily against host bone with acceptable sacrifice of anatomy, then the tertiary goal is achieved. The high hip centre is an example of this [32].

If the loss of bone stock is very severe and the components cannot be stabilized gainst host bone then structural grafts or custom implants must be used to restore anatomy and leg length. This is the quaternary goal [17, 5].

Classification of Bone Defects

It is important to have a functional and relatively simple classification of bone deficits associated with loose hip implants. There are more complicated classifications in the literature [19, 81] but we have found that all of our defects can be fitted into the following classification.

Pelvic Side Defects

a) Protrusio: A contained cavitary defect with the acetabular walls and columns intact. Morsellized bone is usually used for this type of defect.
b) Minor column (Shelf): Loss of part of the rim plus the corresponding acetabular wall but less than 50% of the acetabulum. A structural graft is used but less than half of the acetabulum is replaced. This is called a minor column or shelf graft.
c) Major Column: Loss of one or both columns with its corresponding acetabular wall involving over 50% of the acetabulum. A major column structural graft involving over 50% of the acetabulum is used.

Principles of Resolution of Bone Stock in Revision Surgery of the Hip

Bone grafts are classified into heterografts (bone from another species), allografts (bone from the same species) and autografts (bone taken from one part of the same individual). In the revision situation because of the quantity and quality of bone required allograft is more practical than autograft. There are however certain advantages and disadvantages of each.

Autograft has the advantages of not being immunogenic and even more importantly is best for inducing new bone formation in the host. Its disadvantages are the quantity available, the strength, shape and form which cannot duplicate the deficit.

Allografts on the other hand are available in quantity and can be strong and duplicate the deficit. They are however immunogenic [6, 27, 7] and are not as effective as autografts for inducing new bone formation [15].

Allograft bone can be further classified according to how it is used: (1) morsellized (2) structural—(a) simulated, (b) anatomical.

A simulated structural graft is where bone from another region is shaped to simulate the deficit. For example a distal femur can be sculpted to duplicate an acetabulum.

An anatomical structural graft is when the graft is the actual anatomical part being duplicated. For example an acetabular allograft is used in whole or in part to replace an acetabular defect.

The advantages of a structural graft are restoration of anatomy and they can provide structural support for the implant. The disadvantage of a structural graft is that revascularization and remodelling can lead to resorption and/or collapse and therefore weakens with time.

Structural grafts are indicated for uncontained defects where it is necessary to restore anatomy and leg length and to provide bone support for the implant. Acceptable compromises to the anatomy and leg length are preferable to structural grafts if adequate bone stock is available, i.e., high hip centre [32].

Morsellized bone is indicated for contained defects where it serves as a filler scaffold. It can undergo revascularization and remodelling and strengthens with time. It cannot be used for early structural support.

All reconstructions will eventually fail whether they are synthetic or biological. As surgeons, our role is to prolong the time to failure, and to make sure that when failure occurs further reconstruction is possible. Bone grafts restore bone for future surgery.

Guidelines

1. Do not devascularize host bone.
2. Autograft is best for bone induction and should be used to promote union i.e., as a flying buttress for shelves, at allograft-host junctions.
3. Use rigid fixation that goes from live bone to live bone bridging the graft.
4. Cement can be used in bone grafts because it strengthens them, and delays vascularization and membrane formation.
5. Use strong bone for structural grafts.
6. Trochanteric osteotomy for complex reconstructions.
7. Do not use structural grafts unless definitely necessary:
   a) to provide support for implant
   b) to restore anatomy and leg length

Acceptable compromises to the anatomy and leg length are preferable to structural grafts if adequate bone stock is available, i.e., high hip centre.

Surgical Approach

In our hospital, all revisions requiring the use of allograft bone are done in a laminar flow operating room with body exhaust systems. If there is preoperative evidence of infection or any suggestion at the time of surgery (even with a negative Gram stain), the surgery is staged for any revision requiring the use of allograft bone.

Any allograft bone is brought into the operating room at the beginning of the case, unwrapped, cultured, and immersed in warm Betadine. The bone is obtained from our own bone bank, where it has been deep frozen at −70°C after being irradiated with 2.5 megarads.

The surgical approach is either transgluteal [20] or transtrochanteric. The transtrochanteric approach is used most commonly because of the need for extensive exposure and also because, in many cases, there is a pre-existing trochanteric nonunion.

The large fragment proximal femoral grafts should be done via the transtrochanteric approach and the trochanteric fragment should be kept as long as possible so that it will unite and so it will also reinforce the allograft. The proximal femur is exposed by reflecting the vastus lateralis off the septum anteriorly, being careful not to strip any residual bone off its soft tissue completely.

A Steinmann pin is inserted into the iliac crest as a reference point to adjust leg length. The distance from the pin to the rough line (insertion of the vastus lateralis) is recorded prior to dislocation.

Reconstruction of the Acetabulum in Revision Arthroplasty of the Hip

Restoration of bone stock on the pelvic side in arthroplasty of the hip is a difficult and controversial area. The spectrum of surgical opinion goes from avoiding the use of bone graft if at all possible [32, 25] to the use of morsellized bone only [13, 14] to the use of complex structural grafts [28, 17].

There is no question that structural grafts on the pelvic side have a guarded prognosis and should be avoided if possible [17, 25]. At the same time there are situations where bulk allograft has to be used, and if used properly can yield acceptable results and restore bone stock for future surgery [17].

Surgical Technique (See Figs. 1, 2, 3, 4, 5)

The acetabulum is prepared after the hip has been dislocated. After the acetabular prosthesis and the cement are removed the membrane is excised carefully because of possible complete bony defects avoiding penetration into the pelvis. The defect is then defined by visualization, palpation, and using a trial cup. If the defect is a contained cavity (protrusio) morsellized bone can be used. If the defect is a minor or major column

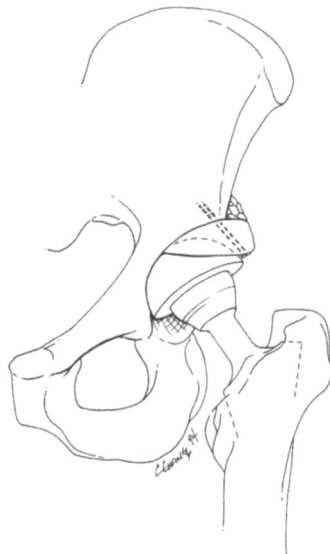

Fig. 1. Minor column (shelf) graft. The cup has been reconstructed at correct level with the support of a minor column graft. The cup is supported by more than 50% host bone. The allograft is fixed by 2 oblique 4.5 mm cancellous screws. Note the flying buttress graft of the junction of allograft and host pelvis

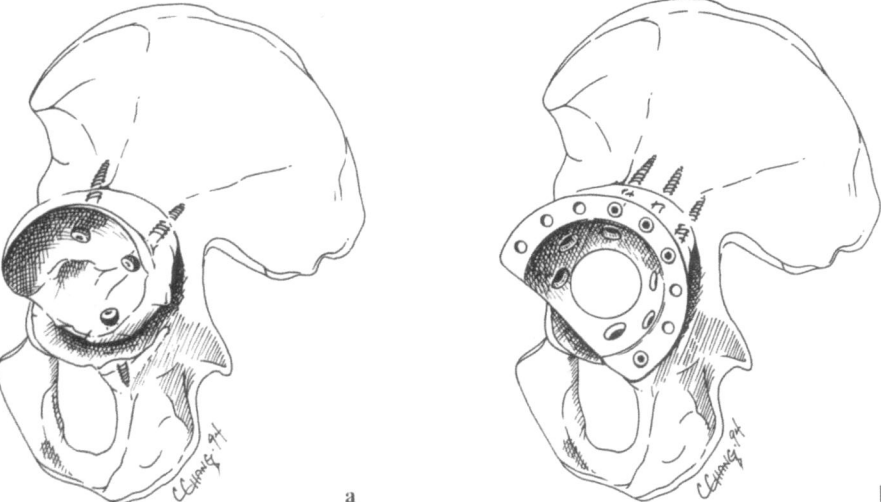

a   b

Fig. 2. Major column graft. **a** A whole acetabular allograft has been fixed to host the pelvis by three cancellous screws; **b** Further fixation and protection of the allograft is provided by a reinforcement ring that goes from host bone to host bone

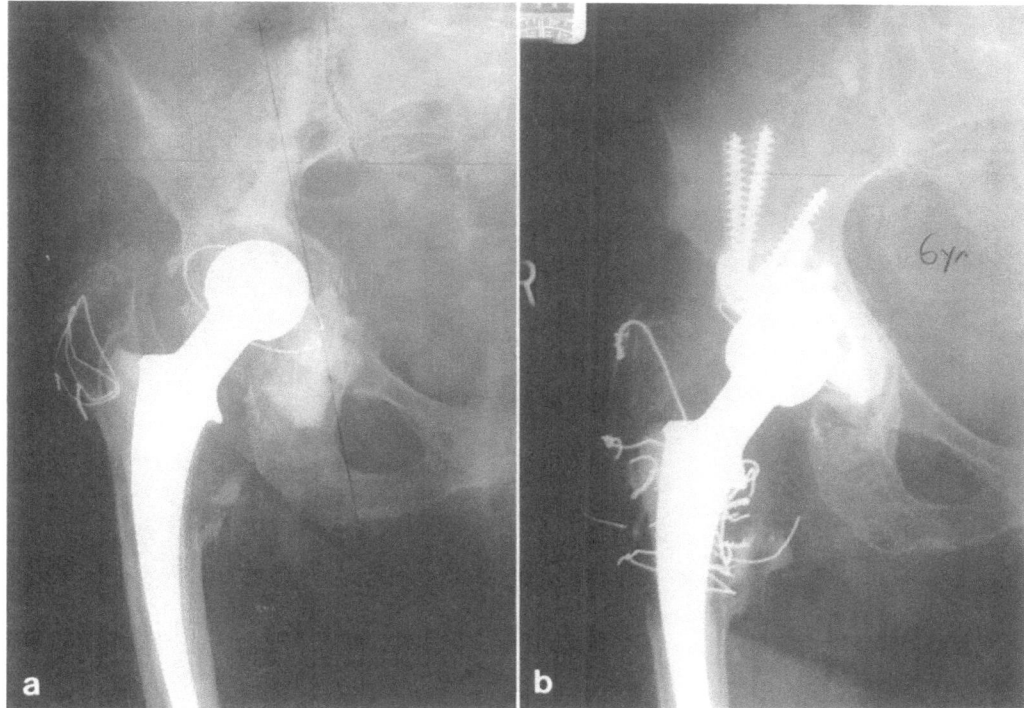

Fig. 3. Contained acetabular defect. **a** AP x-ray of the right hip demonstrating severe superomedial defect 10 years after total hip replacement in a 45 year old female; **b** 6 years after reconstruction with morsellized allograft bone, a roof reinforcement ring and a cemented cup

defect, bulk allograft is indicated. If a bulk allograft can be avoided by raising the acetabulum 1 or 2 cms. to get into better bone stock, then this alternative should be used because better contact with host bone is obtained [25]. Bulk allografts on the pelvic side should be avoided if possible and in the majority of cases, the acetabulum can be seated in host bone supplemented by morsellized allograft (protrusio graft). If a major or minor column defect does exist and cannot be compensated for by raising or centralizing the acetabular bed then a bulk allograft should be used. For bulk allografts we prefer to fashion true acetabular allografts but male femoral heads or even distal femurs can be used. If morsellized bone is needed female femoral heads should be used rather than sacrificing strong structural bone.

We prefer not to use a bone mill because the bone is made too mushy. The bone can be easily morsellized by hand using curretes and rongeurs and is fine enough to pack into cavities but still has some structural integrity.

Morsellized bone can be packed into cavities using the acetabular reamers in reverse.

Minor column grafts can be fixed by two vertical to obliquely oriented cancellous screws (4.5 mm) (Fig. 1). Reinforcement rings or reconstruction pelvic plates are used for the major column grafts (Fig. 2). If possible it is our preference to bridge these major column grafts from host bone to host bone using a plate or a reinforcement ring. It is best not to ream these grafts, but if it is necessary, the cartilage is reamed off leaving the subchondral bone intact. It is done very lightly with the grafts fixed in position.

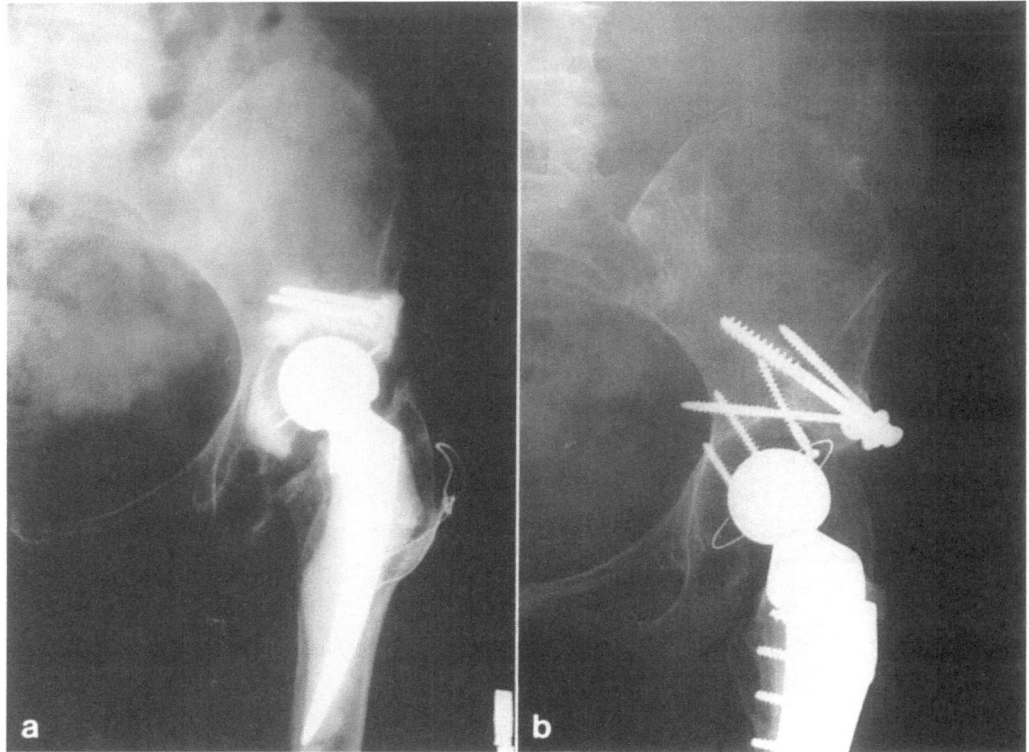

Fig. 4. Uncontained minor column (shelf) defect. **a** Pre-op AP x-ray of left hip in a 50 year old female with cemented acetabular and femoral components 10 years following cemented total hip arthroplasty; **b** Post-op 8 years after reconstruction of acetetabulum with an uncemented press fit cup and a minor column (shelf allograft). Three screws are holding the cup and three the allograft

If possible do not expose cancellous surfaces of the allograft to anything but host bone.

There are several options for the acetabular prosthesis. In the protrusio situation, morsellized bone, a reinforcement ring and a cemented cup is a good reconstruction for the moderate to low demand elderly patient. The best reconstruction for a protrusio defect in the higher demand patient is morsellized bone with an uncemented fixed large diameter, metal backed porous coated cup with direct contact with at least 50% host bone. In most cases screws are necessary to fix the cup. Bipolar or biarticulating cups are only used if nothing else is technically or biologically possible, or because of the patients' health a more extensive procedure is not indicated.

A shelf or minor column defect will allow contact with at least 50% host bone and here we prefer to use an uncemented porous coated cup, press fit or fixed by screws. A cemented cup may however be used.

A major column graft involves more than 50% of the acetabulum which means the cup is mainly in contact with dead allograft bone. Under these circumstances, the cup should be cemented.

We attempt to obtain fixation of the porous coated cups by press fit antirotation lugs if possible. If not we use screws to fix the metal backing in place. We have had no experience with screw-in cups.

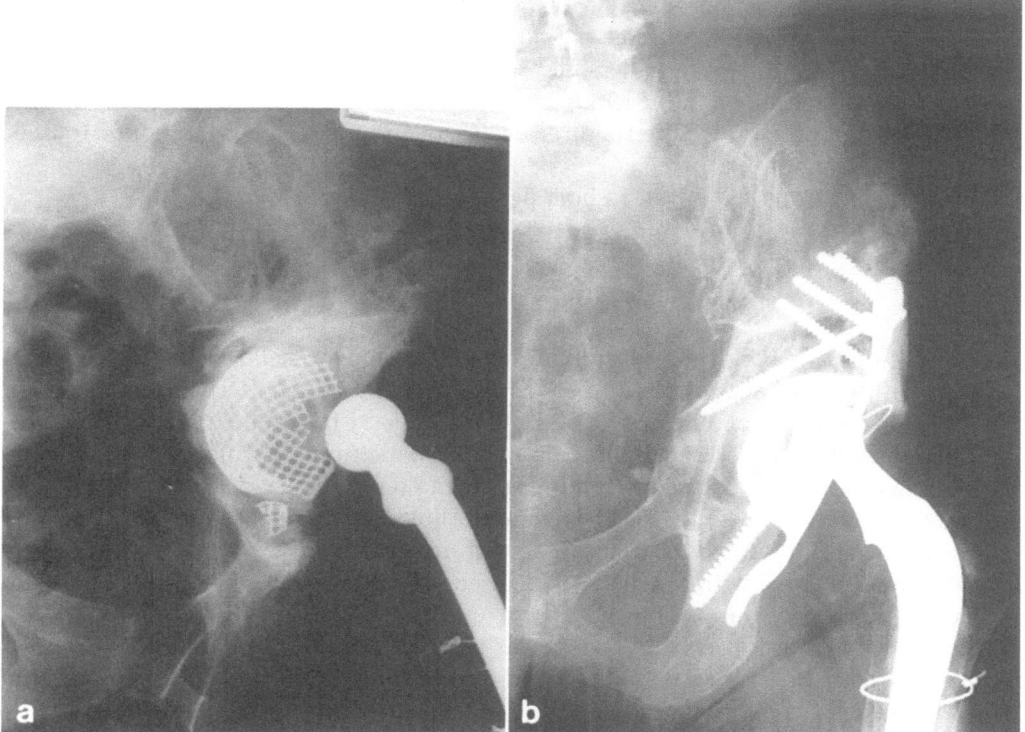

Fig. 5. Uncontained major column defect. **a** Judet view of left hip in a 40 year old female demonstrating anterior column defect 8 years after a cemented total hip; **b** 11 years after reconstruction with major column allograft fixed with cancellous screws and protected by roof reinforcement ring

Postoperative Care

Prophylactic intravenous antibiotics are used for 5 days followed by 5 more days of oral antibiotics. We prefer a cephalosporine. If the patient is catheterized intraoperatively, we use gentamycin during the surgery and for the first 24 hours but then switch to Septra until the catheter is removed. Because of the extent of the surgery, we usually keep the patients on bed rest and in abduction for 5 days. The patients are not allowed any weight bearing until union is obtained between allograft and host, usually at 3–6 months.

Principles of Surgery for Acetabular Grafting

1. Preoperatively decide on type of bone (morsellized or bulk), type of fixation and implant.
2. Use an exposure that allows access to anterior and posterior columns. Trochanteric osteotomy is advantageous in most cases.
3. Use internal fixation that goes from host bone to host bone if a structural graft involving over 50% of the acetabulum is used. Small grafts are fixed by cancellous screws oriented in an oblique to vertical direction.
4. If a structural graft is necessary use strong bone i.e., acetabular allograft, distal femur or male femoral head.

5. If a structural graft involving over 50% of acetabulum is used cement the cup.
6. Do not expose cancellous surface of graft to soft tissue of host if possible.
7. Do not use structural grafts unless necessary: (a) to provide support for the implant (b) to restore anatomy and leg length. Acceptable compromises to the anatomy and leg length are preferable to structural acetabular grafts if adequate bone stock is available, i.e. high hip centre.
8. Autograft junction of allograft to host pelvis.

Results

As of July 1, 1993, we performed acetabular revisions using morsellized allograft bone in 179 hips with an average follow-up of 4.57 years (range 1–11), 56 shelf grafts (minor column) with an average follow-up of 5.12 years (range 1–10), and 67 acetabular grafts (major column) with an average follow-up of 5.23 years (range 1–10).

A follow-up study of 58 reconstructions of contained cavitary defects using morsellized bone was carried out [17, 1]. The average follow-up was 46.4 months (range 26 to 87). Morsellized allograft bone was used with an uncemented porous coated metal backed cup in 32 hips, with a Mueller Ring and a cemented cup in 15 hips, and with a biarticulating device (bipolar) in 11 hips.

A modified Harris hip scoring system was used [21]. Failure was defined as a postoperative increase in score of less than 20 points or the need for further surgery as a result of problems with the allograft.

A successful outcome was seen in 100% of reconstructions with the Mueller Ring and the cemented cup, and 94% of the reconstructions using the uncemented cup. Only 64% of the reconstructions using the biarticulating device were successful.

Radiographic review demonstrates probable loosening (circumferential lucent lines of more than 2 mm) in 57% and definite loosening (migration or change of orientation) in 14% of reconstructions using reinforcement rings (average follow-up, 63 months). Possible loosening was seen in 5% of the uncemented cups at an average follow-up of 39 months. Of the bicentric reconstructions, fifty seven percent showed significant migration and less satisfactory pain reduction. Overall, the average medial migration of the bicentric devices was 3.2 mm (range 0–10 mm) and superior migration averaged 17.0 mm (range 0–60 mm). The superior lateral corner of the obturator foramina served as landmarks utilizing horizontal and vertical lines from the center of the femoral head to determine superior and medial migration. In contrast, cemented implants with reinforcement rings averaged 0.1 mm of medial migration (range −1 to +1 mm) and 1.7 mm of superior migration (range −6 to +12 mm). The fixed noncemented implants averaged 0.9 mm of medial migration (range −3 to +4 mm) and 1.1 mm of superior migration (range −9 to +9 mm).

Remodelling and resorption of the morsellized graft were observed. The final width of the bone graft was noted to be diminished compared with the immediate postoperative width. Percentage resorption was 5.7% (range 0–27%) in the cemented cups, 50.6% (range 17–100%) in the bicentric devices and 26.4% (range 0–83%) in the noncemented cups.

A follow-up study of bulk (major and minor column) acetabular allografts was performed [17, 16]. A modified Harris scoring system was used [21].

In this study there were 19 patients with 22 shelf (minor column) reconstructions with a mean follow-up of 40.8 months (range 29–68). The mean pre-op score was 31 and post-op 72. Two grafts had complete graft resorption. Eight grafts showed a stress shielding type of resorption or remodelling in which the unloaded portion of the graft was resorbed. This affected the most lateral part of the graft and usually involved 3 to 7 mm. Acetabular implant migration occurred in 3 cases, 2 of which were bipolar prostheses. Of the 22 shelf (minor column) grafts there were 3 failures, 2 for deep sepsis requiring further surgery, and 1 for a dislocated cup. The overall success rate was 86%.

In the major column group there were 28 reconstructions in 26 patients with a mean follow-up of 36 months (range 24–71). The mean pre-op score was 29, and the mean post-op score 75.

There was one case of deep sepsis requiring excision in a reconstruction using femoral heads. A patient with flaccid paralysis (myelomenigocele) reconstructed with an acetabular allograft required further surgery for recurrent dislocation.

Six of the remaining 14 true acetabular allografts (i.e. reconstruction with acetabular allograft bone) required further surgery due to fracture or fragmentation of the graft. The subsequent reconstruction was greatly facilitated by the restored bone stock. Five of these six reoperated acetabular allografts have a successful clinical score 2 years after reoperation. The last patient with a bipolar reconstruction remains a failure due to the minimal increase in her clinical score after reoperation. Six allografts were associated with implant migration and five of these cases involved a bipolar prosthesis that had eroded the allograft in varying amounts of 5–15 mm in a proximal medial direction. Only one of the six bipolar reconstructions was not associated with migration. The overall success rate for major column allografts was 71% (20 of 28 cases).

A more recent review of our cases revealed the following data as of July 1, 1993.

Of 179 acetabular reconstructions using morsellized allograft bone, 9 have required revision (inc. 5%) at an average follow-up of 4.57 years. The reasons for revision were: 4 cases for cup loosening and 5 for dislocation. All revisions were successful.

Of 56 minor column (shelf) allografts 4 revisions were necessary (inc. 7%) at an average follow-up of 5.12 years. Two were revised for loose cups, 1 for infection and 1 for resorption. All were revised successfully.

Of 67 major column grafts 25 revisions have been necessary (inc. 37%) at an average follow-up of 5.23 years. Ten were revised successfully and 6 underwent excision arthroplasty. The reasons for revision or excision were as follows: dislocation 4 hips, loose cup 10 hips, non-union 5 hips, fracture 3 hips, infection 2 hips, and nerve injury 1 hip.

The incidence of revisions of major column grafts of 37% is inflated due to the fact that 16 hips had 25 complications. The incidence of patients requiring further surgery was therefore 16 of 60 = 27%.

References

1. Allan GD, Butuk D, Gross AE (1991) Morsellized allograft reconstruction of contained cavitary defects in revision total hip arthoplasty. Orthop Transact 15 (3): 821
2. Amstutz HC, Ma S, Jinnah RH (1982) Revision of aseptic loose total hip arthroplasties. Clin Orthop Rel Res 170: 21–33
3. Bargar WM (1993) Personal Communication
4. Callaghan JJ, Salvati EA, Pellicci PM, et al (1985) Results of revision for mechanical failure after cemented total hip replacement, 1979 to 1982. A two to five year follow-up. J Bone Joint Surg 67A: 1074–1085
5. Chao EYS, Ivins JC (1983) The design and application. In: Tumour prostheses for bone and joint reconstruction. New York: Thieme-Stratton, p 335

6. Czitrom AA (1992) Immunology of bone and cartilage allografts. In: Czitrom AA, Gross AE (eds) Allografts in orthopaedic practice. Baltimore: Williams & Wilkins, pp 15–25

7. Czitrom A, Gross A, Langer F, et al (1988) Bone banks and allografts in community practice. Instructional Course Lectures American Academy of Orthopaedic Surgeons, 37: 13–24

8. D'Antonio JA, Capello WN, Borden LS (1989) Classification and management of acetabular abnormalities in total hip arthroplasty. Clin Orthop Rel Res 243: 126–137

9. Emerson RH Jr, Head WC, Berklacich FM, et al (1989) Noncemented acetabular revision arthroplasty using allograft bone. Clin Orthop Rel Res 249: 30–43

10. Engh CA, Glassman AH, Griffin WL, et al (1988) Results of cementless revision for failed cemented total hip arthroplasty. Clin Orthop Rel Res 235: 91–110

11. Estok DM, Harris WH (1994) Long term results of cemented femoral revision using second generation techniques. An average 11% year follow-up evaluation. Clin Orthop Rel Res 299: 190–203

12. Fuchs MD, Salvati EA, Wilson PD Jr, et al (1988) Results of acetabular revisions with newer cement techniques. Orthop Clin North America 19: 649–659

13. Gie GE, Linder L, Ling RSM, Simon J-P, Sloof TJJH, Timperley AJ (1993) Impacted cancellous allografts and cement for revision total hip arthroplasty. J Bone Joint Surg 75-B (1): 14–21

14. Gie GA, Linder L, Ling RSM, Simm J-P, Sloof TJ, Timperley AJ (1993) Contained morsellized allograft in Revision Total Hip arthoroplasty: Surgical Techniques. Orthop Clin of North America, 24 (4): 717–727

15. Goldberg VM, Stevenson S (1992) Biology of bone and cartilage allografts. In: Czitrom AA, Gross AE (eds) Allografts in orthopaedic practice. Baltimore: Williams & Wilkins, pp 1–13

16. Gross AE, Allen DG: Revision arthoplasty using allograft bone. In: Heckman JD (ed) Instructional Course Lectures, 42. American Academy of Orthopaedic Surgeons. Rosemont, pp 363–380

17. Gross AE (1992) Revision arthroplasty of the hip using allograft bone. In: Czitrom AA, Gross AE (eds) Allografts in orthopaedic practice. Baltimore: Williams & Wilkins, pp 147–173

18. Gross AE, Lavoie MV, McDermott AGP, et al (1985) The use of allograft bone in revision of total hip arthroplasty. Clin Orthop Rel Res 197: 115

19. Gustilo RD, Pasternak HS (1988) Revision total hip arthroplasty with a titanium in growth prosthesis and bone grafting for failed cemented femoral component loosening. Clin Orthop Rel Res 235: 111–119

20. Hardinge K (1982) The direct lateral approach to the hip. J Bone Joint Surg 64-B: 17–19

21. Harris WH (1969) Traumatic arthritis of the hip after dislocation and acetabular fractures: treatment by mold arthroplasty. An end result study using a new method of result evaluation. J Bone Joint Surg (Am) 51-A: 737

22. Harris WH, Krushell RJ, Galante JO (1988) Results of cementless revisions of total hip arthroplasties using the Harris-Galante prosthesis. Clin Orthop Rel Res 235: 120–126

23. Hedley AK, Gruen TA, Ruoff DP (1988) Revision of failed total hip arthroplasties with uncemented porous-coated-anatomic components. Clin Orthop Rel Res 235: 75–90

24. Hunter GA, Welsh RP, Cameron HU, et al (1979) The results of revision of total hip arthroplasty. J Bone Joint Surg 61-B (4): 419–421

25. Jasty M, Harris WH (1990) Salvage total hip reconstruction in patients with major acetabular bone deficiency using structural femoral head allografts. J Bone Joint Surg (Br) 72-B: 63

26. Kavanagh BE, Ilstrup DM, Fitzgerald RH Jr (1985) Revision total hip arthroplasty. J Bone Joint Surg 67-A: 517–526

27. Langer F, Czitrom A, Pritzker KP, et al (1975) The immunogenicity of fresh and frozen allogeneic bone. J Bone Joint Surg 57A: 216

28. Oakeshott RD, Morgan DAF, Zukor DJ, et al (1987) Revision total hip arthroplasty with osseous allograft reconstruction. Clin Orthop Rel Res 225: 37–61

29. Pellicci PM, Wilson PD Jr, Sledge CB, et al (1982) Revision total hip arthroplasty. Clin Orthop Rel Res 170: 34–41

30. Pellicci PM, Wilson PD Jr, Sledge CB, et al (1985) Long-term results of revision total hip replacement. A follow-up report. J Bone Joint Surg 67-A: 513–516

31. Pierson JL, Harris WH (1994) Cemented revision for femoral osteolysis in cemented arthroplasties. J Bone Joint Surg 76-B (1): 40–44

32. Russotti GM, Harris WH (1991) Proximal placement of the acetabular component in total hip arthroplasty. A long-term follow-up study. J Bone Joint Surg (Am) 73-A: 587–592
33. Wilson-MacDonald J, Morscher E, Masar Z (1990) Cementless uncoated polyethylene acetabular components in total hip replacement. A review of five to 10 year results. J Bone Joint Surg 72-B (3): 423–430

Author's addresses: A.E. Gross, M.D. FRSC(C), Chief, Division of Orthopaedic Surgery, Mount Sinai Hospital, 600 University Avenue, Suite 476A, Toronto, ON, M5G, IX5, Canada; D. Garbuz, M.D., FRSC(C), Clinical Fellow Mount Sinai Hospital, Toronto, Ontario, Canada; E.S. Morsi, MBBCH, MS (Orth), Mount Sinai Hospital, Department of Orthopaedic Surgery, University of Menoufyia, U.S.A.

Major Loss of Acetabular Bone Stock at Revision Total Hip Arthroplasty

K. B. Otto, E. Nieder, and D. Klüber

Endo-Klinik, Hamburg, Federal Republic of Germany

The surgeons at the Endo-Klinik have been performing joint replacement operations since the mid-nineteen-sixties—at first in cases of femoral neck fractures and arthritis, and then for severe hip dysplasia [1, 10, 13]. At that time small defects in the secondary acetabulum were closed using cement, which was often reinforced by screws. But in the following years we observed in more and more cases that these cement wedges were pressed out of position and the acetabular cup became loose.

In the mid-nineteen-seventies, Harris proposed that the femoral heads resected in hip replacement operations should be used for the reconstruction of the acetabular roof [5, 6]. We followed this proposal at the end of the seventies. However, in contrast to Harris's method in which the femoral head was implanted in the physiological direction and fixed with bolts and intrapelvic nuts, we turned the head around, fitted the cancellous side into the acetabular defect and used the sclerosed side of the head as a buttress for screws without nuts. With this method we treated at first small defects, and later also large defects in the acetabular roof region. In cases of arthrosis with extreme protrusio acetabuli we were also able to achieve good bony reconstruction by filling the defects with autologous cancellous bone [7].

In revision arthroplasty we at first used only autologous bone for transplants. If a hip had to be revised and primary hip arthroplasty was necessary on the contralateral hip as well, we used the femoral head of the contralateral side as a graft in the revised hip. If this was not possible, we used bone blocks taken from the iliac wing.

The good results achieved with autologous bone grafts prompted us in 1983 to establish a bank for allogeneic bone grafts [2, 3, 4, 11, 12, 14]. In view of more than 3000 joint replacement operations and more than 1000 exchange operations per year it was logical to use the femoral heads removed during primary arthroplasty for reconstruction purposes.

After removal, the head is immediately washed in Neomycin solution, sealed in three-ply plastic foil and frozen to a temperature of −70°C. Tissue material taken from the head is sent for bacteriological and serological examination and if the results are negative, the head can be used for grafting. The possibility of transferring disease from the donor to the recipient of a graft, and especially the HIV problem, led us a few years ago to subject harvested femoral heads to additional heat treatment before using them. After cleaning, the grafts are replaced in sterile containers and heated to +80°C in a water bath for about one hour. The liquid is then removed, material samples are taken for bacteriological examination and the bone is sealed and frozen again to −70°C. Again, if the results are negative the material can be used for grafting.

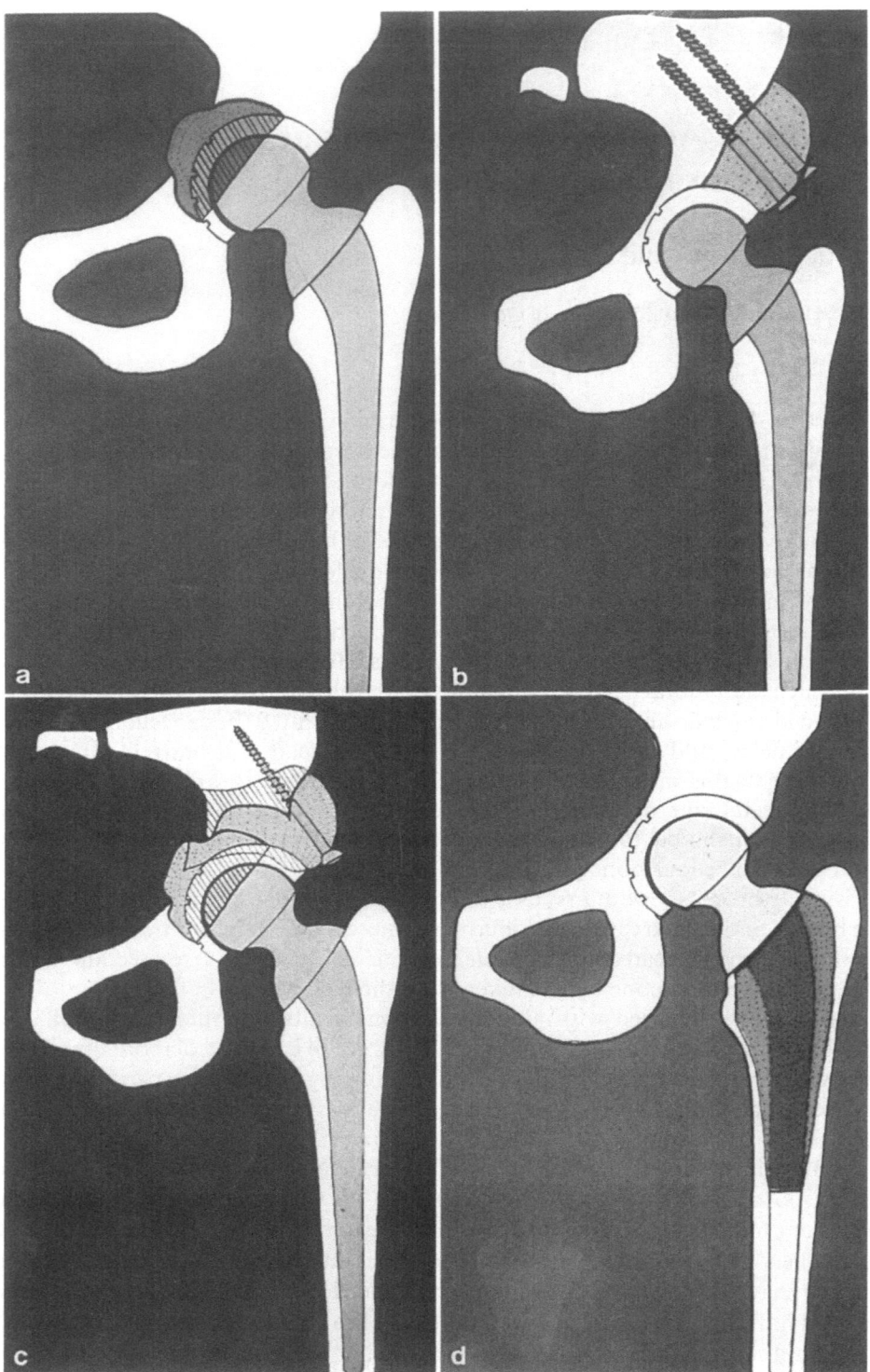

Fig. 1. a Acetabular floor graft; **b** Acetabular roof graft; **c** Combined Y-graft of acetabular roof rim and mushroom-shaped floor graft; **d** Reconstruction of the femoral shaft using homologous bone graft

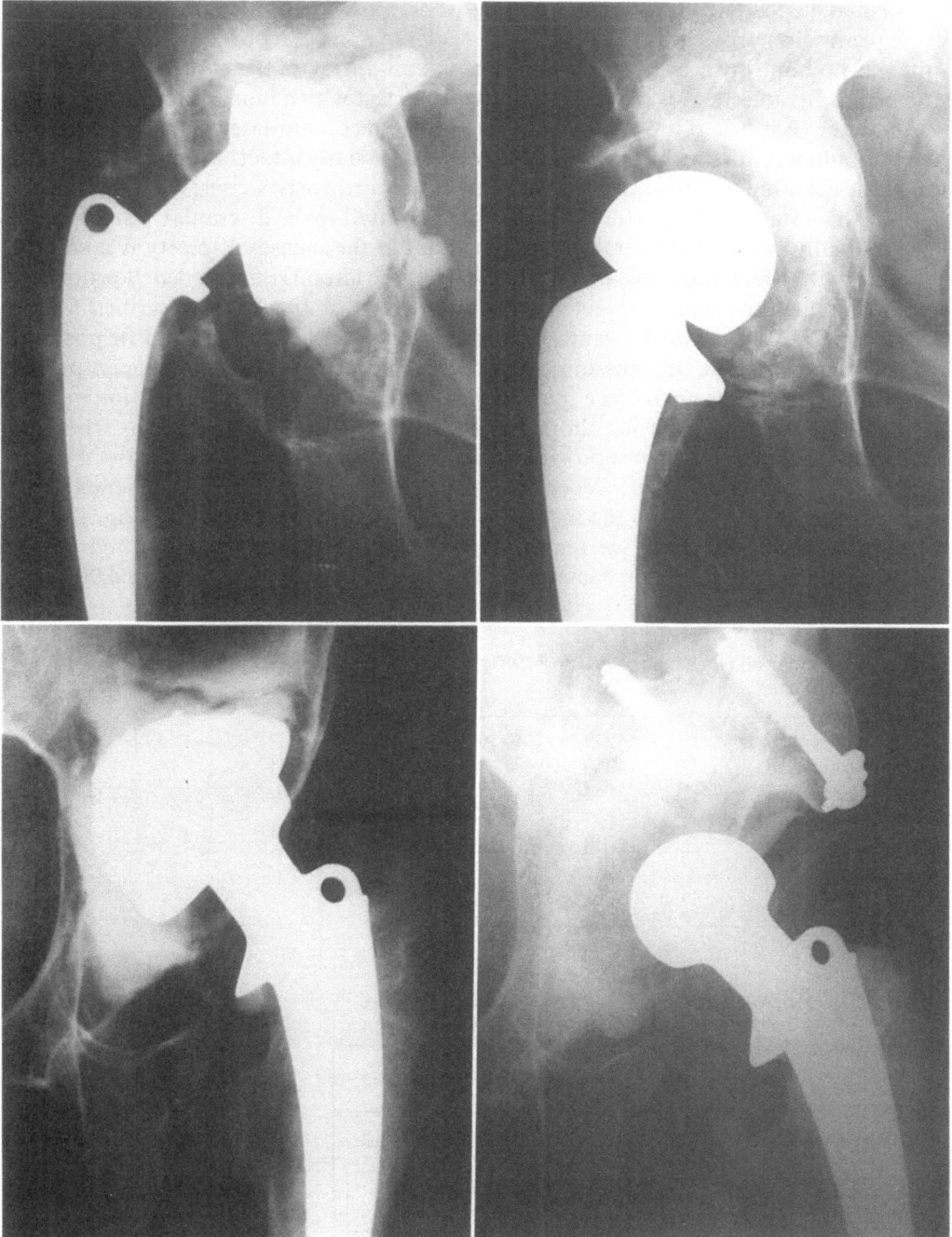

Fig. 2. Reconstruction of the acetabulum using homologous bone graft. Radiographic follow-up after 8 years

After reconstruction of the acetabulum we always fix the new cup with cement as it affords better primary stability. The different types of loss of bone stock make different reconstruction techniques necessary (Fig. 1).

If the acetabulum is only moderately enlarged on all sides but without large defects in the floor, it can be reinforced with a bed of cancellous bone meal upon which the new cup is cemented, instead of a large-size cup being implanted. This is also possible in cases of severe protrusion provided there is still a thin layer of bone as a border to the true pelvis. If there is no bone layer left due to cranio-medial migration of the cup, i.e. there is open protrusion, an attempt must be made to close the defect with a mushroom-shaped block of solid bone (Fig. 1a). If the cup has migrated towards cranio-lateral, the lateral rim of the acetabulum is missing but the acetabular floor is usually intact. As in the reconstruction of the acetabular roof in cases of dysplastic osteoarthrosis, we screw a femoral head on from the outer side (Fig. 1b). If the cup has migrated towards cranial, a smaller and more cranially positioned acetabular roof forms. In these cases Y-plasty is a suitable technique with which the roof can be distalised and the lateral rim widened. If protrusion is also present, this is reconstructed with bone chips or blocks as described for the migration of the cup towards cranio-medial (Fig. 1c). If either the anterior or posterior circumference, or both, are missing—as usually happens in the case of open protrusion—and the pelvis is unstable, a metal cup with additional bands for fixation must be implanted in combination with allogeneic grafts . Particularly in situations where the pelvic ring is open, it is often not possible to reconstruct the pelvis. In these cases a saddle prosthesis is the alternative [8]. When the proximal femur is thinned and widened we try to reconstruct it according to the method proposed by Gie and Ling [5] (Fig. 1d).

Between 1983 and 1993 we removed 6,339 femoral heads during primary joint replacement operations. After bacteriological and serological examination 4,909 were

Table 1. Acetabular allogeneic bone grafting 1983–1993

Femoral heads excised	6339
Femoral heads used	4909
No. of patients	3843
Patients followed	447
Follow-up period	8–11 years
Age of patients	27–86 years
Mean age	57 years

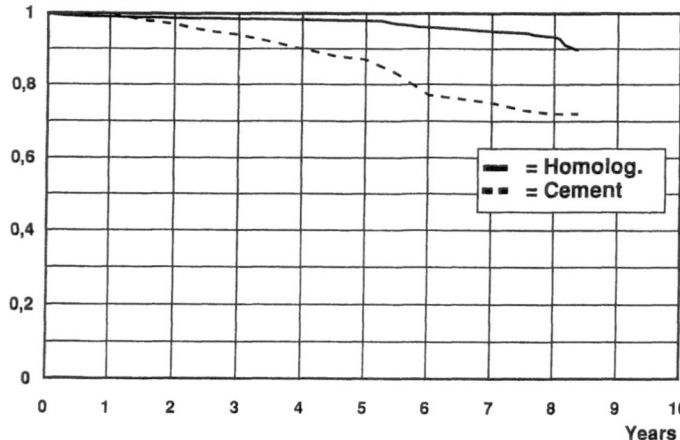

Fig. 3. Survival curves. Comparison of allogeneic (homologous) transplant with cement reconstruction

used for grafting in 3,843 patients. A follow-up examination was made of 447 patients who had undergone arthroplasty with acetabular reconstruction between 1983 and 1985 (Fig. 2). The follow-up period was eight to eleven years. The patients' ages ranged from 27 to 86 years, mean 57 years. All the reconstruction types described here (cf. Fig. 1a–c) were more or less equally represented (Table 1).

We compared these 447 acetabular reconstructions with 102 operations in which only cement or cement in combination with screws had been used for reconstruction. The survival rates analysis shows that aseptic loosening of the cup occurred in 7% after 8 years when the acetabulum was reconstructed using bone grafts, but that loosening occurred much more often, namely in 28%, when cement had been used for reconstruction. This shows clearly that reconstruction using allogeneic bone is superior to reconstruction using cement (Fig. 3).

References

 1. Buchholz HW, Baars GW, Dahmen G, Behrend R (1985) Früherfahrungen mit der Mini-Hüftge-lenkstotalendoprothese (Modell "St. Georg-Mini") bei Dysplasie-Coxarthrose. Z Orthop 123: 829
 2. Bürkle de la Camp H (1954) Über die Kältekonservierung von Knochengewebe und dessen Verwendung zur homoisoplastischen Verpflanzung. Zentralbl Chir 79: 163
 3. Dick W, Morscher E (1982) Homologe Spongiosa als Werkstoff bei Problemfällen der Hüftchirur-gie. In: Hackenbroch M, Refior H-J, Jäger M (eds) Osteogenese und Knochenwachstum. 4. Münchner Symposium für Experimentelle Orthopädie. Stuttgart, New York: Thieme, pp 226–230
 4. Friedlaender GE (1982) Current concepts review bone banking. J Bone Joint Surg [Am] 64: 307–311
 5. Gie GA, Linder L, Ling RSM, Simon J-P, Slooff TJJH, Timperley AJ (1993) Impacted cancellous allografts and cement for revision total hip arthroplasty. J Bone Joint Surg [Br] 75: 14
 6. Harris WH, Crothers O, Oh I (1977) Total hip replacement and femoral-head bone-grafting for severe acetabular deficiency in adults. J Bone Joint Surg [Am] 59: 752
 7. Harris WH (1982) Allografting in total hip arthroplasty. Clin Orthop 162: 150
 8. Heywood AWB (1980) Arthroplasty with a solid bone graft for protrusio acetabuli. J Bone Joint Surg [Br] 62: 332–336
 9. Nieder E, Engelbrecht E, Steinbrink K, Elson RA, Kasselt MR, Keller A (1990) The saddle prosthesis for salvage of the destroyed acetabulum. J Bone Joint Surg [Br] 72: 1014
10. Otto KB (1982) Verwendung des Hüftkopfes als zusätzliche Pfannendachplastik bei Versorgung schwerer angeborener Hüftgelenksdysplasien mit einer totalen Hüftgelenksendoprothese. In: Hackenbroch M, Refior H-J, Jäger M (eds) Osteogenese und Knochenwachstum. 4. Münchner Symposium für Experimentelle Orthopädie. Stuttgart, New York: Thieme, pp 266
11. Otto KB (1984) Lokaler Substanzverlust im Bereich der Hüftgelenk Beckenregion bei Implantat-lockerung. Versorgungsmöglichkeiten mit autologen und homologen Knochentransplantaten. Acta Med Austr [Suppl] 32: 25
12. Otto KB, Baars GW, Nieder E (1987) Beckenknochendefekte in der Alloarthroplastik. Orthopäde 16: 261
13. Otto KB, Baars GW, Nieder E (1989) Alloarthroplastische Therapie der kongenitalen Hüftgelenks-dysplasie. Orthopäde 18: 470
14. Tscherne H, Trentz O (1981) Transplantation von Knochen. In: Pichlmayr R (ed) Transplantations-chirurgie. Berlin, Heidelberg, New York: Springer, pp 923–950

Authors' address: K. B. Otto, E. Nieder and D. Kluber, Endo-Klinik, Holstenstrasse 2, D-22767 Hamburg, Federal Republic of Germany.

Allograft Reconstruction of Acetabular Bone Defects Combined with Reinforcement Ring in Revision Total Hip Arthroplasty

M. Itoman and M. Sekiguchi

Department of Orthopaedic Surgery, Kitasato University School of Medicine, Japan

Introduction

Reconstruction of bone defects in revision total hip replacement (THR) after loosening of the prosthesis is often difficult, because of the size of the bone defect [1, 2, 3]. In revision THR, a large amount of autogenous bone is difficult to obtain. The femoral head has already been removed and many of these patients are elderly so that the cancellous bone of the ipsilateral iliac crest is remarkably porotic. For these reasons it would be attractive, where it is possible and clinically successful, to use allografts from the bone bank. Particularly in middle-aged patients, where the possibility of the next revision surgery has to be strongly considered, high placement of the acetabular component should be avoided. Accordingly, by generous use of frozen allograft, we repaired the bone defects and mounted the acetabular component in an anatomical position for such patients [3, 5]. This paper presents a retrospective study on repair of bone defects with allografts and the fate of the grafts.

Materials and Methods

Since 1980 to 1992, 59 prostheses of 53 patients were revised in our department because of aseptic loosening. The underlying diseases requiring primary THR were osteoarthritis (OA) in 38 hips, rheumatoid arthritis (RA) in 9 hips and avascular necrosis (AN) in 12 hips. Age of the patients at revision surgery ranged from 34 to 82 (mean: 63.3) years. Eleven cases were males and 42 females. The patients with AN were relatively younger (mean: 41.8 years). The prostheses used in primary surgery were of the surface replacement type in 7 hips, the Mueller type with cement in 39 hips, Moore hemiarthroplasty without cement in 9, Isoelastic uncemented in 3 and Lord uncemented in 1. In revision surgery, Isoelastic uncemented cups were used for 8 cases and cemented cups with reinforcement ring were used in 51 cases. Duration of follow-up was 2 to 13 years after revision surgery (mean: 5.9 years).

When our classification system [3] was applied to the present series, 41 cases belonged to Type-D, that is cranio-central defects. While the central wall of the acetabulum was retained in 16 cases, small penetrations were observed in 18, and large central wall defects in 7. In all cases, the technique of allografting was uniform. To optimize apposition and allow secure bony union at the graft-recipient junction, crushed or morsellized bone with fibrin glue was grafted by impaction onto the irregular and sclerotic acetabular wall after reaming and making numerous drill holes until active bleeding was visible from them. Then, a cancellous block was grafted onto the crushed bones.

To clarify the usefulness of the reinforcement ring, patients were divided into 2 groups. In 8 cases, that is group I, the acetabular component was installed directly onto the allograft. In group II, including 51 cases, a reinforcement ring was placed between the allograft and the high density polyethylene (HDP) cup. The position of the acetabular cup on each radiograph was measured with a transparent MEM template. The template was specially designed for determining the position and migration of an acetabular component. This template is available from the Mueller foundation. Using this template, the position of the cup was measured on radiographs, taken immediately after revision surgery and again at the latest follow-up. The thickness of the graft that was maintained at the latest follow-up was calculated as a percentage of the initial thickness following Wilson's report in 1989 [6].

Results

Results of measurements are presented in Tables 1 and 2. In almost all cases classified into group I, there was evidence of both cranial and/or central migration of the components. The magnitude of cranial migration in 8 cases of group I ranged from 1 to 8 mm (mean value was 3.6 mm in cranial direction and 2.9 mm in central direction). However, bone union at the graft recipient junction was achieved in all cases within 6 months postoperatively. On the other hand, no cranial or central migrations were found in 48 cases of group II, except in 3 cases. The magnitude of migration in these three cases was less than 4 mm. Mean value was 0.2 mm in both directions. A statistical significant difference was noted both in the cranial and central migration between group I and II ($p < 0.01$). The percentage of initial thickness of the graft that was maintained at the latest follow-up was also compared between those two groups. In group II, almost 100% of the initial thickness was maintained both in cranial and in central directions. In comparison, only 60% in cranial direction and 75% in central direction was maintained for cases of group I ($p < 0.01$). While asymptomatic and minimal partial resorption of the allograft at the lateral aspect during incorporation was found in 2 cases of group II, no evidence of loosening was noted at the latest follow-up.

Table 1. Radiological evaluation of cranial and central migration of the acetabular components

Group	No. of cases	Migration of the cup (mm) mean ± SD		Significance of difference
		Cranial	Central	
Group I	8	3.6 ± 2.9	2.9 ± 2.1	$p < 0.01$
Group II	51	0.2 ± 0.1	0.2 ± 0.1	

Table 2. Radiological evaluation of maintenance of the thickness of the grafts

Group	No. of cases	Maintenance of thickness of the graft (%) mean ± SD		Significance of difference
		Cranial	Central	
Group I	8	60.6 ± 31.9	75.0 ± 15.8	$p < 0.01$
Group II	51	98.2 ± 18.1	98.5 ± 15.7	

Discussion

For successful THR, the acetabular component should be placed in anatomical position in both revision and primary surgery. However, revision of the acetabular component is often difficult, because of the amount of the bone defect and the quality of remaining acetabular bone [1, 2, 3, 5, 6]. A minimum requirement for successful revision THR is to understand the site and magnitude of bone defect to be restored prior to surgery. From this point of view, we classified the acetabular bone defects into type A through D, based on site and magnitude [1]. Type A bone defects, that is lateral defects, were common in dysplastic hips. Type B (central defect) was common in RA, type C (cranial defect) in RA and so called rapidly destructive coxarthropathy (RDC). In type D, bone defects were shown both in central and cranial directions. The defects in which the central wall was retained were classified as type D-1, defects with minor penetration which can be restored with femoral head as type D-2. The most serious bone defects were classified as type D-3. In the last type, there was complete deficiency of the central wall and sometimes disruption of the anterior and/or posterior column of the acetabulum [3].

In revision THR, the procedure is much more difficult compared with the primary surgery for several reasons. The most difficult task with revision surgery consists of preparing the remaining bone bed that securely receives an acetabular component in an anatomical position, following reconstruction of the bone defect. Usually, the remaining acetabular bone is thin, sclerotic and has an irregular surface. Sometimes it is necrotic with poor vascular supply so that the incorporation of the graft tends to be prolonged. Moreover, the quality of the allograft is inferior in osteoinductive property and mechanical strength compared with that of an autograft [4, 7]. However, allograft reconstruction of the acetabular bone defect in revision THR is a beneficial procedure, because the ipsilateral iliac crest is remarkably porotic so that adequate volume and quality of autograft to restore a huge bone defect is not available.

The allografts that were most frequently used were cancellous bone blocks with crushed bone which had been stored in a deep freezer under sterile conditions. To obtain optimal apposition and to allow secure bony healing at the graft-recipient junction, crushed or morsellized bone with fibrin glue was grafted by impaction onto the irregular and sclerotic acetabular wall, after reaming and making numerous drill holes until active bleeding is visible [5, 6]. Then the cancellous bone block was grafted by compression on the crushed bone layer.

In this series, 6 out of 8 cases of group I in which a cementless cup was installed directly onto the allograft block, showed certain cranial and/or central migration. On

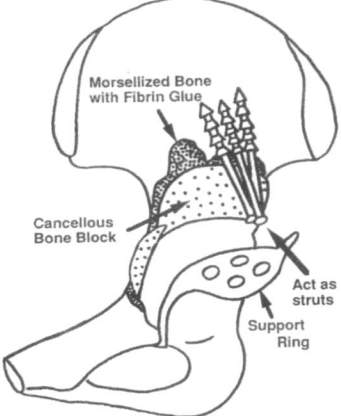

Fig. 1. Schematic representation of placement of the allografts and insertion of screws

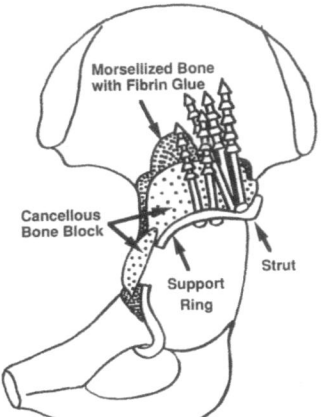

Fig. 2. Schematic representation of installation of the reinforcement ring onto the allograft and screw heads by compression

the other hand, negligible migration was noted in group II in which a reinforcement ring was used. The amount of cup migration and the thickness of the graft were statistically different between those two groups. These results indicate that the time after revision surgery required for the entire graft to become incorporated into the recipient site is considerably prolonged. Consequently, the combined use of reinforcement devices with allografts is necessary for enforcement of primary stability. From the technical point of view, particularly in the case of bone defects in the weight bearing area, the cancellous bone block should be fixed with 2 or 3 cancellous screws prior to installation of the reinforcement ring (Fig. 1). These screws must be inserted from the lateral corner of the cancellous bone block, to act as struts for the support ring. Then, the reinforcement ring should be installed by compression onto the allograft and the screw heads. The screws which are inserted under the reinforcement ring act as struts for the ring and the HDP cup (Fig. 2). The utilization of the reinforcement ring is essential to provide primary fixation of the cup and to prevent mechanical collapse of the allograft until secure incorporation of the allograft is achieved. Furthermore, once incorporation and re-modelling of the graft has been achieved, long-term stable fixation of the acetabular component in an anatomical position is obtained. In our 13 year experience of revision THR, using reinforcement rings in a manner described above, no loosening of the components was noted.

Conclusion

A radiological study was carried out on 59 hips of 53 patients in whom allograft reconstruction was performed in combination with an acetabular revision THR. In 8 hips where the acetabular component was installed directly on the allograft (group I), significant cranial and central migration was noted. On the other hand, in 51 hips where the reinforcement ring was used combined with the allograft (group II), migration was negligible. Utilization of the reinforcement ring is essential to provide primary fixation, particularly in cases in which allograft is placed on the weight bearing area, until secure incorporation of the allograft is achieved. Once incorporation and remodelling has been achieved, long-term stable fixation of the component in anatomical position has been obtained.

References

1. Harris WH (1982) Allograft in total hip arthroplasty. Clin Orthop 162: 150–164
2. Harris WH (1990) Salvage total hip reconstruction in patients with acetabular bone deficiency using structural femoral bone allografts. J Bone Joint Surg 72-B: 63–67
3. Itoman M, et al (1990) Bone defect and its repair in total hip replacement—A new classification of the bone defect. J West Pacif Orthop Assoc 27: 1–5
4. Itoman M, et al (1991) Experimental study on allogeneic bone grafts. Intern Orthop (SICOT): 161–165
5. Itoman M, et al (1992) Radiological evaluation on allograft reconstruction of the acetabulum combined with supporting device in revision total hip replacement. J Jpn Orthop Assoc 66: 23–30
6. Wilson MG, et al (1989) The fate of the acetabular allografts after bipolar revision arthroplasty of the hip. J Bone Joint Surg 71-A: 1469–1479
7. Yamazaki M, et al (1992) Effects of preservation procedures on the biomechanical and osteoinductive properties of rabbit bone. Kitasato Med 22: 478–484

Authors' address: M. Itoman and M. Sekiguchi, Department of Orthopaedic Surgery, Kitasato University School of Medicine, Kitasato 1-15-1, Sagamihara, Kanagawa 228, Japan.

Impaction Grafting and Cement in Acetabular Revision Arthroplasty

T. J. J. H. Slooff[1], P. Buma[2], J. W. Schimmel[1], J. Gardeniers[1], and R. Huiskes[2]

[1]Institute of Orthopaedics, University Hospital Nijmegen, The Netherlands
[2]Institute of Orthopaedics, Laboratory of Experimental Orthopaedics, University Hospital Nijmegen, The Netherlands

Summary

Animal experiments were performed to restore bony defects with morsellized allograft chips. Acetabular defects were created in the Dutch milk goat and impacted with fresh frozen allograft bone chips. The speed of consolidation with the host bone bed, the mechanism and completeness of incorporation and the processes at the graft cement interface were studied in detail with histological and biomechanical procedures.

Histology showed that the graft had consolidated with the trabecular host bone bed within three weeks. In the subsequent period a front of vascular sprouts infiltrated the graft. Graft resorption, new bone formation and bone remodelling resulted in a new trabecular structure with optimal trabecular orientation for load bearing. After twelve weeks only scarce remnants of the original dead graft material remained in the incorporated area of the graft. At revascularized areas of the graft-cement interface, graft resorption and new bone formation had resulted in direct vital bone-cement contact sites and in areas with a soft tissue interface. After longer follow-up periods progressive interface formation and loosening of the cup was found in most of the animals.

The histological results were confirmed by biomechanical stability tests. In the first postoperative weeks the stability of the reconstruction increased, but at later follow-up periods, interface formation at the new bone-cement layer compromised the stability of the reconstruction.

The results indicated that reconstruction with morsellized graft material leads to rapid consolidation, incorporation and remodelling of the graft. Problems at the graft-cement interface are probably not related to the use of the morsellized graft, but to the goat model used.

Introduction

Without doubt it can be stated that bone transplantation was already performed in the early centuries. However, it takes a deep and extensive study of all historical reviews to distinguish the truth from fairy-tales. From sporadic use of autogenous grafts and allografts in the past, bone grafting has gained in popularity during the last decades. As laboratory and clinical work on bone transplantation was introduced by Ollier [28] in

France, MacEwen [25] in Scotland, Barth [4] and Axhausen and Lexer [3, 24] in Germany and Curtis [13] in the USA. The development of preservation techniques by Bush and Wilson in 1947 [12] and in 1950 the foundation of the National Naval Tissue Bank in Bethesda (U.S.A.) made it possible to use allografts clinically on a larger scale.

In general it can be stated that with regard to graft incorporation most of the current data are related to animal experiments [1, 2, 3, 5, 10, 12, 15, 16, 18, 19, 22, 26, 29, 30, 40]. Heiple, Herndon and Chase [23], Burwell [9, 10] and Campbell [12] demonstrated an immune response in animals receiving allograft bone. In 1953, Urist and coworkers [41–43] developed the theory of osteoinduction. A substantial part of allograft studies was also activated by the development of modern surgical methods in orthopaedic oncology [7, 8, 14].

An important clinical application which started in the 70th's, was the repair of major acetabular bone deficiencies in association with primary and revision total hip arthroplasties. Initial reports by Hastings and Parker [21] and Harris and Crothers [20] about these acetabular reconstructions with morsellized and structural cortico-cancellous bone graft set a stage in this field. In the human situation this process has been usually evaluated on radiographs which are in our opinion only a crude parameter.

Summarizing the data in the literature about the reconstruction methods of failed total hip arthroplasties, it is essential to distinguish the use of different types of grafts. In all grafts there can be several processes occurring such as union, incorporation, rejection, infection and remodelling. With special regard to union and incorporation, these processes are different for the various grafts. In our clinical series we define successful graft incorporation as complete revascularization and concurrent substitution of the graft with new bone without significant loss of strength. The new bony structure can bear physiologic loads and remodel itself in response to changes in load and fatigue damage.

Compared to cortical grafts, cancellous grafts do have a more open structure, which in theory allows a more uniform, a more complete and a more rapid vascular invasion. Cortical grafts incorporate irregularly, incompletely, slowly and with mechanical weakening due to fatigue damage.

The difference between solid and morsellized cancellous grafts is less clearly understood. When using femoral head allograft, the stiffness, quality and size of the structural graft may lead to stress protection of any new bone that is formed within it. Finally, it must be mentioned that the incorporation process depends on the security of fixation (stability), the degree of contact, the vascularity of the host bone bed, the strain pattern and the degree of antigen matching.

In summary, the use of bone grafts for primary acetabular reconstruction and revision is nowadays a generally accepted procedure. Union of the graft to the host bone bed is nearly always achieved. However, the incorporation and remodelling processes of the various types of grafts are quite different and are not well understood. This distinction in behaviour is clearly demonstrated, particularly during longer follow-up, when cortical, solid or morsellized grafts are used. Clinical success does not necessarily reflect the fate of the grafts. Plain radiographic imaging does not unequivocally prove the solidity of the reconstructed acetabulum. Plain radiographs are, at best, difficult to interpret. Therefore, histologic evidence of the viability and incorporation of the graft is crucial.

In 1984 and subsequently in 1992 we published our acetabular method [38, 39] with a modification of the techniques of Hastings and Parker [21] and McCollum et al. [27]. We used morsellized chip allograft, impacted the graft firmly and pressurized the cement on the graft. With this technique it was possible to treat extensive and serious defects in primary and revision total hip arthroplasty.

Animal Experiments

To support scientifically our surgical reconstruction technique the acetabular method using impaction grafting and cement was developed and tested on an animal model [6, 31–35]. The animal of choice was the goat.

The aims of these experiments were:

A. To make a histological evaluation of the different processes involved in the incorporation of the graft.
B. To evaluate the initial mechanical stability (in vitro) of the graft and the stability of graft incorporation 12 weeks after implantation.

Materials and Method

All the trabecular bone grafts were harvested from the sternum of donor goats under sterile conditions. The grafts were freshly frozen and stored at −80°C ready for implantation. In adult goats, the right hip was operated on under general anaesthesia using standard aseptic techniques. A dorsal lateral incision was used, followed by dislocation of the hip and resection of the femoral head. The acetabular cartilage was removed and a cavitary defect was made in the anterior-superior segment of the acetabulum using hand reamers. Impaction-grafting of the resulting defect was performed in the same way as during clinical application to patients. The acetabular component was cemented. Three specimens were used to analyze the initial stability (in vitro). Six goats were sacrificed at intervals of 6, 12, 24 and 48 weeks. After the operation all the goats were kept in a hammock for 2 days. Antero-posterior and lateral radiographs were taken immediately after the operation. The goats were kept in cages which allowed free walking or in the open field. Three of the 6 cases from each interval were used for histology and three for biomechanical analysis.

Histological Procedures

The goats received different types of fluorochrome to enable the qualitative evaluation of bone ingrowth into the graft. The acetabula were harvested after perfusion of the lower extremity with Micropaque (R) as described by Rhinelander and Baragry. After fixation in a buffed paraformaldehyde solution the acetabula were contact-radiographed and sectioned with a water cooled saw into slices of 2–3 mm. Radiographs were taken of the slices. Calcified and decalcified bone sections of various thickness were subsequently stained according to routine protocols.

Biomechanical Procedures

For mechanical testing of the grafted acetabulum tantalum pellets were fixed to the component prior to insertion. The 3-D displacement of the component relative to the bone (rotation and translation) was measured using Rontgen-Stereophotogrammatic Analysis (RSA), developed by Selvik [36, 37].

The acetabula for the mechanical study were freshly harvested and stored at −80°C ready for testing. After thawing, the bone specimens were embedded in polymethylmethacrylate (PMMA). Tantalum pellets were inserted into small holes drilled into the pelvic bone in standard positions. Furthermore, small PMMA rods containing tantalum

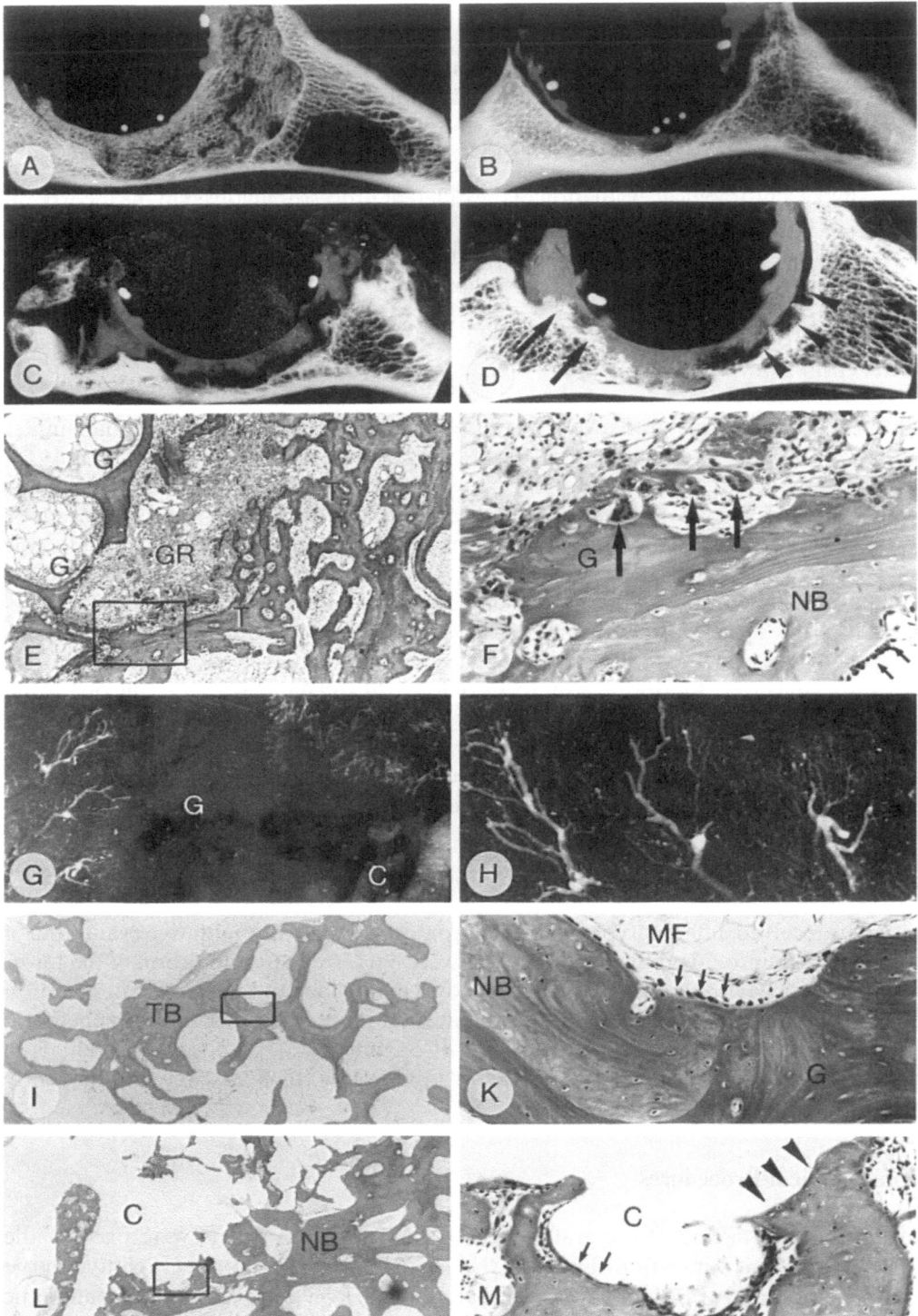

Fig. 1. A–D Roentgenograms of thick sections through the acetabulum of the goat taken at 0 (A), 12 (B), 24 (C) and 48 weeks (D) after surgery. **A**. Note large pieces of graft and the clear transition zone to the host bone-bed. **B**. Complete consolidation of the graft with the host bone. The incorporation of the

(continued)

pellets were inserted into the acetabular component. The prosthesis-bone structures were then loaded into a MTS-testing device in a physiological way. A pelvic load was applied stepwise from zero to 350 and to 700 N and again unloaded. Stereoroentgenograms were taken before loading, after each loading step and ten minutes after the final unloading. Each loading period lasted 10 minutes.

All stereoroentgenograms were evaluated on an Aristomat digitizer, and the 3-D pellet positions were determined with the RSA computer programme. Relative rotations and translations around and along the coordinate axes were calculated. To increase the accuracy of the results, all the stereoroentgenograms were measured 5 times and the results were averaged.

Histological Evaluation or the Grafted Acetabulum

The impacted graft consisted of fairly large pieces of trabecular bone (Fig. 1A), which displayed small micro-fractures at all levels. Generally, the bone graft was devoid of any well-preserved osteocytes, the osteocytes had completely disappeared, or if they were still present, they had a pycnotic appearance (Fig. 1K). Most of the medullary fat in the pieces of graft had been squeezed out during the process of impaction and had been replaced by a fibrin clot. Owing to surgical trauma, a circumferential necrotic zone of circa 1–4 mm was found in the host bone. After revascularization of the host bone, a front of vascular sprouts accompanied by loose connective tissue with many macrophages, penetrated into the graft at a speed of circa 70 µm per day (Fig. 1G, H). A very high dynamic bone turnover was observed in the graft in association with this granulation reaction, comprising bone graft resorption by osteoclasts and bone apposition by osteoblasts (Fig. 1E, F). This is resulted in a new trabecular structure which consisted of a mixture of the remnants of the graft and newly formed, mainly woven bone (Fig. 1B, I, K). Subsequently the percentage of graft in the new trabecular structure decreased further by bone remodelling. Radiographic and histological evaluation demonstrated that the orientation of the newly formed trabecular bone was such that load transfer was possible from the cement layer to the host bone bed (Fig. 1B, D). After 12 weeks, the amount of bone graft was minimal and lamellar bone was found in the new structure. A fibrous tissue membrane of varying thickness had developed at the cement-graft interface (Fig. 1C, D). However, all the animals showed local areas where vital bone was in intimate contact with the cement layer, without the interposition of such a soft tissue interface (Fig. 1L, M). Between 24 and 48 weeks after surgery, the graft in the defect of the

◄──

graft is almost completed. **C.** A radio-lucent zone is present between the cement layer and the bone, indicating that a soft tissue interface has been formed. **D.** Note local contact areas between bone and cement (arrows) and a radio-lucent zone (arrow heads). Note also the dense bone adjacent to the cement layer. **E.** Granulation tissue (GR) in the transition zone between avital graft (G) and newly formed trabecular bone (T) three weeks after surgery. **F.** Enlargement of encircled area in E. Many osteoclastic bone cells (large arrows) resorb the graft (G) and osteoblasts (small arrows) synthesize new bone (NB). **G.** Vascularization front penetrates into the graft (G) 12 weeks after the surgery. Cement (C) had penetrated into the graft. **H.** Enlargement of left part of G. **I.** Structure of new trabecular bone after 12 weeks. **K.** Enlargement of encircled area in I showing active osteoblasts (arrows) and new bone (NB). Remnants of the graft (G) can be recognized by the empty osteocyte lacunae. **L.** Transition between new bone (NB) and the cement 48 weeks after surgery. Cement (C) that was removed during processing of the tissues, had penetrated deeply into the graft. **M.** Enlargement of encircled area of K shows that locally a very thin, one cell layer thick (arrows) soft tissue interface is present, while at other locations the new bone is in direct contact with the cement layer (arrowheads). A–D × 1. E, G, I, L × 12.5; F, H, K, M × 125 acetabulum and femur had become completely revascularized. The percentage of the dead graft present in the new bony structure was very low. Direct bone-cement contact sites were still present, but particularly at later follow up periods the interface had thickened and showed signs of loosening.

Mechanical Evaluation of the Acetabulum

All the specimens seemed to be firmly fixed when tested manually. Coordinate axes were chosen as follows: X-axis dorso-ventral, Y-axis cranio-caudal, Z-axis medial-lateral. In most of the specimens, elastic recovery was observed after unloading. Initial stability was considered by testing the specimens immediately after implantation. Maximum persistent translation in this group was found in craniocaudal direction (0.6 mm) (Fig. 2H).

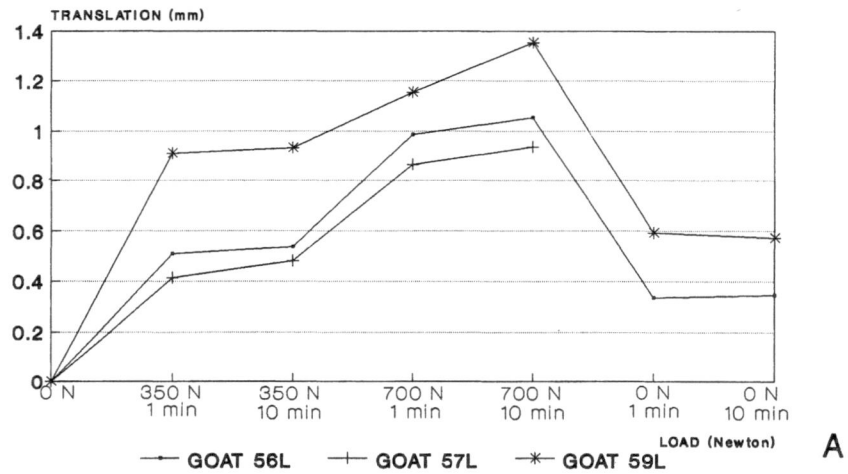

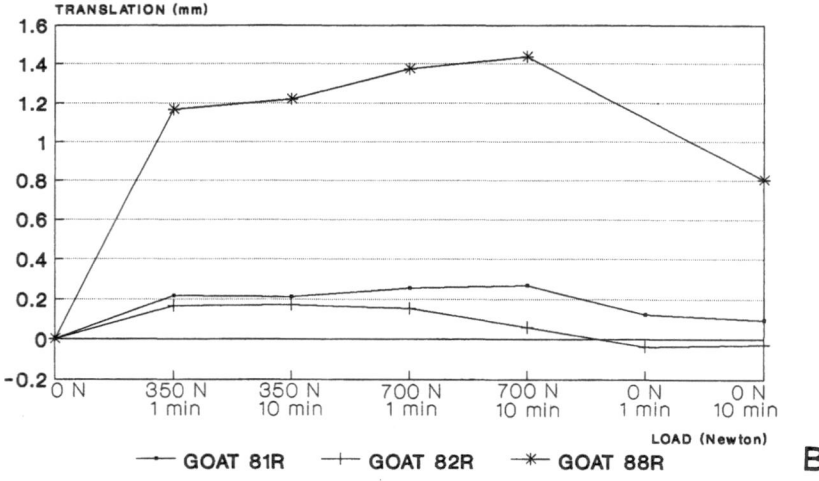

Fig. 2. Translations found in cranio-caudal direction (Y-axis) immediately after implantation (**A**) and 12 weeks after implantation (**B**). Implant in goat 88R showed excessive translations and rotations in all directions and was considered loose

Maximum rotation was measured around the X-axis (-3.1 degrees). In course of time a rather consistent pattern was observed showing increasing stability 12 weeks after implantation. Persistent translation in all directions declined from the zero group to the 12 weeks group, as was the case for rotations. At 12 weeks maximum persistent translation was measured in a medial-lateral direction (0.2 mm) (Fig. 2) with maximum persistent rotation around the Z-axis (-2.1 degrees).

Conclusions from the Animal Experiment

The reconstruction technique resulted in rapid union between the graft and the host bone. From 12 weeks onwards, very little of the impacted bone graft remained. Instead, a new trabecular bony structure of lamellar bone had formed. Although a fibrous tissue membrane of modest thickness had formed in some areas at the bone-cement interface, direct contact sites remained between the cement and newly formed bone.

Our histological and mechanical results showed that the reconstruction technique provided sufficient initial stability to enable the incorporation of the impacted acetabular grafts. Although the follow-up period in these animal experiments was limited to 48 weeks and the surgically prepared host bone was far less compromised than in the real clinical situation of humans with failed total hip arthroplasties, the results of this study encouraged us to continue to apply this biological reconstruction in small and large acetabular deficiencies.

References

1. Albee FH (1923) Fundamentals in bone transplantation. Experiences in three thousand bone grafts. J Am Med Assn 81: 1429–1432
2. Albee FH (1912) Discussion of the preservation of tissues and its application in surgery. J Am Med Assn 59: 527
3. Axhausen G (1911) Arbeiten aus dem Gebiet der Knochenpathologie und Knochenchirurgie.1. Kritische Bemerkungen und neue Beiträge zur freien Knochentransplantation. Arch Klin Chir 94: 241–281
4. Barth A (1908) Ueber Osteoplastik. Arch Klin Chir 86: 859–872
5. Brooks DB, et al (1963) Immunological factors in homogenous bone transplantation. IV. The effect of various methods of preparation and irradiation on antigenicity. J Bone Joint Surg 45-A: 1617–1625
6. Buma P, Schreurs BW, Versleyen D, Huiskes R, Slooff TJ (1992) Histologic evaluation of allograft incorporation after cemented and non-cemented hip arthroplasty in the goat. In: Older J (ed) Bone implant grafting. London: Springer, 12
7. Burchardt H, Busbee OA, Enneking WF (1975) Repair of experimental autologous grafts of cortical bone. J Bone Joint Surg 57-A: 814
8. Burchardt H (1989) Biology of cortical bone graft incorporation. In: Aebi M, Regazzoni P (eds) Bone transplantation. Berlin: Springer, pp 23–29
9. Burwell RG, Gowland G (1962) Studies in the transplantation of bone. The immune response of lymph nodes draining components of fresh homogenous bone treated by different methods. J Bone Joint Surg 44-B: 131–148
10. Burwell RG (1969) The fate of bone grafts. In: Apley GA (ed) Recent advances in orthopaedics. London: Churchill, pp 115–207
11. Bush LF (1947) The use of homogenous bone grafts. A preliminary report on the bone bank. J Bone Joint Surg 29: 620–628
12. Campbell CJ (1953) Experimental study of the fate of bone grafts. J Bone Joint Surg 35-A: 332–346
13. Curtis BF (1892) Bone transplantation for nonunited fractures. Medical Record, Jan 2

14. Enneking WF, Mindell ER (1991) Observation on massive retrieved human allografts. J Bone Joint Surg 73-A: 1123–1142
15. Friedlaender GE (1991) Bone allografts: the biological consequences of immunological events. J Bone Joint Surg 73-A: 1119–1123
16. Friedlaender GE (1987) Current concepts review on bone grafts. The basic science rationale for clinical applications. J Bone Joint Surg 69-A: 780
17. Goldberg VM, Powell A, Shaffer JW, Zika J, Stevenson S, Davy D, Heiple K (1989) The role of histocompatibility in bone allografting. In: Aebi M, Regazzoni P (eds) Bone transplantation. Berlin: Springer, 126
18. Goldberg VM, Stevenson S (1987) Natural history of autografts and allografts. Clin Orthop 225: 7
19. Greco F, De Palma U, Spechia A, Santucci A (1989) Biological aspects of repair osteogenesis in cortico-spongy homologous grafts. Ital J Orthop Traumatol 23: 491
20. Harris WH, Crothers O, Oh I (1977) Total hip replacement and femoral head bone grafting for severe acetabular deficiency in adults. J Bone Joint Surg 59-A: 752
21. Hastings DE, Parker SM (1975) Protrusio acetabula in rheumatoid arthritis. Clin Orthop 108: 7684
22. Heiple KG, Chase SW, Herndon CH (1963) A comparative study of the healing process following different types of bone transplantation. J Bone Joint Surg 45-A: 1593–1612
23. Herndon CH, Chase SW (1954) The fate of massive autogenous and homogenous bone grafts including articular surfaces. Surg Gynec Obstet 98: 273–290
24. Lexer E (1908) Über Gelenktransplantation. Med Klin 4: 817
25. MacEwen W (1881) Observations concerning transplantation of bones: Illustrated by a case of interhuman osseous transplantations, whereby over two-thirds of the shaft of a humerus was restored. Proc Roy Soc London 32: 232–247
26. Mankin HJ, Friedlaender GE (1989) Bone and cartilage allografts: physiological and immunological principles. In: Chandler HP, Penenberg BL (eds) Bone stock deficiency in total hip replacement. Thorofare, NJ: Slack, chapter 1
27. McCollum DE, Nunley JA, Harrelson JM (1980) Bone grafting in THR for acetabular protrusion. JBJS 72-A: 248–252
28. Ollier L (1867) Traite experimental et clinique de la regeneration des os et de la production artificielle du tissue osseux. Victor Masson et Fils: Paris
29. Ottolenghi CE (1972) Massive osteo and osteoarticular bone grafts. Technique and results of 62 cases. Clin Orthop 87: 156–164
30. Scales JT, Wright KWJ (1983) Major bone and joint replacement using custom implants. In: Chao EYs, Irin IC (eds) Tumor prothesis for bone and joint reconstruction, the design and application. Stuttgart: Thieme, pp 149–168
31. Schreurs BW, Huiskes R, Slooff TJJH (1990) Proceedings 7th Meeting European Society of Biomechanics, Aarhus, DK, A14
32. Schreurs W, Huiskes R, Slooff TJJH, Buma P (1992) A method to estimate the initial stability of cemented and non-cemented hip stems fixated with a bone grafting technique. In: Older J (ed) Bone implant grafting. Berlin: Springer, chapter 18, pp 131–134
33. Schreurs BW, Buma P, Huiskes R, Slagter JLM, Slooff TJJH (1993) Transactions ORS, 452, San Francisco, USA
34. Schreurs BW, Buma P, Huiskes R, Slagter JLM, Slooff TJJH (1994) A technique for using impacted trabecular allografts in revision surgery with cemented stems. Acta Orthop Scand 65: 267–275
35. Schreurs BW, Huiskes R, Slooff TJJH (1994) The initial stability of cemented and noncemented femoral stems fixated with a bone grafting technique. Clin Mater 16: 105–110
36. Selvik G (1989) Roentgen stereophotogrammetry. Acta Orthop Scand 60 [Suppl 232]
37. Selvik G (1974) A roentgenstereophotogrammatic method for the study of the kinematics of the skeletal system. Thesis, University of Lund, Lund, Sweden
38. Slooff TJ, Van Horn J, Lemes A, Fluiskes R (1984) Bone grafting for total hip replacement for acetabular protrusion. Acta Orthop Scand 55: 593–596
39. Slooff TJJH (1992) Acetabular augmentation in cemented arthroplasty: pre-operative assessment and surgical technique. In: Older J (ed) Bone implant grafting. Berlin: Springer, chapter 8, pp 51–55

40. Stevenson S, Xiao Qing Li, Martin B (1991) The fate of cancellous and cortical bone after transplantation of fresh and frozen tissue-antigen-matched and mismatched osteochondral allografts in dogs. J Bone Joint Surg 73-A: 1143–1157
41. Urist MR (1953) The physiological basis of bone graft surgery, with special reference to the theory of induction. Clin Orthop 1: 207
42. Urist MR (1965) Bone: formation by auto-induction. Science 150: 893–899
43. Urist MR, De Lange RJ, Finerman GA (1983) Bone cell differentiation and growth factors. Science 220: 680

Author's addresses: Tom J.J.H. Slooff, J.W. Schimmel and J. Gardeniers, Institute of Orthopaedics, University Hospital Nijmegen, P.O. Box P101, NL-6500 HB Nijmegen, The Netherlands; P. Buma and R. Huiskes, Institute of Orthopaedics, Laboratory of Experimental Orthopaedics, University Hospital Nijmegen, The Netherlands.

Acetabular Reconstruction Technique

H. Winkler[1], F. Bohmann[2], and W. Schwägerl[2]

[1] Department of Orthopaedics, Donauspital, Vienna, Austria
[2] Department of Orthopaedics, Pulmologisches Zentrum, Vienna, Austria

Introduction

Acetabular bone deficiencies are an increasingly frequent problem in revision total hip arthroplasty. As long as there is enough host bone available to grant stable fixation for a new implant, defects can easily be filled with milled or morsellized bone. Whenever the remaining bone cannot support a prosthesis, structural allografting will be necessary. Known techniques for such cases generally are considered to be very demanding and results often seem to be unpredictable. The fate of the reconstruction depends on several factors, which can be summarized to four major areas of interest:

1. Biomechanical principles
2. Host Bone
3. Graft
4. Implant

Since there is constant interaction, successful reconstruction can only be expected when harmonized techniques are applied, fulfilling the demands of all sites.

Biomechanical Aspects

Functional Loading

Bony ingrowth into implant surfaces is significantly accelerated by load bearing stresses [4, 8]. This relationship is governed by Wolff's Law, which implies that the structure and strength of bone is directly influenced by the mechanical environment it is subjected to [16]. The fate of bone allografts is also correlated with the amount and patterns of stress acting on the graft [13, 15]. Unloaded parts of the grafts incorporate very slowly or are even resorbed, grafts therefore should be loaded functionally as soon as possible to favour rapid incorporation.

On the other hand, excessive loading of grafts, which usually are weaker than living bone, leads to their collapse. Allografting seems to be a tightrope walk. One must keep a balance between too much and too little pressure on the graft.

Anatomical Reconstruction

While in primary cases the correct positioning of the implant is pregiven, anatomical conditions are usually changed during revision. The loose implant often migrates cranially and dorsally, setting a defect of varying extent. Implanting the new cup into that defect creates a non-anatomical center of rotation, which may be the cause of recurrent dislocation and early re-loosening [1, 10]. Grafting defects without restoring the original anatomy will lead to non-physiological stress flow through the graft and may be related with delayed incorporation. Therefore, all possible efforts should be undertaken to reconstruct the anatomically correct center of rotation.

Host Bone

After loosening of a prosthesis the remaining bone is usually sclerotic, regardless of the amount of deficiencies. There is no cancellous structure which would allow cement to interdigitate [3]. There is also minor vascularization, compromising secondary ingrowth into an uncemented cup or a bone-graft. Although there are multiple gaps and cavities, the surface's microstructure is relatively even. The bone therefore requires special treatment. The irregularly shaped surface should be trimmed to a smooth level to provide uniformly balanced stress distribution to as many contact-points as possible. At the same time the even sclerotic micro-surface should be roughened to provide for better friction with the graft to be implanted. Preparation to a certain percentage of bleeding bone surface improves vascularization, thus accelerating the incorporation of a graft. Sacrifice of bone exceeding those purposes should be avoided.

Graft

Following the biomechanical principles, protection of the graft against load bearing by using rings or plate constructs should be avoided. Such constructs remain stable, as long as the implants do. As soon as the implants fail, sudden failure of the whole reconstruction may occur. The non-loaded allograft becomes weaker rather than stronger while protected by internal fixation. The proper grafting technique therefore should concentrate on providing immediate weight bearing capability to the graft.

Structure

Morsellized allografts may be incorporated faster but are less capable of immediate weight bearing. Bulk allografts initially show similar strength as original bone and therefore, seem to be more appropriate for the use under weight bearing conditions. Loss of strength in the following months and years must be expected, but should simultaneously be compensated by consistent formation of new bone inside the graft, triggered by dynamic loading. Revascularization should proceed in a directed way from the host bone to the implant's surface, thus consistently revitalizing the entire graft.

Treatment

Several modes of treating the allografts (sterilization, radiation, freeze-drying, etc.) have shown to decrease their antigenicity. At the same time they are decreasing their mechanical strength. For clinical use immunology seems to be of little relevance, while under loaded conditions mechanical strength is of significant importance. Fresh frozen allografts seem to be the strongest, but treated grafts may perform as well, provided that a proper grafting technique is used.

Surface

Edges and spikes always produce local stress peaks which easily can exceed the load bearing capability of allograft bone. Loading an incongruent surface results in local over-loading of contact areas and under-loading of areas without primary contact. Only after the graft has settled due to local collapse of overloaded areas, incorporation of the allograft becomes homogenous. The implant subsequently migrates cranially and thereby often gets loose. The load on the graft should be distributed on the whole surface in a balanced way and should show a jointless contact with the host bone, avoiding any edges. A concave surface seems to be preferable to provide for balanced stress distribution. The graft's surface adjacent to host bone ideally should be purely cancellous. For contact to soft tissue cortical or sclerotic bone seems to be more favourable because of increased strength and slower remodelling. Primary stability and balanced stress distribution should be achieved by shaping a jointless contact between graft and host bone, preferably a press-fit [14].

Fixation

The stability of an allograft determines its fate. Only a stable allograft has a chance to be incorporated, in particular, loading is only possible if primary stability has been achieved.

Rigid Fixation

For rigid fixation the graft is bolted to the host bone as firmly as possible, not allowing any movement. Usually screws are placed through the graft in various directions, wherever hold can be found in the underlying host bone. This kind of reconstruction will stay "rigid" as long as no changes occur on the allograft. As soon as only small parts of the graft are resorbed at the interface or around the screws, micromotion between graft and host bone must be expected. Under loading conditions this will occur when screws cross the lines of natural load transfer. Such screws then act as a pivot or axis with the graft rotating around it. Micromotion caused by rotatory and shearing forces will avoid incorporation and lead to failure within some years [9].

Dynamic Fixation

Dynamic fixation does not compromise physiological stress flow through the graft. Primary stability ideally should be granted by press-fit alone, if this is not possible only one or two parallel cancellous lag screws in the loading direction should be enough to secure against rotatory forces [14]. Since a dynamically loaded allograft consistently is pressed against the host bone by constant, physiological forces, stability may be expected to be obtained during the entire time of incorporation. This kind of fixation allows controlled settling within mild ranges in case of local weakening of the graft.

Implant

Design and Surface

Loading of the allograft always originates from the implant's surface. In order to keep local stresses at every single point as low as possible, forces should be distributed as homogeneously as possible. As mentioned before, the best way to provide the desired conditions is to choose a concave surface, i.e., a hemispherical design of the cup [7]. Threaded cups as well as conical or ring-shaped ones produce load peaks at their edges, which consequently may protrude into the allograft [2, 12, 15], (Fig. 1a–c). Their use for reconstructions therefore should be avoided. Loads also should cover a surface as large as possible. Increasing the surface may be obtained either by cement or by porous coating. This ideally should be of a microstructure that stimulates close linking with new bone and increases primary stability through high friction [11].

Cemented versus Non-Cemented

Excellent load distribution in combination with ideal primary stability can be achieved by using cement, provided that a cancellous bed is available. Loosening processes between cement and avital allograft bone are uncommon. However, possible problems have to be expected: 1) Slight condensation of the allograft can lead to moderate migration of the cup. In such a case cement breakage may occur, especially when parts of the cement mantle are firmly attached to host bone (Fig. 1d). 2) The fate of the implant is doubtful, as soon as the allograft is fully revascularized and the cement gets into touch with living bone again. 3) Cement between graft and host bone compromises incorporation.

On the other hand uncemented cups so far could not prove to be more successful in combination with structural allografts [6]. Although such combinations provide for fast incorporation of parts of the allograft, mildest resorption may lead to partial loss of contact and consequent loosening of uncemented implants.

Fixation

Cemented sockets usually do not need additional fixation. Using a metal backed hemispherical implant without cement can offer a lot of advantages, yet rotatory stability compared to other implant designs is diminished. This disadvantage can only partially be compensated through press-fit effect, anatomical positioning and high friction coefficients of porous coated surfaces. Some authors therefore recommend the use of penetrated shells, which can additionally be stabilized by means of screws. This possibility should be considered only with caution. Holes reduce the available surface of the cup, thus compromising ideal stress distribution. They later might act as areas of local contact between polyethylene and bone. Resulting wear might be the cause of repeated loosening [7]. Subsidence of the metal shell will make screw heads more prominent and corrode the back surface of the liner. Common screw systems also cannot completely avoid tilting in case of local graft collapse [6]. On the contrary, a stable screw can even initiate such a process under certain conditions. Using several screws pointing into different directions will also compromise physiological load transfer. This also is shown by the high incidence of screw breakage under such conditions [2].

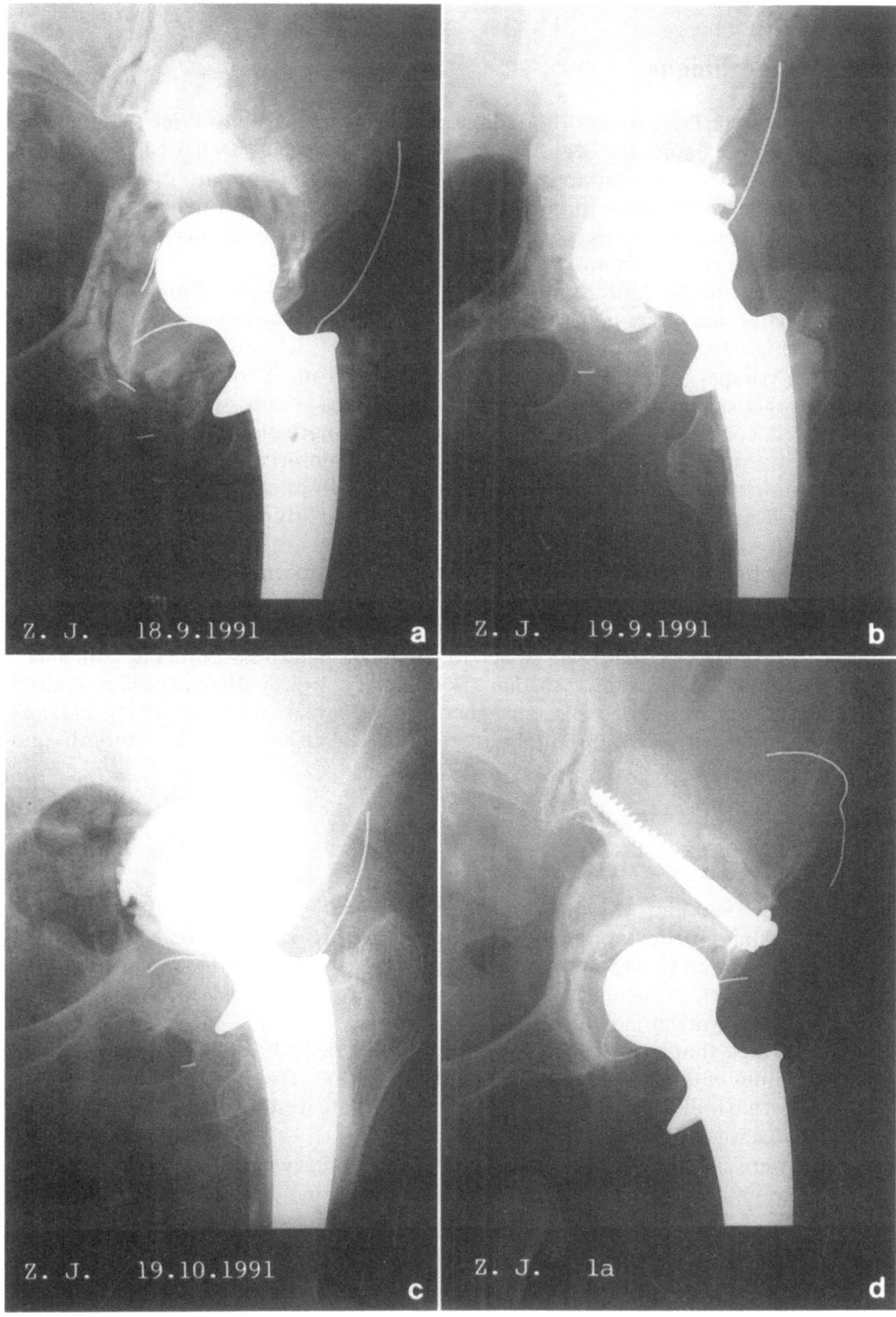

Fig. 1. Failure of reconstruction using morsellized allograft bone and a conical threaded cup. **a** Pre-operative radiograph demonstrating a combined superomedial defect; **b** Post-operative X-ray after reconstruction using three milled femoral heads and a Zweymueller cup (elsewhere's case); **c** Medial edge of cup protruded through the allograft and penetrated into the pelvis one month after surgery; **d** Re-revision using one bulk femoral head, fixed by two screws. Two years postoperatively there is no sign of loosening. Cement breakage visible at 9 o'clock indicates mild subsidence

Operative Technique

At the Orthopaedic Department Pulmologisches Zentrum der Stadt Wien ("Baumgart-ner Höhe Hospital") since the beginning of 1990 a technique has been used, that tries to fulfill all demands mentioned above. Defects larger than 35 mm are prepared, using hemispherical reamers (male) to obtain a smooth concavity and roughen the sclerotic surface. Remaining minor defects can be filled with the gained bone meal. The surface is smoothened by reverse reaming (Fig. 2a).

Fresh frozen femoral heads are then prepared with inverse female reamers of a diameter 0 to 4 mm larger up to a convex surface with a cancellous contact area to the host bone (Fig. 2b). The contact area to soft tissue is left sclerotic or cortical. We use femoral head shapers of 7 sizes with diameters ranging from 38 to 58 mm, which ensure quick and exact spherical preparation. The prepared head's convexity is impacted into the prepared concavity (Fig. 2c). There are no incongruencies and in ideal cases a press-fit can be provided. The graft is fixed either temporarily by means of Kirschner wires or definitely with as few implants as possible. Usually one cancellous lag screw plus washer is sufficient. The screw is oriented cranially and slightly dorsally along the lines of weight-bearing forces (Fig. 2d). When two or more screws are necessary they should be orientated in parallel. The graft then is stable enough to enable preparation of the implant bed as easily as in original bone.

Implantation of the socket, either cemented or uncemented, does not differ from primary arthroplasty. Usually we prefer to cement a Charnley-Cup (Fig. 2d). Post-operative management is similar to that after primary surgery. Patients are mobilized immediately. They are advised to use crutches for 6 to 12 weeks postoperatively. Patients are followed prospectively, radiographs are routinely taken after 2 weeks, 6 months and every year.

Patients

Between April 1990 and March 1994 182 reconstructions were performed using the described technique. Postoperative complications were rare. There were no deep infections. There was 1 dislocation and 2 cases with loosening of the implant required further revision before the end of the first year. Thrombosis and embolism were as frequent as after primary surgery.

Of the 90 hips, that have been reconstructed until March 1992, 72 could be followed with a minimum of two years and a maximum of 4 years. Two patients have deceased before the 2 years follow up, 16 could not be traced. There were 12 males and 60 females, their mean age was 67.7 years.

Defects were classified according to Gross [5] as cavitary in 21, minor column in 35 and major column in 16 cases. The cup was uncemented in 6 and cemented in 66 cases.

Results

Until September 1994 we found seven cases with a change of position of the implant of more than 5 mm, usually together with the graft. All but one showed at least one of three operative mistakes: vertical implantation of the socket, positioning of the socket at a position more than 1 centimeter above the natural center of rotation or a lack of stability against rotatory forces.

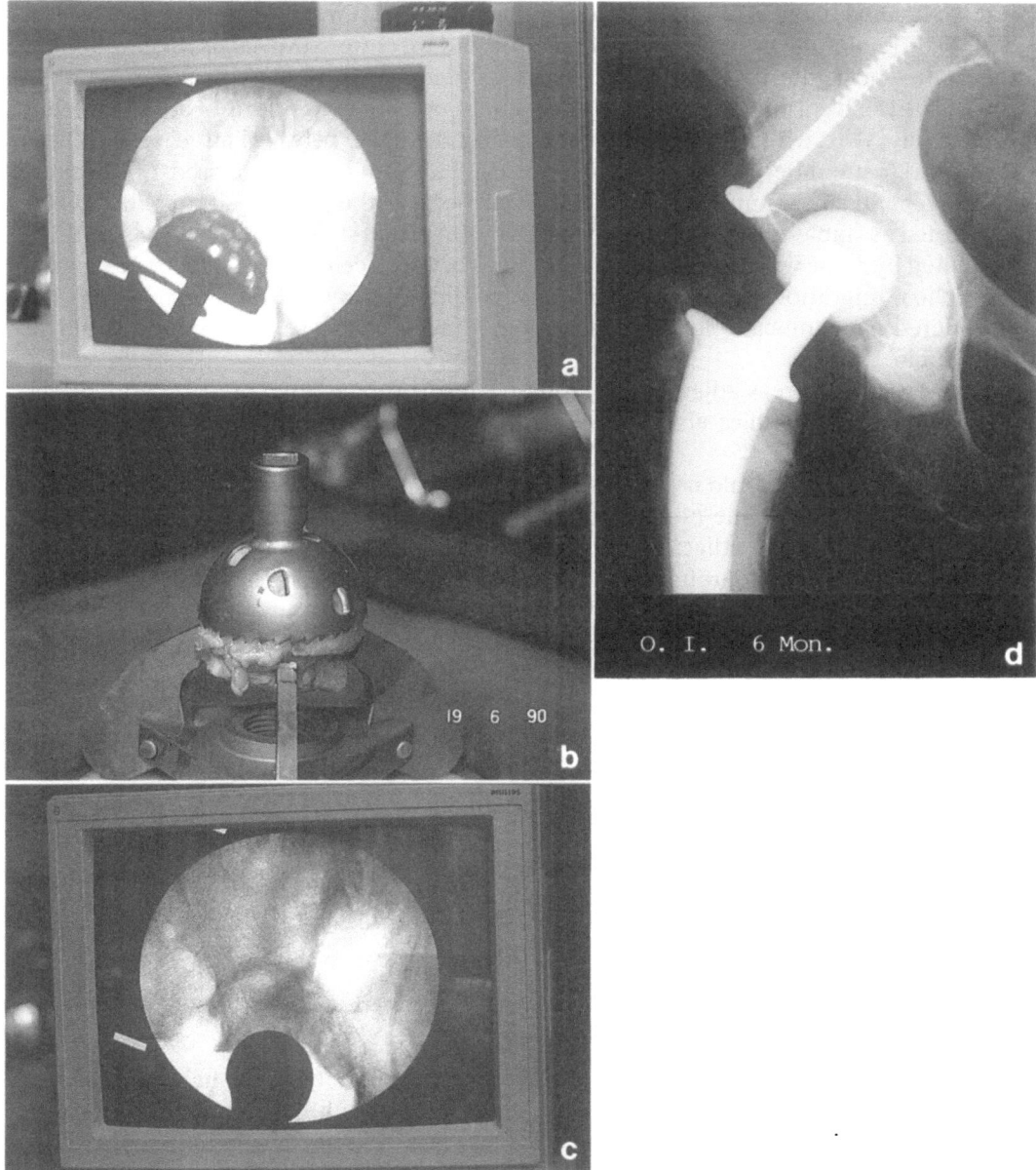

Fig. 2. Operative technique. **a** Defect trimmed with hemispheric reamer (intraoperative fluoroscopy); **b** Femoral head shaped with inverse reamer 2 mm larger; **c** Impaction of graft into defect (intraoperative fluoroscopy); **d** Graft secured against rotation using one traction screw in the loading direction. Cup cemented at anatomically correct level

Six hips meanwhile have been revised a second time. Once a loosened cementless cup had to be replaced and once excessive heterotopic bone formation had to be removed. In both cases the allografts showed good incorporation and were left in place. In three cases progressive tilting of the allograft and the implant lead to early loosening. Dislocation always took place between host bone and graft while the cemented cup always stayed firmly attached to the graft. On revision both cup and graft were without contact to host bone. The remaining graft was mainly necrotic, but there were thin layers of new bone at the graft—host interface. All of those cases could be supplied with a new implant successfully, once using another bulk allograft. In one hip the graft resorbed completely within one year with the implant penetrating into the pelvis. This case has been converted to a saddle-prosthesis. Two loose hips have not yet been revised, one because of bad general condition of the patient and one because the patient felt no pain. 65 hips were rated as stable, although 13 seemed to have migrated slightly superiorly as could be estimated by some widening of radiolucent lines between cement and host bone distally. Since those migrations did not exceed 5 mm and did not show progression they were not considered as significant signs of loosening. Cracks of the cement-mantle could be detected in 12 cases.

In non loaded areas adjacent to soft tissue, resorption as an expression of remodelling was observed 17 times, always within the first year and without change of position of the implants (Fig. 3).

Radiolucent lines could never be seen between graft and implant. On the other hand they were observed at the junction of graft to host bone in most of the cases. Those usually were visible immediately after the operation and showed progression in 10 cases.

Incorporation of allografts usually is estimated by evaluating the obliteration of the gap between host bone and graft as well as the appearance of new structures inside the graft. We are very reserved in interpreting these signs since we think they might be an expression of condensation of the allografts. After the end of the second year this interface commonly was no longer detectable in the loaded zones 1 (lateral) and 2 (superior) while in the less loaded zone 3 (inferior) the gap mostly was still visible.

Similarly the appearance of new structures inside the graft continuously increased faster in zones 1 and 2, filling the loaded parts of the graft completely at the end of the second year. In zone three structuring did not yet reach the inner third of the allograft at that time.

The mean Harris hip score improved from 42 points preoperatively to 91 points after two years. 48 hips were rated as excellent, 14 as good, 8 as fair and 2 as poor.

Discussion

Loading of allografts seems to enhance their incorporation, but only balanced loading can avoid early collapse. Press-fit-grafting seems to be a suitable method to reconstruct deficient acetabuli in an anatomical way, rendering increased primary stability without additional implants. Dynamic loading and balanced stress distribution on the whole graft surface may be provided, resulting in accelerated incorporation and significantly less resorption. Patients are capable of immediate weight bearing. Short time results therefore are significantly improved. Expectation of better long time results seems to be justified.

Partial collapse of the allograft followed by subsidence of the implant can be reduced significantly, yet it cannot be expected to be completely prevented during the period of incorporation. In particular, treated grafts are likely to show moderate condensation. We often had the impression that lucent lines between cement and host bone of the inferior parts of the acetabulum showed progression, but since the amount rarely exceeded 2 mm it has not been considered as a significant sign of subsidence. The fact that there has been some migration could be concluded from a few cases, where cement breakage was found. As we could observe, subsidence did not necessarily lead to

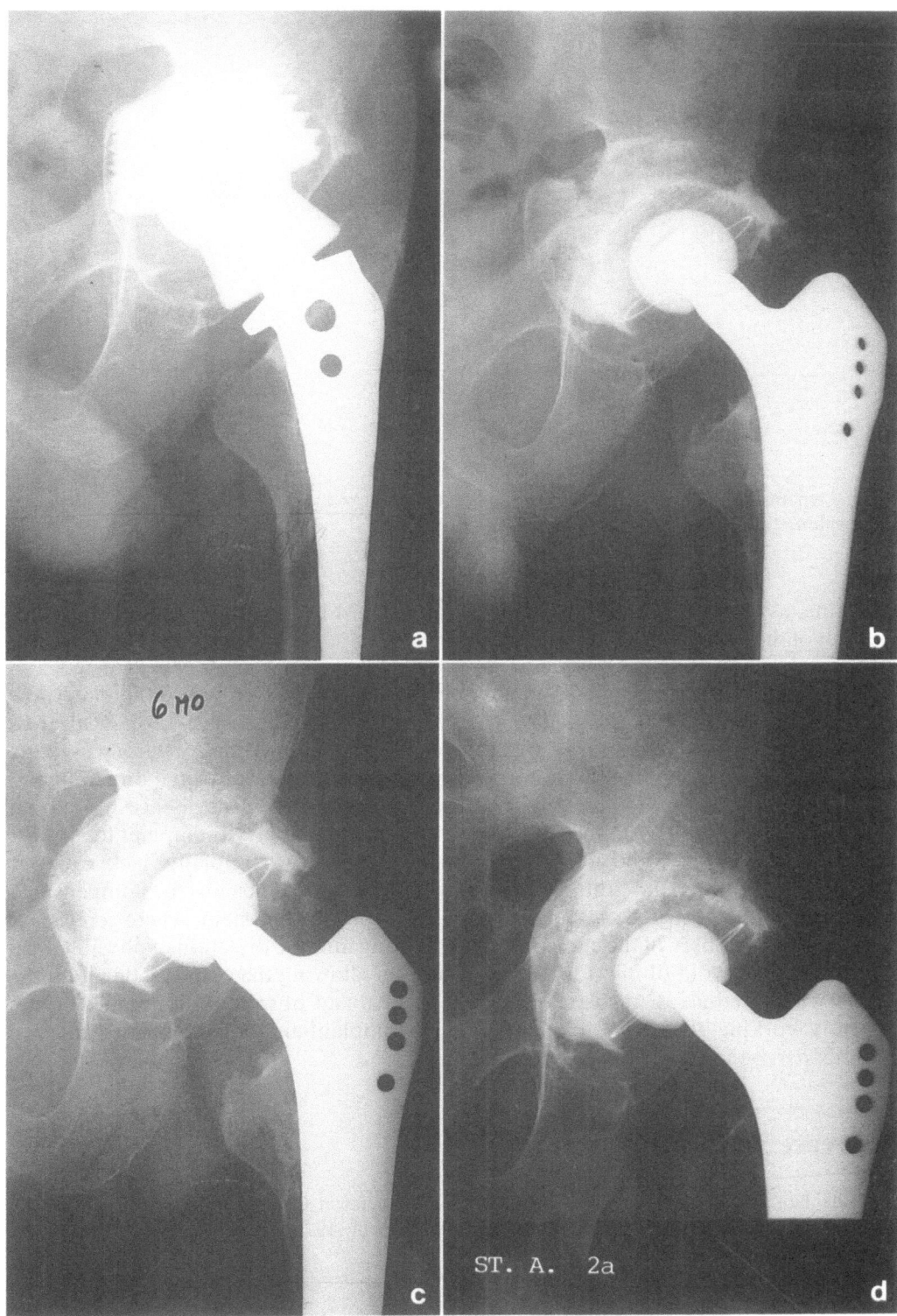

Fig. 3. Resorption of non loaded bone. **a** Preoperative radiograph demonstrating a large protrusio type defect; **b** Reconstruction using two femoral heads; **c** Resorption of non loaded medial parts of the graft is visible 6 months postoperatively; **d** No more resorption is visible 2 years later. Good incorporation of the allograft with unchanged position of the implant

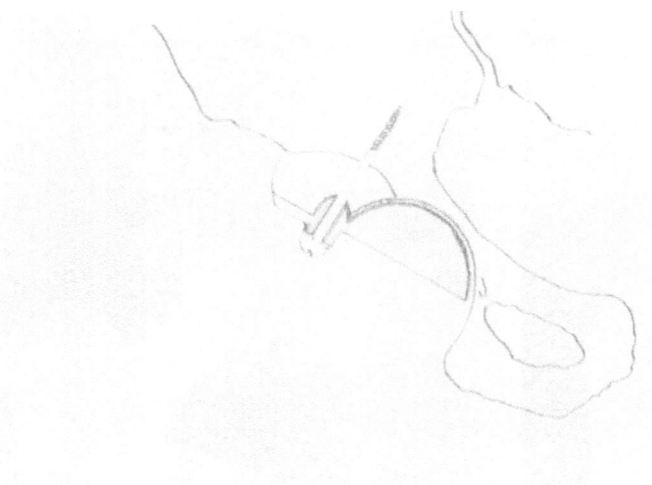

Fig. 4. Dynamically stabilized socket. The implant may follow eventual partial collapse of the graft. Sliding along two parallel screws avoids tilting or rotating

loosening, as long as the implant and the graft did not tilt or rotate during migration. Five out of the seven failures among our cases were associated with tilting, while in cases with purely axial migration usually no signs of loosening could be detected and migration did not show progression after the end of the first year. We therefore now recommend to secure grafts against rotation without compromising physiological stress flow by using one or more parallel traction screws in the loading direction (Fig. 2d). A cemented cup then follows an eventual movement of the graft in axial direction and both stay untilted. However, cement breakage may occur during subsidence and should be considered with concern, since this sign usually is correlated with implant loosening. Uncemented systems could avoid this problem, but known implants lack rotatory stability in case of partial graft resorption, which cannot sufficiently be compensated with common screws [6, 7]. A possible solution could be a system, where screws are placed at the periphery of the cup, uniformly pointing into the direction of physiological load transfer to avoid tilting (Fig. 4). A mechanism allowing the cup to slide along the screws would reduce disturbance of stress flows to an absolute minimum. We are currently working on the development of such an implant and hope to further improve our already good results.

References

1. Callaghan JJ, Salvati EA, Pellici PM, Wilson PD, Ranawat CS (1985) Results of revision for mechanical failure after cemented total hip replacement, 1979 to 1982. A two to five—year follow-up. J Bone Joint Surg (Am) 67-A: 1074–1085
2. Engh CH, Griffin WL, Marx CL (1990) Cementless acetabular components. J Bone Joint Surg (Br) 72-B: 53–59
3. Flechter T, Weber GG (1993) Excessive cementing of acetabular components in total hip revision. 1er Congress European d'Orthopèdie (EFORT). Revue de Chirurgie Orth Nr, 504
4. Goldstein SA, Matthews LS (1991) The response of trabecular bone to implant load. Orthopaedics and Related Sciences, German 2G: 185–190

5. Gross AE (1992) Revision arthroplasty of the hip using allograft bone. In: Czitrom AA, Gross AE (eds) Allografts in orthopaedic practice. Baltimore: Williams and Wilkins, pp 147–176

6. Hooten JP jr, Engh CA Jun, Engh CA (1994) Failure of structural acetabular allografts in cementless revision hip arthroplasty. J Bone Joint Surg (Br) 76-B: 419–422

7. Huk Olga L, Bansal M, Betts F, Rimnac CM, Lieberman JR, Huo MH, Salvati EA (1994) Polyethylene and metal debris generated by non-articulating surfaces of modular acetabular components. J Bone Joint Surg (Br) 76-B: 568–574

8. Jasty M, Harris WH (1990) Experience with cementless porous-surfaced acetabular components. Orthopaedics and Related Sciences, German 1G: 52–60

9. Jasty MJ, Harris WH (1990) Salvage total hip reconstruction in patients with major acetabular bone deficiency using structural femoral head allografts. J Bone Joint Surg (Br) 72-B: 63–67

10. Linde F, Jensen J (1988) Socket loosening in arthroplasty for congenital dislocation of the hip. Acta Orthop Scand 59: 254

11. Paprosky W (1993) Allograft reconstruction in massive acetabular defects. Techniques Orthop 7(4): 44–57

12. Silber DA, Engh CA (1990) Cementless total hip arthroplasty with femoral head bone grafting for hip dysplasia. J Arthroplasty 5(3): 231–240

13. Trancik TM, Stulberg BN, Wilde AH, Feiglin DH (1986) Allograft reconstruction of the acetabulum during revision total hip arthroplasty. J Bone Joint Surg (Am) 68-A: 527–533

14. Winkler H, Bohmann F, Lintner F, Schwägerl W (1992) Gleichmässige Belastung allogener Knochentransplantate durch fugenlose Einpassung. Osteologie 1 [Suppl 1]: 82

15. Winkler H, Bohmann F, Schwägerl W (1992) Einheilverhalten tiefgefrorener Femurköpfe bei Kombination mit zementfreier Schraubpfanne. Orthop Praxis 1: 47–53

16. Wolff J (1892) Das Gesetz der Transformation der Knochen. Berlin: Hirschwald

Authors' address: Dr. H. Winkler, Department of Orthopaedics, Donauspital, SMZO, Langobardenstrasse 122, A-1220 Wien, Austria.

Tumor

Indications for Combined Grafts (Allografts + Vascularized Fibula) after Intercalary Resections for Bone Tumor

D. A. Campanacci[1], R. Capanna[1], M. Ceruso[2], R. Angeloni[2], M. Innocenti[2], G. Lauri[2], M. Manfrini[2], A. Gasbarrini[3], and C. Bufalini[2]

[1]Department of Orthopaedic Oncology and Reconstructive Surgery, Centro Traumatologico Ortopedico, Firenze, Italy
[2]Department of Hand Surgery and Reconstructive Microsurgery, Centro Traumatologico Ortopedico, Firenze, Italy
[3]University Clinic, Istituto Ortopedico Rizzoli, Bologna, Italy

Introduction

During the last decades, massive bone allografts have been largely employed for reconstruction after resection of bone tumors. In the case of an intercalary resection for a diaphyseal tumor, the reconstructive alternatives are: massive allografts, autogenous bone grafts, Ilizarov technique (bone transportation) and vascularized fibular autografts.

After massive allograft reconstruction, a prolonged immobilization period is required and, despite strong and rigid fixation, the risk of nonunion at the allograft-host junctions is high, and allograft fracture is a frequent complication. Reconstruction with autogenous bone grafts alone is rarely adopted for short skeletal defects, because of the low mechanical strength, the poor stability of the implant and the slow healing. The Ilizarov technique is a valid alternative to reconstruct small bone defects (<10 cm), although it is not easy to manage for the patient, and the regenerate takes a long time to form. Moreover, postoperative chemotheraphy in tumor patients may have a negative effect on bone formation during distraction.

During the seventies, the vascularized autogenous graft was firstly described by McKee (1970), and subsequently Taylor et al. (1975) reported the first cases of vascularized fibular autograft employed to reconstruct a skeletal defect after bone tumor resection. The reconstruction with a vascular fibula alone does not provide sufficient stability, and is too weak to allow early weight bearing.

In 1988, Capanna et al. [2] described the association of a massive allograft with a vacularized fibular autograft for the intercalary reconstruction of diaphyseal skeletal defects. In the present paper, we present the results in a series of patients who received the combined allograft as a primary reconstruction after resection for bone tumors. The surgical technique is briefly described and the indications for this innovative reconstructive technique are discussed.

Table 1. Histologic diagnosis of treated patients

Diagnosis	N° of cases
Osteosarcoma	26
Ewing's sarcoma	8
Adamantinoma	4
Fibrosarcoma	3
Malignant fibrous histiocytoma	3
Dedifferentiated chondrosarcoma	1
Angiosarcoma	1
Desmoplastic fibroma	1
Total	47 cases

Materials and Method

At the "Centro Traumatologico Ortopedico" of Florence, between 1988 and 1994, 47 patients received a combined graft (massive allograft + vacularized fibular autograft) as reconstruction after resection of diaphyseal bone tumors. The series consisted of 29 males and 18 females, with an average age of 16.5 years, range 4–48 years. The surgeries were performed for malignant tumors in 46 cases and for a benign lesion in one case. The histological diagnoses are reported in Table 1. The reconstruction was done in the lower limb in all cases, 16 involving the femur and 31 the tibia.

The vascularized fibula was assembled either concentrically with the massive allograft or parallel in a dual position . Tibial reconstruction was concentric in 28 cases and parallel in 3 cases, while femoral reconstruction was concentric in 2 cases and dual in 14 cases. Patients were followed at an average of 31 months with a range of 2-72 months.

Surgical Technique

The surgical field is prepared to allow two surgical teams to work simultaneously. While the oncologic team performs the resection, on the contralateral leg the fibula and its vascular pedicle are prepared according to the surgical technique described by Taylor [6]. The fibula, covered by the periosteum, is sized prior to osteotomy to exceed the length of oncologic resection by at least five centimeters.

Concentric Assembling

This technique is recommended for tibial reconstructions where soft tissue closure is difficult (Fig. 1a, 1c). If the biopsy tract excision causes a large skin defect, the fibula may be transplanted together with a pedicled skin island. Otherwise, a medial gastrocnemius flap may be rotated to cover the implant, and a split thickness skin graft is applied.

An oversized deep frozen proximal tibial allograft is preferred because the wider medullary canal can contain the transplanted fibula. The allograft is cut in a frontal plane and the medullary canal is curetted until the fibula fits in. The vascularized fibula is inserted into the distal tibial medullary canal for at least three centimeters. The allograft

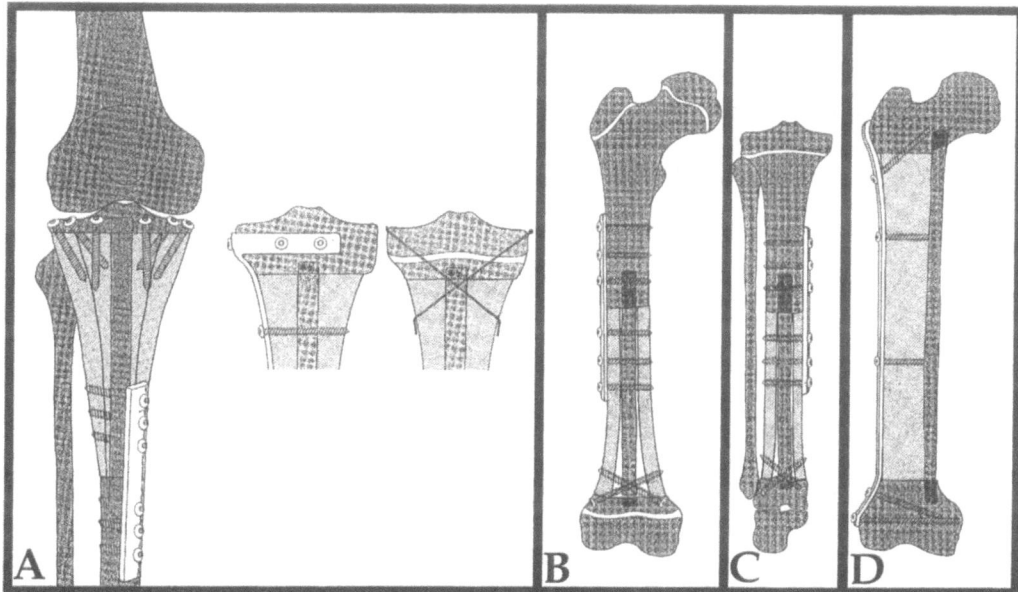

Fig. 1. A Concentric assembling for intraepiphyseal or metaphyseal resections of proximal tibia. A minimal proximal synthesis and a rigid distal fixation is performed after intraepiphyseal resections. After metaphyseal resection, a rigid plate fixation is feasible in adult patients, while smooth Kirschner wires allow to preserve the growth plate in children; **B** Concentric assembling with minimal distal fixation for metaphyseal distal femur resection; **C** Concentric assembling for ankle arthrodesis with minimal distal fixation preserving the subtalar joint; **D** Parallel dual assembing with long plate rigid fixation after extensive femoral diaphyseal resection

shell is positioned around the fibula taking care to avoid damage to the vascular pedicle. The host tibial plateau is curetted to receive the fibular stump.

Minimal proximal osteosynthesis is required for intraepiphyseal resection, where just a thin part of the epiphysis and articular surface is saved (Fig. 1a). When the growth plate is preserved, Kirschner wires passing through the epiphysis are used to avoid epiphysiodesis (Fig. 1a). In all cases the distal osteotomy is fixed with a plate and screws crossing the fibula. If there is enough bone to perform a rigid fixation, a long plate crossing both osteotomies is preferred (Fig. 1a).

Parallel Dual Assembling

In case of extensive femoral diaphyseal resections, our policy is to perform a combined allograft and vascularized fibular autograft with parallel dual assembly fixed with a long rigid plate crossing both the osteotomies (Fig. 1d). This technique provides biological augmentation and offers a medial cortical support for the allograft. In all femoral reconstructions, parallel dual assembling is preferred because the vascular pedicle is medial (allowing anastomosis with a branch of the profunda femoris artery). Since the mechanical axis is medial there is an advantage in reinforcing the medial cortex. When the resection is performed very close to the growth plate (Fig. 1b) or to the articular surface, minimal osteosynthesis with concentric assembling is preferred in the femur also.

The level of the vascular pedicle may be modified, by turning the fibula upside-down. A termino-terminal anastomosis is preferred using one artery and two veins. Commonly, in the leg, anastomosis is performed with the anterior tibial vessels. When the vascularization of the foot is not optimal, a termino-lateral anastomosis with the anterior tibial artery may be performed. In some cases, for oncologic reasons, the anterior tibial vessels are resected with the tumor. In this situation, the vascular pedicle of the fibula may be anastomosed with the distal stump of the anterior tibial vessels, obtaining a retrograde blood flow. When all these alternatives are not feasible, a termino-lateral anastomosis with the posterior tibial artery may be performed.

Results

We observed three local recurrences (6%), and in two cases one angiosarcoma and one dedifferentiated chondrosarcoma a distal skip metastasis in the same bone appeared at a later time (4%). Three patients developed pulmonary metastases (6%), two of them died of disease, while one patient is disease free after metastasectomy.

In two cases (4%) a postoperative wound slough occurred, and both of them healed after surgical debridment. One patient (2%) had a deep infection requiring amputation.

Ten patients had a fracture of the implant (21%), but in 90% of cases spontaneous healing was observed. In 10% of cases minor revision surgery was necessary (autogenous bone grafting), while no case required a major revision .

Delayed union was observed in two cases (4%), and both healed after autogenous bone grafting.

Discussion

The basic theory of the combined allograft reconstructive procedure is the association of mechanical resistance given by the massive allograft with the biologic capacity of a vascularized fibula.

In intercalary allograft reconstructions, the graft acts as a spacer with osteoconductive capacities. Although rigid fixation is achieved, the healing of osteotomies takes a long time and the internal repair continues in 20% of the graft for several years after implantation (3).

Allograft healing and internal repair take place by the process of creeping substitution, consisting in continuous resorption and new bone formation. During the initial period of time after implantation (2 to 3 years), the resorption process is predominant and the allograft's mechanical strength decreases progressively. As a matter of fact, other authors [1, 7] reported a higher incidence of allograft fractures after 2 years from implantation. On the other hand, the vascularized fibular autograft has osteogenetic and osteoinductive properties, which allow an early union at the osteotomies (as a normal fracture callus), which may encourage allograft union and internal repair. Furthermore, after union and weight bearing activity, the fibular autograft becomes hyperthrophic, and may support the allograft, which is weakened by creeping substitution.

There are general and special indications for this reconstructive procedure. In intercalary diaphyseal resections, a general indication to combined allografts is the chance to decrease the recovery time of the patient and to decrease the complication rate.

After a combined allograft procedure, the patient is immobilized in a cast for one month. After cast removal, the knee and the hip are mobilized for a few days, and a new cast is applied for another month. Then, a brace is worn until union is achieved, and at that time progressive weight bearing is allowed. In our experience, the osteogenic capacity of the vascularized fibula provides early union and allows a quick functional recovery.

A fracture of the graft occurred in 21% of cases, which is a higher rate compared to reports of other authors on large allograft series [1, 4, 5, 7]. Nevertheless, in the vast majority of cases (90%) the fractures in this series were undisplaced stress fractures of the vascularized fibula, which went on to spontaneous healing with hyperthrophic callus formation after cast immobilization. In 10% of cases the fractures healed after autogenous bone grafting, and a major revision (allograft substitution or new fixation) was never performed. In some cases, the fracture callus was an additional osteogenic stimulus for fibular hypertrophy and internal repair of the allograft.

Nonunion of osteotomies has been reported as a common complication in allograft surgery [4, 5]. In this series, a nonunion was observed in 4% of cases, and perfect healing was always achieved after autogenous bone grafting. The osteogenic properties of the vascularized fibula proved effective in promoting an early union.

Special indications to combined allograft procedure are the chances to preserve important anatomical structures. Metadiaphyseal tumors of the knee joint are commonly treated by intra-articular resection even when the articular surface and the subchondral bone are not involved by the tumor. In these cases, an intraepiphyseal resection can be performed, preserving a thin fragment of articular surface, and intercalary reconstruction is feasible with the combined allograft procedure. Minimal fixation is necessary at the epiphyseal osteotomy, while a rigid osteosynthesis is required at the diaphyseal level. In our experience, the union of osteotomies is quickly achieved. Initial stability of the

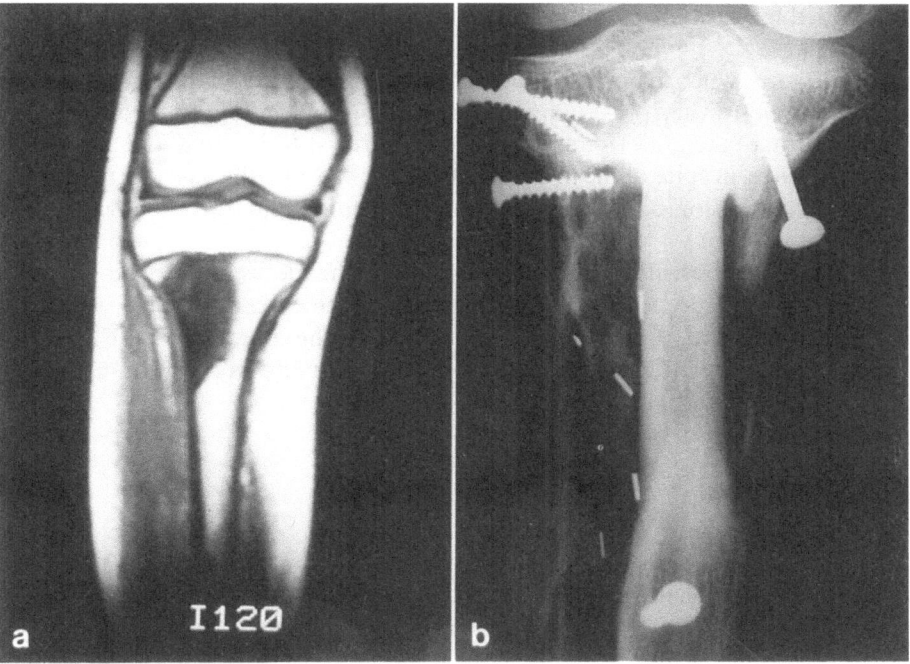

Fig. 2. a MRI of metaphyseal osteosarcoma in a 9 years old boy; **b** An intraepiphyseal resection was performed, and reconstruction was done with a concentric combined allograft. X-ray follow-up, five years later, shows union of osteotomies, hypertrophy of the fibula and partial resorption of the allograft shell

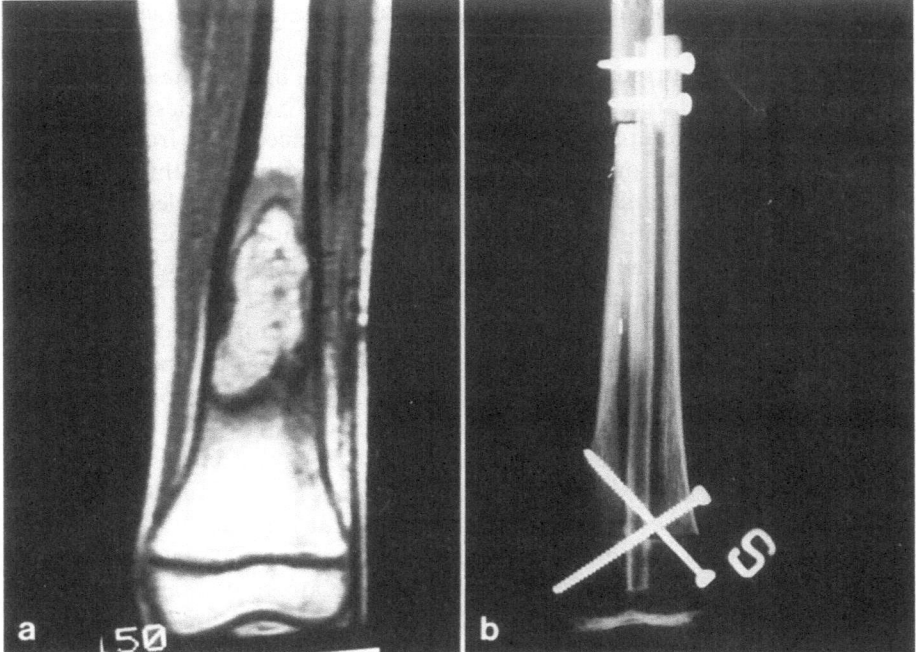

Fig. 3. a Distal femur osteosarcoma in a 12 years old boy; **b** Metaphyseal resection was performed preserving the growth plate. No leg length discrepancy was present at last follow-up 5 years later

implant is provided by the allograft, and late stability is supplied by the hyperthrophied fibula (Fig. 2a, b).

In growing patients, when a metadiaphyseal tumor does not involve the growth plate and resection can be performed preserving the physis, combined allograft reconstruction with minimal fixation of the graft (Kirschner wires or screws) allows to avoid epiphysiodesis. In our experience, in spite of the low stability of the fixation, the vascularized fibula provides the necessary biologic activity to achieve early union and quick recovery of the patient (Figs. 1b and 3a, b).

When a distal tibial resection is performed, an arthrodesis reconstruction with combined allograft procedure is feasible. With minimal screw fixation of the grafts it is possible to achieve an arthrodesis with the talus preserving the subtalar joint (Fig. 1c). In this situation, expecially in children, subtalar joint function allows a flexion-extension range of up to 60° degrees.

References

1. Berrey BH Jr, Lord CF, Gebhardt MC, Mankin HJ (1990) Fractures of allografts. Frequency, treatment and end-result. J Bone Joint Surg 72-A: 825–833
2. Capanna R, Bufalini C, Campanacci M (1993) A new technique for reconstructions of large metadiaphyseal bone defects—a combined graft (Allograft Shell plus Vascularized Fibula). Orthop Traumatol 2 (3): 159–177
3. Enneking WF, Mindell ER (1991) Observations on massive retrieved human allografts. J Bone Joint Surg 73-A, 8: 1123–1142
4. Gebhardt MC, Flugstad DI, Springfield DS, Mankin HJ (1991) The use of bone allograft for limb salvage in high-grade extremity osteosarcoma. Clin Orthop 270: 181–196

5. Mankin HJ, Doppelt S, Tomford W (1982) Clinical experience with allograft transplantation. The first ten years. Clin Orthop 174: 69–86
6. Taylor GY, Miller GDH, Ham FJ (1975) The free vascularized bone grafts. Plast Reconstr Surg 55: 533
7. Zehr RJ, Enneking WF, Heare T, Liang TS (1991) Fractures in large structural allografts. In: Brown KLB (ed) Complication of limb salvage. International Symposium on limb Salvage, Montreal, pp 3–8

Authors' addresses: D.A. Campanacci and R. Capanna, Department of Orthopaedic Oncology and Reconstructive Surgery, Centro Traumatologico Ortopedico, Firenze, Italy; M. Ceruso, R. Angeloni, M. Innocenti, G. Lauri and C. Bufalini, Department of Hand Surgery and Reconstructive Microsurgery, Centro Traumatologico Ortopedico, Largo Palagi 1, I-50139 Firenze, Italy; M. Manfrini and A. Gasbarrini, University Clinic, Istituto Orthopedico Rizzoli, Via Pupilli 1, Bologna, Italy.

Allografts in Malignant Bone Tumors

M. San Julian, S. Amillo, and J. Cañadell

Department of Orthopaedic Surgery, University Clinic of Navarre, School of Medicine, University of Navarre, Pamplona, Spain

Introduction

In order to cure primary malignant bone tumors it is necessary to perform en bloc resection of all macroscopic disease. The available surgical procedures give two main options: amputation and limb-sparing techniques. Over recent years the introduction of modern diagnostic techniques and the widespread use of preoperative chemotherapy, radiotherapy and multiagent adjuvant chemotheraphy have aided in the development of limb preserving techniques.

With the development of bone banks [1, 6], reconstructive surgery with massive allografts represents a successful alternative to prosthetic implants in young patients with long life expectancy. Allografts offer advantages over metallic implants such as the ability to replace articulating joint surfaces, allowing union to host bone and attachment of soft tissues [7]. From June 1986 to October 1994 at the University Clinic of Navarre we used 142 massive bone allografts in the conservative treatment of malignant bone tumors. The purpose of this study is to analyze the clinical results, the complications and the consolidation time of these allografts and to analyze the factors which influenced the outcome.

Patients and Methods

We have reviewed the first 142 allografts used in limb preserving therapy of bone tumors implanted in 128 patients (14 patients had their allografts removed due to infection, fracture or recurrence and a second allograft was implanted; and in 5 of these cases the allograft was removed and substituted for a third). The histological diagnosis of the resected specimens was: 74 osteogenic sarcomas, 19 Ewings's sarcomas, 10 chondrosarcomas, 7 malignant fibrous hystocytomas, 6 fibrosarcomas, 3 aggressive giant cell tumors, 3 metastatic tumors and 1 myeloma.

The preoperative staging studies included: conventional radiology, digitalized angiography, radionuclide scan, CT scan, MRI, and biopsy by percutaneous puncture. In the surgical indication we did not take into account Enneking's criteria regarding intra or extra compartmental involvement. We also took an X ray and CT scan of the lung to rule out metastatic disease.

Allografts were harvested under sterile conditions from cadaveric donors, and they were cryopreserved, following the guidelines of the American Association of Tissue

Banks [6]. Laboratory exams included cultures for anaerobic and aerobic bacteria, the VDRL test, and serology for hepatitis B and C virus and HIV.

When dealing with a primary, non metastatic tumor, we performed en bloc resection including the biopsy scar. The level of osteotomy was determined on the basis of the intramedullary spread of the tumor as revealed by the CT scan and the MRI. Our tumor safe margin was 5 cm. We performed intraoperative biopsy of the resection margins. Every patient received prophylactic cephalosporins. Chemotherapy and radiotherapy were performed following the University Clinic of Navarre Cancer Protocol [16, 17].

The allograft type depended on the involvement of the cartilage growth plate and the possibilities of preserving the joint near the tumor. The following reconstructions were performed:

- 48 composite allograft-prostheses (41 knee prostheses, 3 total hip and 2 partial hip prostheses, and 1 shoulder prostheses into a fresh frozen allograft (in the same patient we used an osteoarticular elbow allograft because we performed the replacement of the whole humerus)
- 46 intercalary allografts (in 20 cases we used Canadell's technique to preserve epiphysis [3])
- 27 osteoarticular allografts
- 8 arthrodesis with corticocancellous allografts
- 6 pelvic allografts
- 4 anterior spinal fusions with femoral allografts
- 2 sternal reconstructions with iliac allografts.

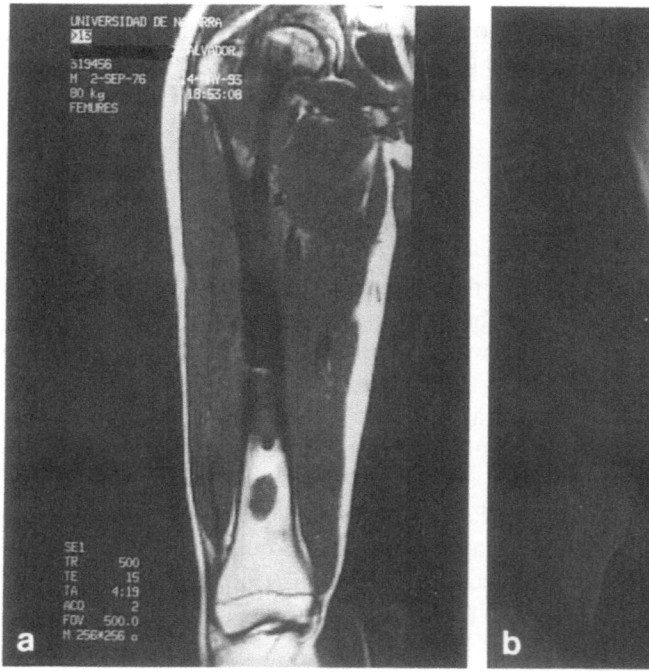
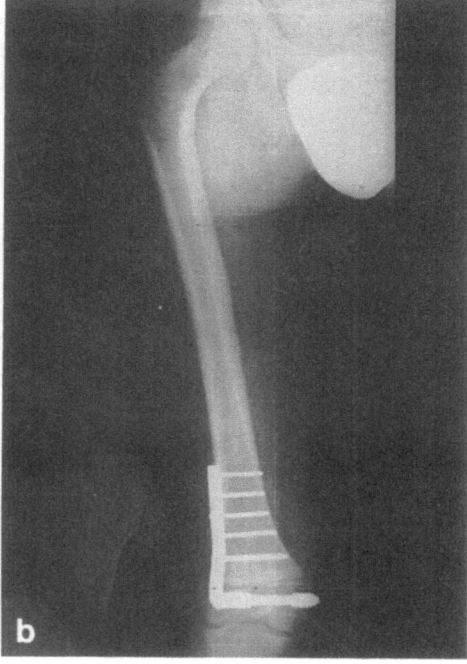

Fig. 1. a Osteosarcoma involving almost the whole femur, with a skip metastasis in the distal metaphysis; **b** In this case we used the longest osteoarticular allograft of the series (42 cm) from the proximal epiphysis to the distal metaphysis

The mean allograft length was 18 cms (range, 4 to 42) (Fig. 1a and 1b) and the mean age of the group was 19.6 years (range, 4 to 69). The mean follow-up time was 33.7 months (range, 3 to 78).

We did monthly follow-ups during the first year of systemic chemotherapy, with diagnostic studies to assess the local and systemic control of disease. Afterwards, follow-ups were carried out every three months for another year, and then every six months.

Results

Functional Results

The functional results rated according to Mankin's classification [7] were excellent in 37.29%, good in 42.37%, fair in 16.95% and poor in 3.39%. The results were excellent or good in about 80% of the cases (87.8% in intercalary allografts, 82% in endoprostheses of the knee, 73% in arthrodeses, and 40% in pelvic allografts).

Allograft Consolidation

The mean consolidation time of metaphyseal osteotomies was 6.5 months, and we did not find any statistically significant influence of the studied factors. We observed one nonunion, without clinical significance, in a patient in whom we used a tibia allograft to perform an ankle arthrodesis. Consolidation was achieved in many cases with minimal osteosynthesis.

The mean consolidation time of diaphyseal osteotomies was sixteen months. We found statistically significant differences with: the use of systemic chemotherapy ($p < 0.05$), the use of external radiotherapy ($p < 0.01$), (both factors delayed consolidation), and recipient age ($p < 0.01$), (the older the patient, the worse the consolidation results). We have not found statistically significant differences with: the use of intra-arterial chemotherapy, intraoperative radiotherapy, donor's age, osteosynthesis type (plates vs. intramedullary devices), osteotomy type (horizontal vs. oblique), type of tumor, or location of the tumor. There were seven diaphyseal nonunions (5.5%).

In 15 diaphyseal osteotomies reosteosynthesis and autogenous iliac bone grafting was needed. Most of these were osteosyntheses performed with plates, some of them deficient ones performed in children with the osteosynthesis "ad minimum" law.

Infection

Nineteen patients (13.3%) suffered infection of their allograft. The treatment of the infections was as following:

In 3 cases, surgical debridment and antibiotics was the only treatment. In 16 cases, the allograft was removed. In these cases we used external fixation during the antibiotic treatment. The status of these 16 cases is as follows:

− In 9 cases we performed an allograft replacement after the infection was cured with antibiotics.
− In 5 cases, we removed the allograft and used a plastic spacer, cement or endoprosthesis without allograft.
− The other 2 cases are waiting for allograft replacement with an external fixation system in place.

Fracture

We observed eight allograft fractures (5.8%). Five of these consolidated with standard treatment of the fracture (osteosynthesis and autologous bone grafting). In the other three cases we performed an allograft replacement.

Discussion

The functional results were excellent or good in 80% of the cases. The best results were obtained with the use of intercalary allografts. The negative results clearly depended on complications (nonunion, fracture or infection) or the use of external radiotherapy. In every particular case we used the most adequate option for the patient.

In diaphyseal tumors with five centimeters safe margin on both sides of the tumor, we used intercalary allografts.

In metaphyseal tumors without invasion of the epiphysis, we performed physeal distraction following Canadell's technique [3], and reconstruction with intercalary allografts.

In tumors involving the epiphysis in the knee, osteoarticular allografts resulted in poor results in our experience, and therefore we prefer composite allograft-prostheses (Fig. 2a and 2b) if the patient is not too young.

In the ankle, shoulder, elbow and in some cases in the hip, the results with osteoarticular allografts have been very good.

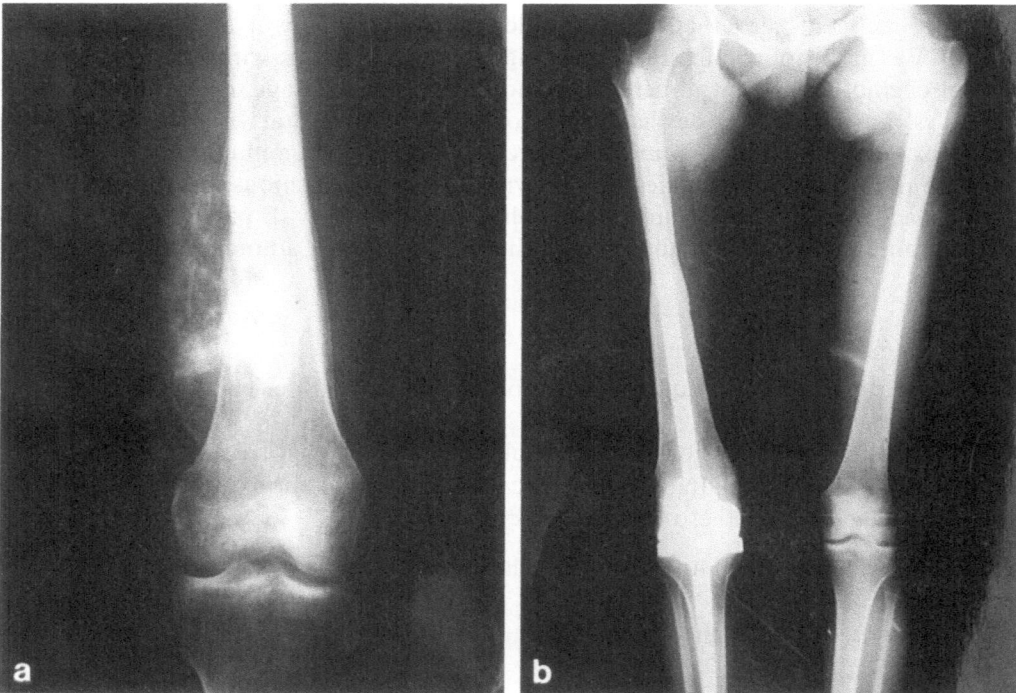

Fig. 2. a, b Osteosarcoma in the distal femur treated with composite allograft-prosthesis

In tumors involving vertebral bodies, femoral allografts give strong support in anterior spinal fusion. In extremities, arthrodesis with allograft has been used only in a few cases, when the condition of the limb did not allow another possibility.

In our patients metaphyseal osteotomies consolidated after a mean time of six months, which is similar to the time reported by Vander Griend [22]. While the mean consolidation time of diaphyseal osteotomies was 16 months in our series, the mean consolidation time was 9 in Vander Griend's (even though he does not give the criteria to determine consolidation) and 18 months in Mankin's [11]. In both series, almost half of the patients did not receive chemotherapy (giant cell tumors, low grade chondrosarcomas, etc.), while in ours, most of the patients (86%) received chemotherapy after the implantation of the allograft. We think that systematic chemotherapy plays an important role in delaying consolidation. In our series we found statistically significant differences between those patient who had intensive adjuvant chemotherapy for a year after the operation and those who did not. Our finding is supported by clinical data from other series [4, 5, 12, 18]. Shinohara found that all grafted bone in patients receiving chemotherapy failed to heal primarily [19]. Experimental studies [9, 24] have also proved that chemotherapeutic agents impair bone healing and that allogeneic cortical bone grafts incorporate more slowly when chemotherapy is administered.

In our series external radiation also delayed consolidation. Ionizing radiation is known to have a deleterious effect on skeletal growth, which results from alteration of chondroblastic, and periosteal activity [8, 15]. Radiation also damages small and medium blood vessels that supply nutrients to the bone, reducing the chances for irradiated bone to heal [18].

Our percentage of nonunion was similar to the one reported in other series [7, 11, 13, 14, 22]. Seven of the eight nonunions occurred in diaphyseal osteotomies. Some authors advocate routine autogeneic bone graft supplementation at the allograft-host junction, at the time of graft implantation [2, 23]. We only used autogenous graft in patients with delayed consolidation, to avoid morbidity at the donor site.

We thought that oblique osteotomies would heal faster than transverse ones, due to the larger contact area between allograft and host bone, as other authors suggest [25]. However, we did not find any statistically significant difference in the consolidation time between the two osteotomy types. Therefore, presently we use the oblique osteotomies only to avoid rotation when we use non-locked intramedullary systems.

Another important factor in our study has been the type of osteosynthesis. Although we did not find statistically significant differences in the consolidation time and the rate of union, we prefer to use intramedullary devices over plates whenever possible. Intramedullary stems allow weigh bearing immediately after surgery [10, 22], contrary to plates which require partial weight until consolidation is achieved. In our study fixation with a plate was associated with a higher rate of fracture of the allograft, as reported by others [22] and with the need for reosteosynthesis, particularly in diaphyseal osteotomies following the osteosynthesis "ad minimum" principle which we followed at the beginning in children.

In fractures through the shaft of the allograft, some authors favour replacement [11, 22] of the allograft or even amputation [7], because of the limited intrinsic healing potential of allografts. In our series we achieved graft fracture consolidation with conventional treatment in five cases, as found by others [20].

Our infection rate was 13.3%. It appears very high, but it is important to take into account that in our series most of the patients were immunodeficient because of the chemotherapy treatment. In other series the infection rate varied between ten and thirty percent [5, 11, 12, 21], and the lower rates were reported in patients without chemotherapy treatment where the allografts were implanted after resection of benign tumors. Bacterial infection is considered to be the most devastating complication after transplantation of large bone allografts. In all cases in our series the infection was cured without the need for amputation.

References

1. Amillo S, Cara J A, Valenti JR (1990) Banco de tejidos del sistema musculoesqueletico. Aplicaciones clinicas. Rev Med Univ Navarra 227–234
2. Aro HT, Aho AJ (1993) Clinical use of bone allografts. Ann Med 25: 403–412
3. Cañadell J, Forriol F, Cara JA (1994) Removal of methaphyseal bone tumors with preservation of the epiphysis. Physeal distraction before excision. J Bone Joint Surg 76-B: 127–132
4. Delépine N, Delépine G, Hernigou PH, Desbois J (1989) Bone union of allografts and chemotherapy considerations about 55 consecutives cases. 5th International Symposium on Limb Salvage. St Malo 5
5. Dyck H, Malinin T, Mnaymneh W (1988) Massive allograft inplantation following radical resection of high grade tumours requiring neoadjuvant chemotherapy treatment. Clin Orthop 197: 88
6. Friedlander GE, Mankin H (1981) Bone banking: current methods and suggested guidelines. AAOS Instr Course Lect 30: 36–48
7. Gebhardt M, Flugstad D, Springfield D, Mankin H (1991) The use of bone grafts for limb salvage in high-grade extremity osteosarcoma. Clin Orthop 270: 181–196
8. Goldwein JW (1991) Effects of radiation therapy in skeletal growth in childhood. Clin Orthop 262: 101–107
9. Khoo DB (1992) The effect of chemotherapy on soft tissue and bone healing in the rabbit model. Ann Acad Med Singapore 21: 217–221
10. Kohler R, Lorge F, Brunat-Mentigny M, Noyer D, Patricot L (1990) Massive bone allografts in children. Int Orthop (SICOT) 14: 249–253
11. Mankin H, Springfield D, Gebhart M, Tomford W (1992) Current status of allografting for bone tumors. Ortopedics 15: 1147–1154
12. Mnaymneh W, Malinin T, Lackman R, Hornicek J, Ghandur-Mnaimneh L (1994) Massive distal femoral allografts after resection of bone tumors. Clin Orthop 303: 103–115
13. Ottolenghi CE (1972) Massive osteo and osteoarticular bone grafts: technic and results of 62 cases. Clin Orthop 87: 156–164
14. Parrish FF (1973) Allograft replacement of all or part of the end of a long bone following excision of a tumor. Report of twenty one cases. J Bone Joint Surg 55-A: 1–22
15. Rubin P (1975) Radiation biology and radiation pathology syllabus. Chicago, Illinois American College of Radiology
16. Sierrasesumaga L, Antillon F, Canadell J (1991) Treatment of Ewing's sarcoma. Protocol, description, applications and results. In: Canadell J, Sierrasesumaga L, Calvo F, Ganoza (eds) Treatment of malignant bone tumors in children and adolescents. Servico de Publicaciones de la Universidad de Navarra S.A., Pamplona
17. Sierrasesúmaga L, Antillón F, Cañadell J (1991) Treatment of osteosarcoma. Protocol, description, applications and results. In: Cañadell J, Sierrasusúmaga L, Calvo F, Ganoza (eds) Treatment of malignant bone tumors in children and adolescent. Servico de publicaciones de la Univesidad de navarra S.A., Pamplona
18. Silverman EN (1948) The skeletal lesions in leukemia: clinical and roentgenographic observations in 103 infants and children, with a review of the literature. AJR 59: 818
19. Sinohara N, Sumida S, Masuda S (1990) Bone allografts after segmental resection of tumours. Int Orthop 14: 273–276
20. Thompson RC, Pickvance EA, Garry D (1993) Fractures in large-segment allografts. J Bone Joint Surg 75-A: 1663–16673
21. Tomford WW, Tohongphasuk J, Mankin JH, Feraro MJ (1990) Frozen musculoskeletal allografts: A study of the clinical incidence and causes of infection associated with their use. J Bone Joint Surg 72A: 1137–1141

22. Vander Griend R (1994) The effect of internal fixation in the healing of large allografts. J Bone Joint
    Surg 76A: 657–664
23. Wong JW, Shih CH (1993) Allograft transplantation for aggressive or malignant bone tumors. Clin
    Orthop 297: 203–209
24. Zart DJ, Miya L, Wolff DA, Mackley JT, Stevanson S (1993) The effects of cisplatin on the
    incorporation of fresh syngeneic and frozen allogeneic cortical bone grafts. J Orthop Res 11:
    240–249
25. Zatsepin ST, Burdygin VN (1994) Replacement of the distal femur and proximal tibia with frozen
    allografts. Clin Orthop 303: 95–102

Authors' address: M. San-Julian, S. Amillo and J. Cañadell, Department of Orthopaedic Surgery,
University Clinic of Navarre, School of Medicine, University of Navarre, Avda. Pio XII s/n, E-31080
Pamplona, Spain.

Allograft Prosthetic Reconstruction: Review of 120 Composite Prostheses (1984–1992), A Monocentric Study

G. Delepine[1], N. Delepine[2], and D. Goutallier[1]

[1]Hôpital Henri Mondor, Service d'Orthopédie, Créteil, France
[2]Hôpital Robert Debré, Service d'Oncologie Pédiatrique, Paris, France

Introduction

Adequate excision of malignant bone tumors often results in a large osteoarticular defect which needs to be suitably replaced in order to restore a functional limb. The lost bone can be replaced with a massive prosthesis, but the extensive loss of muscle attachments increases stress at the interface between the bone and the prosthesis and reduces the range of active movement. Unless a modular prosthesis is used, it is difficult to adapt the size of a custom-built prosthesis implant during surgery. For these reasons, replacement with a bone graft is now preferred in many situations in spite of the risk of infection, nonunion, secondary fracture and resorption when immunodepressive chemotherapy and/or high dose radiotherapy are used [2, 3, 9, 10].

For these cases, we developed [4, 8] long stem titanium prostheses combined with massive bank allografts. We analyse here the results of our 12 year experience in a single institution.

Rationale for Using a Composite Prosthesis

Composite prostheses have at least four functions:

- Facilitating muscle and ligament reattachment to the implant and thus improving stability and active motion.
- Preventing loosening by changing the lever arm of the large prosthesis to a short one of a common prosthesis as soon as bone healing occurs.
- Restoring bone stock after tumor resection.
- Limiting bone resorption due to stress shielding by transmitting some of the forces applied to the graft to the remaining part of the host bone.

Satisfactory function of composite prostheses is achieved when these functions are satisfied. Bone fusion is mandatory to accomplish all these functions.

Methods and Patients

Patients

From 1984 to 1992, we used 120 long stem prostheses combined with massive bank allografts to reconstruct bone defects secondary to en bloc resection for bone tumors. The age of patients ranged from five years to 87 years (median 18 years). The histological examination revealed 65 cases of osteosarcoma, 18 cases of Ewing's sarcoma, 12 cases of chondrosarcoma, 10 cases of fibrosarcoma or malignant fibrous histiocytoma, and 15 others. According to Enneking's classification, the stage was IA in 8, IB in 24, IIA in 1, IIB in 73 and IIIB in 14 cases.

The tumor location was the distal femur in 59 cases, proximal tibia in 33, upper femur in 16 and proximal humerus in 12 cases. The average length of the bone defect after resection was 21 cm (minimum 6 – maximum 37 cm).

Prosthesis

All implants were custom-made prostheses with individualized sizes according to the author's designs. Forged titanium alloy was chosen for its better mechanical properties (almost twice as light and twice as plastic as stainless steel). The average fabrication time was ten days.

The knee prosthesis was a hinge prosthesis with a titanium axis and polyethylene bearings. The femoral stem had a 5° valgus alignment. The size of the epiphyseal part of the prosthesis was small enough to be inserted from the age of five years and its smooth edges limited soft tissue trauma. No trochlea was necessary. A patellar component was used only in 4 cases of extra-articular resection.

The proximal femoral prosthesis had a metaphyseal part similar to the Merle d'Aubigné model C with modular heads allowing the choice of head material and size.

The proximal humeral prosthesis had a metaphyseal antirotation part, an individualized epiphyseal part and a stem permitting a good fit with the scapula and distal humeral diaphysis.

Allograft

The allografts were all provided by the bone bank of Hospital Henri Mondor in Creteil (Pr Goutallier) [6]. They were removed from organ donors under sterile conditions in the operating room and immediately frozen to −30°. They were stored at −30° for a period not less than three months and not exceeding one year. All allografts were preoperatively sterilized by beta irradiation (2.5–3.5 Mrads) [1, 6].

Operative Technique

The graft was removed from the freezer three hours before operation, cut with an oscillating saw, and then smoothly reamed with special tools in order to permit an excellent fit at the junction between the allograft and host bone. Before implantation, the stem of the prosthesis was cemented into the allograft and the composite prosthesis was cemented into the host diaphysis. In 30 cases the preserved tendons of the host were reattached directly to the allograft. In 13 cases, the en bloc resection could preserve some periarticular tendon reattachments with their bony insertions (e.g.: trochanter, tibial tuberosity) that were reattached to the graft. In other 18 cases, the tibial allograft was harvested with the adjacent patellar tendon and the patella permitting a bony suture of the patella of the patient to the patella of the graft. A fresh autogenous graft harvested from the opposite epiphysis (proximal tibia for distal femoral tumor and distal femur for proximal tibial tumor) was put around the allograft-host junction.

Postoperative Care

Weight bearing was immediate (except in two cases) but active motion was restricted for 45 days in the upper tibial and humeral reconstructions to help muscle reattachment. 88 patients underwent postoperative chemotherapy (average duration: ten months) and 31 radiotherapy (35–45 grays).

Follow Up

All patients were followed up by the same physicians with clinical examination, anteroposterior and lateral radiographs, lung and local computerized tomographies and bone scan every three months for two years, then every six months for three years and then every year. The resection follow up was 5.5 years.

The functional result was rated according to the Enneking evaluation system taking into consideration pain, mobility, deformity, stability, cosmetic appearance and patient acceptance.

The radiologic evaluation followed the EMSOS four-grade rating system as follows:

- *Bone remodelling* is evaluation as 4 grades:
  - No change (Fig. 1)
  - Osteopenia, hypertrophy, sclerosis, bone angulation
  - Resorption of the fixation area <50% cortical thickness and <2 cms length
  - Resorption of the fixation area >50% cortical thickness or >2 cms length (Fig. 2)
- *Interface* is evaluated in 4 grades:
  - No radiolucent line
  - <2 mm thick and incomplete radiolucent line
  - >2 mm incomplete or complete <2 mm radiolucent line, axial migration <5 mm
  - Complete >2 mm radiolucent line, axial migration <5 mm, loosening (Fig. 3).
- *Fusion* is evaluated in 4 grades:
  - osteotomy line no longer visible (Fig. 4)
  - Fusion >or =75%
  - Fusion 25–75%
  - Fusion <25% or no evidence of callus (Fig. 5)
- *Resorption* is evaluated in 4 grades:
  - No resorption or geometric change periostal new bone
  - Resorption <25% and no fracture
  - Resorption 25–50% and no fracture
  - Resorption >50% one fracture with graft dissolution.
- *Fracture* of the graft is evaluated as 4 different degrees:
  - No fracture
  - Incomplete fracture
  - Simple fracture without displacement (Fig. 6)
  - Simple fracture with displacement or comminuted fracture (Figs. 5 and 7)

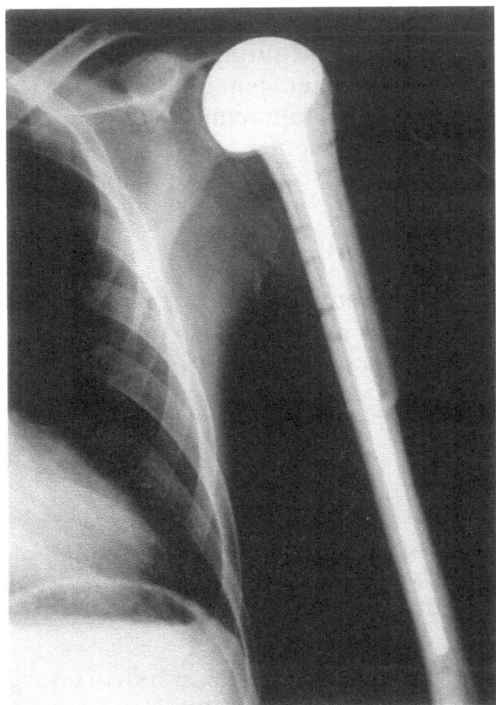

Fig. 1. Composite prosthesis 4 years after resection of upper humeral osteosarcoma. Good functional result. No bone remodelling

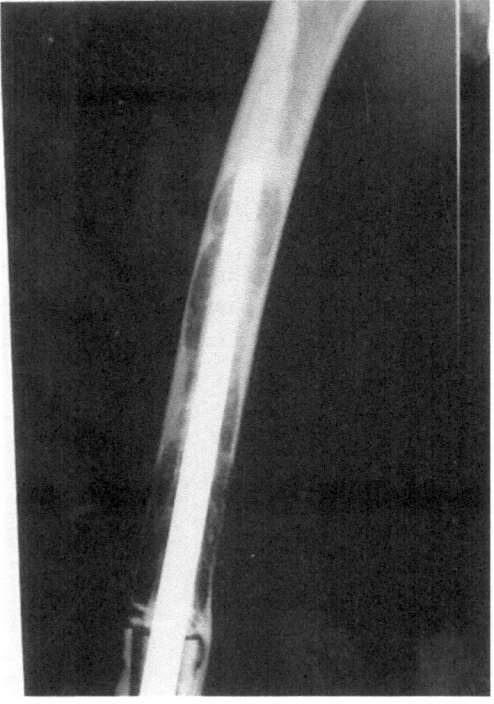

Fig. 2. Distal femur reconstruction with composite prosthesis. Peripheric fusion (grade 2) but severe resorption of fixation area 7 years after operation. Evolution to complete loosening compelling to reoperate

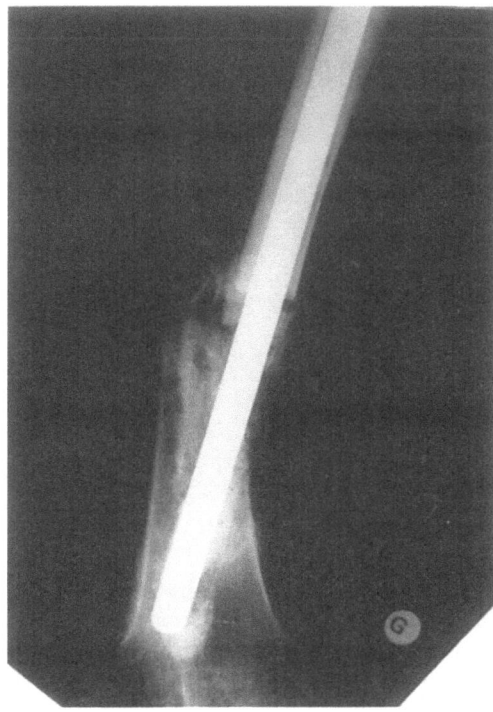

Fig. 3. Osteosarcoma of proximal femur. Bad responder to preoperative chemotherapy. Resection of 27 cms or proximal femur with composite prosthesis, postoperative radiotherapy (45 Gys). 4 years after implantation, no evidence of callus and loosening

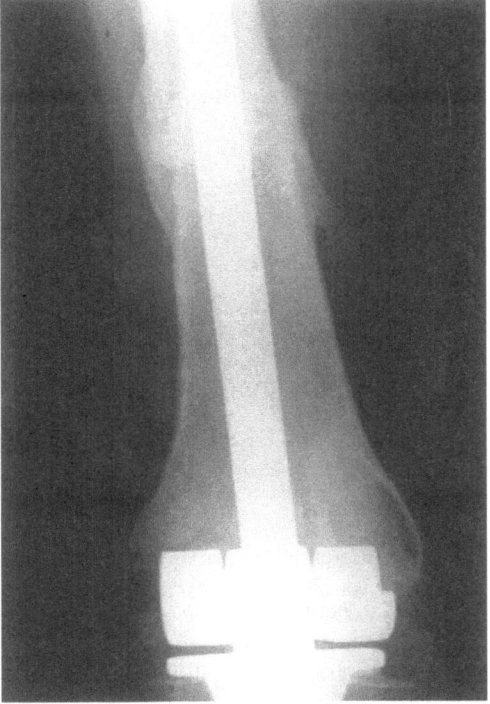

Fig. 4. Low grade chondrosarcoma of distal femur treated by resection and composite prosthesis without adjuvant therapy. Good fusion, no bone remodelling 4 years after implantation

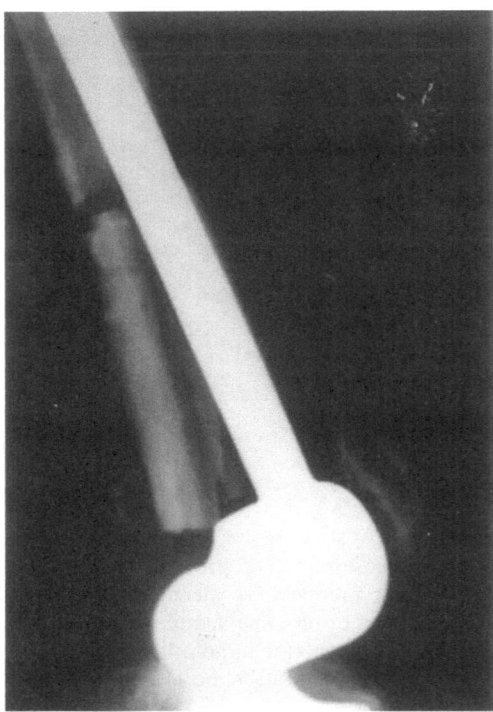

Fig. 5. Osteosarcoma previously treated by high dose radiotherapy (75 Gys) secondary fracture treated by composite prosthesis. 3 years after implantation, no fusion and comminuted fracture of the allograft

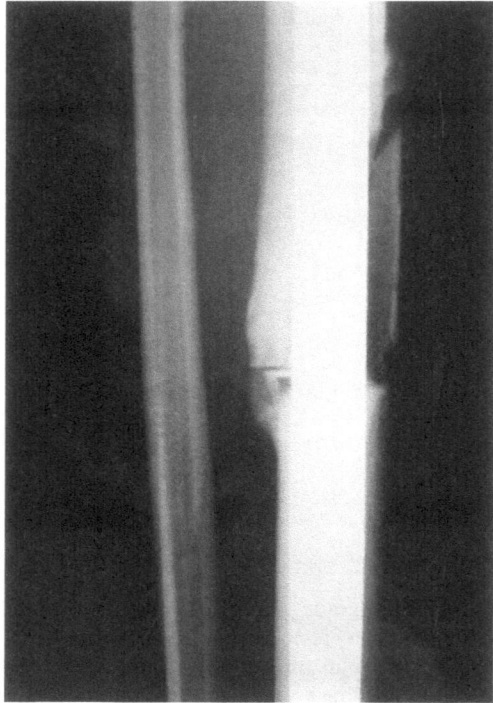

Fig. 6. Osteosarcoma of proximal tibia treated by multidrug chemotherapy and low dose radiotherapy (bad responder to preoperative chemotherapy) five years after implantation fracture of the graft without displacement. Good clinical evolution

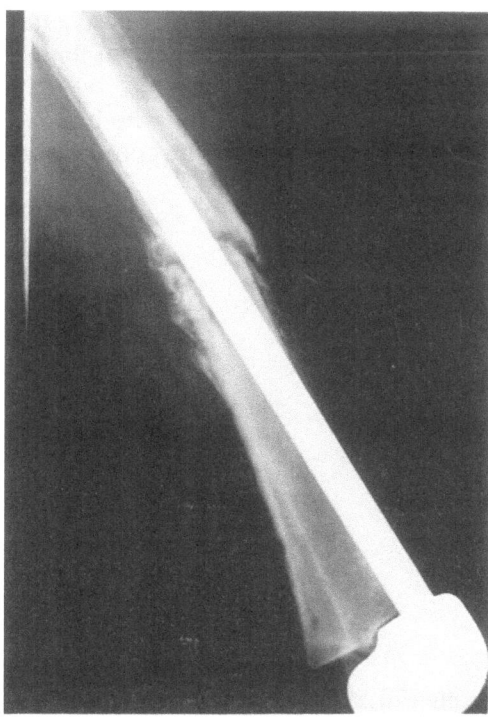

Fig. 7. Osteosarcoma of distal femur treated by chemotherapy and high dose radiotherapy (65 Gys). Comminuted Fracture 2 years after implantation

Results

Postoperative Complications

Infection

Deep infection remains the worst complication. Ten infections (8%) were observed. Nine of these ten occurred in the 88 patients (10%) who had chemotherapy and/or radiotherapy while only one was seen in the 32 patients (3%) who did not receive adjuvant treatment.

Deep infections were seen mostly on upper tibia composite prostheses performed without gastrocnemius flaps (1984–1989). The risk was dramatically reduced by the systematic use of gastrocnemius flaps as advocated by Malawer.

The prognosis of deep infection is poor. In spite of multiple reoperations, the infection could be cured in only 4 patients and amputation had to be performed in six other patients. Among the prognostic factors for deep infection, the preoperative value of radiotherapy must be underlined. 89 patients were not irradiated. Four of these developed deep infection. Three of these could be cured and one leg was amputated. Of thirty-one patients irradiated, six had deep infection. Five of these limbs were secondarily amputated.

Other complications were wound slough (25 cases), phlebitis, hip dislocation (5 cases).

Functional results rated following the Enneking EMSOS criteria for the 120 composite prostheses were as follows: excellent in 30, good in 52, fair in 28, poor in 10.

If we compare the results of composite prostheses with those observed after massive prostheses, the functional improvement is spectacular for the upper femur. and quite clear for the proximal tibia.

The functional results were better in patients without chemotherapy who had less postoperative complications than others. This is shown in the following comparison:

Results in 32 low grade sarcomas treated without chemotherapy:
– Excellent in 18 (55%)
– good in 8 (25%)
– fair in three (9%)
– poor in one (3%)

Results in 88 patients treated, with adjuvant chemotherapy:

– Excellent in 12 (14%)
– good in 44 (50%)
– fair in 25 (27%)
– poor in 9 (10%).

Radiological Evaluation

- *Implant body*:
  There was no change of the implant body in our 120 cases.

- *Bone remodelling*
  – No change: 75
  – osteopenia: 25
  – Resorption of fixation area: 20

- *Resorption*:
  – No resorption or periosteal new bone: 105
  – Resorption <25% and no fracture: 10
  – Resorption 25–50%: 5
- *Fusion*:
  – No visible line: 75
  – Fusion >75%: 17
  – Fusion 25–75%: 16
  – Fusion <25: 12

- *Nonunion* is defined by the persistence of a radiolucent line at the allograft host junction. We observed twelve nonunions (10%) in composite prostheses, most of them in humeral prostheses that had no significant autografting of the junction or in patients treated with chemotherapy and radiotherapy.

  Nonunion was less frequent in children (2/35: 5%) compared to adults (10/85:12%). The complication of nonunion are poor bone remodelling, and a higher risk of implant loosening (7 of 12). The treatment of nonunion was autograft packing (effective if no chemotherapy).

- *Fracture of the allograft*:
  – No fracture: 88
  – incomplete: 23
  – single without displacement: 4
  – Complete with displacement and loosening: 5

Complete fractures of allografts combined with prostheses were seen in nine cases (7.5%) at an average time of 21 months. Four fractures healed spontaneously, five required reoperation for loosening. In these nine cases, five fractures were seen in the irradiated field (four loosened and were reoperated, two of these were secondarily amputated). Four fractures were in patients who were not irradiated (only one loosening was cured by reoperation).

- *Interface*:
  - No radiolucent line: 85
  - <2 mm and complete <2 mm radiolucent line: 10
  - complete >2 mm radiolucent line: 18
  - Loosening: 7

- *Anchorage*:
  - No change: 103
  - Cement fracture: 10
  - Cement fracture with motion of stem: 7
- *Loosening* of composite prostheses was seen in 13 cases out of 120. Seven cases were loosenings of the massive part (6%), all following non-union, five of seven with allograft or host fracture. Six were loosenings of the standard part (5%), all in hinge prostheses. We didn't observe any prosthesis fracture.

Conclusion

1. A more rapid recovery and a better functional result occurs in patients treated with composite prostheses compared to allograft alone or massive prostheses.
2. The long stem prosthesis does not completely abolish the risk of fracture of an allograft cemented around its stem and a massive allograft does not avoid loosening in all cases.
3. There is an increased risk of deep infection, nonunion, allograft fracture and implant loosening when high dose chemotherapy and radiotherapy are used.

Recommendations

1. The prostheses must be specially designed for tumor surgery and feature modular systems, high fatigue resistance, high elasticity modulus, stress-shielding limiting designs.
2. Allografts should include tendons including the patellar tendon and the patella for extensor apparatus reconstruction, the rotator cuff for shoulder reconstruction, and the greater trochanter with gluteal tendon for hip stabilisation.
3. The surgical procedure must be adapted to adjuvant chemotherapy which delays bone union by using strong fixation of the allograft to the prosthesis (cement), precise fitting of the allograft to the host bone (size selection and special tools), autografting of the host-graft junction and good muscular coverage (flap).

References

1. Bright R, Samarsh J, Gambill V (1983) Sterilization of human bone by irradiation; in osteochondral allografts. Boston, Toronto: Little, Brown and Co, pp 223–232

2. Brooks DB, Heiple KG, Herndon CH, Powell AE (1963) Immunological factors in homogeneous bone transplants. Effect of various methods of preparation and irradiation on antigenicity. J Bone Joint Surg (Am) 45: 1617–1628
3. Delepine G, Delepine N (1988) Résultats préliminairos de 79 allogreffes osseuses massives dans le traitement conservateur des tumeurs malignes de l'adulte et de l'enfant. Int Orthop (SICOT) 12: 21–29
4. Delepine G, Delepine N (1985) Titanium new prostheses combined with bone graft. In: Coombs R, Friedlander G (eds) Bone tumour management. London: Butterworths, pp 211–219
5. Eckardi JJ, Eilber FR, Mirra JM (1987) Kinematic rotating hinge knee-distal femoral replacement. In: Ennecking WF (ed) Limb salvage in musculoskeletal oncology. New York: Churchill Livingstone, pp 392–399
6. Hernigou Ph, Delepine G, Goutallier D (1986) Allogreffes massives cryoconservées et stérilisées par irradiation. Revue de Chirurgie Orthop (Paris) 72: 403–413
7. Kaufer H, Matthews JS, Sonstegard DA (1976/1978) Total knee loosening A.A.O.S. symposium on the reconstructive surgery of the knee. Rochester, New York, May 1976, St. Louis C.V. Mosby Cie 1978, p 378
8. Langlais F, Delepine G, Dubousset JF, et al (1991) Composite prostheses in malignant tumors. Rationale and preliminary results of 42 cases. In: Langlais F (ed) Limb salvage. Berlin: Springer, pp 387–394
9. Mankin HJ, Dopplet S, Tomford W (1983) Clinical experience with allograft implantation. The first ten years. Clin Orthop 174: 69–86
10. Ottolenghi CE (1972) Massive osteo and osteo-articular bone grafts. technic and results of 62 cases. Clin Orthop 87: 156–164

Authors' addresses: G. Delepine, M.D., 8 rue Eugène Varlin, F-93700 Drancy, France; N. Delepine, M.D., Hôpital Robert Debré, Service d'Oncologie Pédiatrique, Paris, France; D. Goutallier, M.D., Hôpital Henri Mondor, Service d'orthopédie, F-94000 Géteil, France.

The Importance of Allograft with Patellar Tendon in Prosthetic Reconstruction of the Upper Tibia after en bloc Resection for Bone Tumors

G. Delepine[1], P.G. Harris[2], N. Delepine[3], and D. Goutallier[1]

[1] Orthopaedic Service, Hospital Henri Mondor, Créteil, France
[2] Service de Chirurgie Plastique et Orthopédique Département de Chirurgie, Hôpital Notre Dame, Université de Montréal, Montréal, Québec, Canada
[3] Oncologic Paediatric Service, Hospital Robert Debré, Paris, France

Introduction

The proximal tibia is the third most common site for bone sarcomas and represents 12% of the tumors in our series of limb salvage.

After prosthetic reconstruction following en bloc resection of the upper tibia for bone sarcomas, the functional results depend mostly on the strength of patellar tendon reattachment and the quality of skin healing [2, 3, 5, 6].

This monocentric retrospective study's goal was to determine the role of composite allografts in preventing extensor lag.

Material

From January 1983 to December 1994, 49 patients (36 males, 13 females) aged 4.8 to 63 years old (mean 20.5 years) underwent upper tibial prosthetic reconstruction following en-bloc resection for tumor. There were 36 cases of osteosarcoma, 5 Ewing sarcomas, three chondrosarcomas, three fibrous histiocytomas and fibrosarcomas, one aggressive giant cell tumor and one solitary metastasis. 23 patients presented initially to our institution while 26 were seen either after biopsy or preoperative chemotherapy at another institution. The mean length of bony resection was 16.5 cm (8–27 cm).

At the first work up the tumor was purely intra-osseous (intracompartmental), in three cases, with extra-osseous spread (extracompartmental) in 37 cases and metastatic in 9 patients. One tumor was ulcerating the skin, three were invading the joint, two showed regional bony metastases (one tibial and one condylar). Six patients had massive tumor that was blocking knee flexion requiring in three of these cases a femoral resection and in the other three a fibular resection.

Methods

The surgical technique usually requires three steps performed most commonly in two operations: the biopsy, the resection and the reconstruction.

The reconstruction, depending of the extent of bony and soft tissue resection, intends to re-establish the skeletal continuity, the solidity of the extensor apparatus and preserve the medial skin vascularisation.

Over the years, several types of prostheses have been used by the authors. In the first cases [5], a Guepar type knee with polyethylene bearings was used. Later, we developed a specific titanium prosthesis that allows MRI for follow up. The femoral component has a hinge with axle and bigger polyethylene elements. The tibial component is custom made according to preoperative X-rays, which determine the length and the diameter of the anchoring stem. In young patients, in order to preserve the femoral growth plate, a smaller femoral non-cemented component is used. After four or five years, the sliding tibial prosthesis is replaced with a hinge type growth prosthesis.

The defect of the bony resection was filled with sleeves of various materials. Seven patients received sleeves of polyethylene or methylmetacrylate. Eight patients received massive banked bone allografts. Thirty four patients received composite allografts including not only the tibia, but also the patellar tendon and the extra articular part of the donor's patella (Fig. 1). In this last technique [1] the extra-articular part of the patient patella is resected (keeping the tumor free parts of the patellar tendon and the patellar wings). Two parallel tunnels are drilled to place the sutures. The tip of the allograft patella is fixed anatomically to the patient's patella with metallic transosseous cerclage (Fig. 2). The stump of the patient patellar tendon and wings are sutured onto the allograft tendon at the surface.

The protection of the medial knee skin evolved over time. The first 17 patients had a direct skin closure. The next 32 underwent coverage by gastrocnemius flap. [4, 5]. The medial gastrocnemius muscular flap was harvested through the same incision that was used for the tumor resection and the placement of the prosthesis. The muscular flap is only held on its vascular pedicle and can be rotated 90° allowing a satisfactory coverage

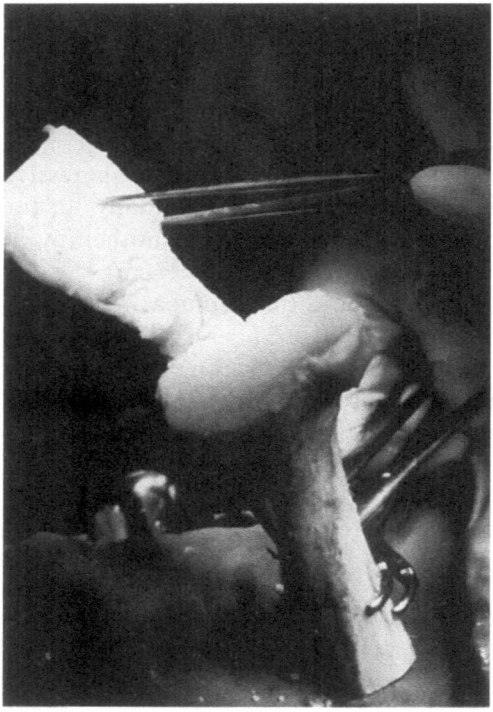

Fig. 1. The composite allograft with patellar tendon, patella and patellar wings of the donor

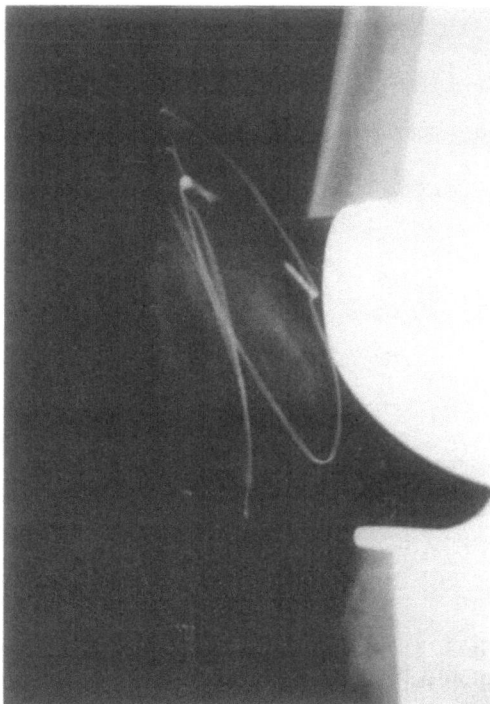

Fig. 2. Osteosynthesis of distal patella of the graft to the articular part of the patella of the receiver

of the articular component of the prosthesis up to the distal part of the tibial tubercle of the graft. The gastrocnemius fascia is sutured proximally to the wings of the patella and distally to the tibial crest of the graft with transosseous sutures. The remaining part of the flap is spread and fixed around its periphery with facial sutures.

Postoperative care includes prophylactic systemic antibiotics. Deep venous thrombosis prevention is achieved with low molecular weight Heparin since oral anti-coagulants have proved to be risky when chemotherapy is required. Weight bearing is allowed immediately with a bivalved knee brace. Reeducation is initiated immediately in bed with the electrical passive motion apparatus set for progressive knee flexion (figure 3); 60° to 80° of flexion are usually obtained at the end of the first month.

Post Operative Adjuvant Therapies

Forty five patients received postoperative chemotherapy. In cases of high grade sarcoma, perioperative chemotherapy was given on the first or second postoperative day.
Forteen patients received postoperative radiation therapy. They included patients with high risk biopsy and poor responders to preoperative chemotherapy.

Monitoring and Follow-Up

The patients were jointly followed by the medical oncologist and surgeon every three month for the first two years, then every six month for two years and eventually yearly.

The survival is calculated from the time of biopsy to the last examination. Deep infections were diagnosed every time the clinical presentation (fever, fistula, unexplained

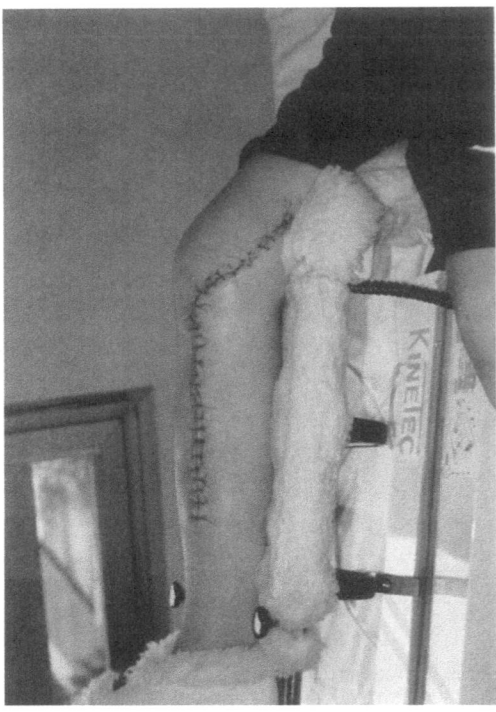

Fig. 3. The use of composite allograft and bony suture permits immediate postoperative mobilisation

pain) was accompanied by positive cultures. The mean follow-up is 63 months (minimum 9 months, maximum 130 months).

Results

Oncologic Results

No local recurrence has been noted even with very large tumors or some (18) marginal resections. 13 patients are dead from metastatic spread, most commonly from pulmonary involvement. One patient died from marrow aplasia due to the toxicity of chemotherapy. The remaining 35 patients are alive in total remission with a mean follow-up of 70 months.

Orthopaedic Results

Early complications have been numerous, especially at the beginning of the series. One patient required reoperation for evacuation of an expanding hematoma.

Intermediate complications included skin necrosis (10 cases) and deep infection caused by the large size of the tumors, the marrow aplasia secondary to the chemotherapy and/or the radiation therapy. The 10 cutaneous complications were associated with early deep infection of the prosthesis is six cases.

Two other patients presented with deep infection 1 to 6 months after surgery during septic episodes while in marrow aplasia. Four additional patients presented with late deep infections beyond two years, one occurring spontaneously, three following surgery for loosening of the prosthesis. Deep infection is therefore the most serious complication [7]. When it occurs during chemotherapy, it postpones treatment and might necessitate an immediate amputation. In all cases, it threatens the salvage of the limb. In fact, eight amputations followed twelve infections.

Late complications included mostly extensor apparatus ruptures, loosening of the prosthesis and mechanical complications of the allograft.

Twelve secondary ruptures of the extensor apparatus have been seen characterized clinically by a loss of extension against gravity and radiologically by an increased tibial tuberosity-patella distance.

Twelve loosenings of the prosthesis occurred. Three involved only the femoral (standard) component and were cured by a secondary cementing procedure. Nine cases involving the massive tibial component required more difficult procedures. Three of these patients were infected at a secondary operation and ultimately required amputation to control chronic infection.

Overall, the functional results at last follow-up based on Enneking's criteria are excellent in 22 cases, good in 13 cases, fair in 5 and poor in nine cases.

Analysis of the prognostic factors reveals the important role of the immediate medial gastrocnemius muscular flap in preventing infection. In 17 patients without flaps, 9 suffered deep infection and six required amputation, while only 3 out of 32 patients who

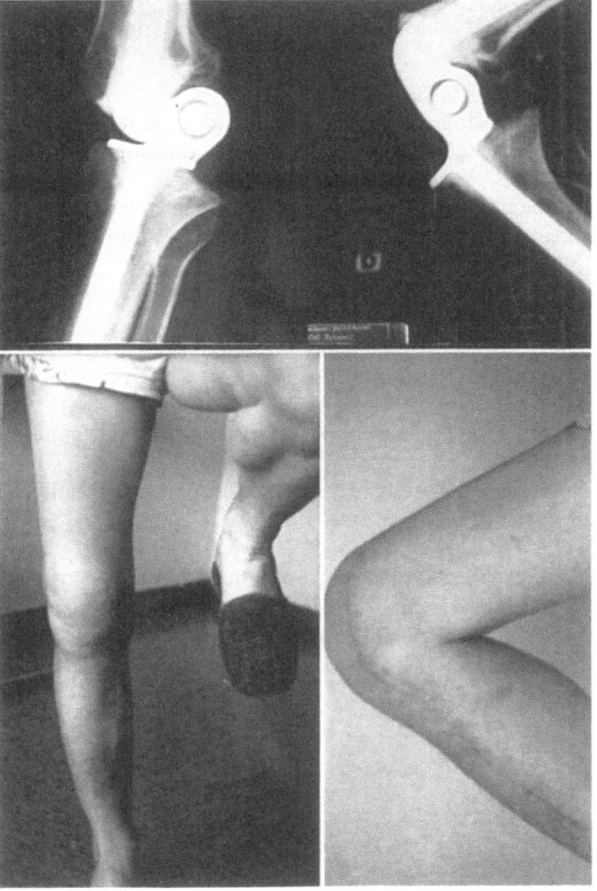

Fig. 4. Radiological and clinical result 2 years after implantation

received immediate gastrocnemius flaps developed infection and only 2 required amputation. This difference is statistically significant.

Massive stainless steel prostheses coated with polyethylene don't provide a reliable reattachment of the patellar tendon and extension lag appeared in all 5 cases after 6 to 10 months.

Composite prostheses with bone allografts permit a real reinsertion of the patellar tendon, but require shortening of the tendon which limits flexion (if the oncologic safety requires resection of a part of the patient's tendon) and are threatened by secondary fracture of the tibial tuberosity.

The best results were obtained with bony suture of the extensor apparatus with the composite allograft including the tibia, patellar tendon and patella. This procedure provides a good length of patellar tendon and permits bony suture through the patella and immediate mobilization (Fig. 4).

Conclusion

Upper tibia composite allograft reconstruction permits a much better reconstruction of the patellar tendon, avoiding extensor lag while allowing acceptable knee flexion. The allograft should be harvested with the patella and the patellar tendon to permit bone to bone reattachment of donor to host patella.

Gastrocnemius flaps help to power extension and decrease the risk of deep infection requiring secondary amputation. Flap coverage should be performed in all cases.

References

1. Delepine G, Delepine N, Hernigou Ph (1991) Allograft with patellar tendon in recontructive procedure after upper tibia resection. In: Limb salvage. Major reconstruction in oncologic and non-tumural conditions. Berlin: Springer, pp 435–437
2. Jenbon JS (1983) Resection arthroplasty of the proximal tibia. Acta Orthop Scand 54: 126–130
3. Koiz R (1983) Possibilities and limitations of limb-preserving therapy for bone tumors today. J Cancer Res Clin Oncol 106: 68–76
4. Malawer MM, Price WM (1984) Gastrocnemius transposition flap in conjunction with limb-sparing surgery for primary bone sarcoma around the knee. Plast Reconstr Surg 73: 741–750
5. Malawer MM, McHale KC (1989) Limb-sparing surgery for high-grade tumors of the proximal tibia: Surgical technique and a method of extensor mechanism reconstruction. Clin Orthop Rel Res 239: 231–248
6. Sim FH, Chao EYS (1979) Prosthetic replacement of the knee and a large segment of the femur or tibia. J Bone Joint Surg 61A: 887–891
7. Tomford NW, Starkweather RS, Goldman MH (1981) A study of the clinical incidence of infection in the use of banked allograft bone. J Bone Joint Surg (AM) 63: 244

Authors' addresses: G. Delepine, M.D., D. Goutallier, M.D., Henri Mendor, Avenue Delattre de Tassigny, Créteil 94000, France; P.G. Harris, M.D., Service de Chirurgie Plastique et Orthopédique, Département de Chirurgie, Hâpital Notre Dame, Université de Montréal, Montréal, Québec, Canada N. Delepine, M.D., Oncologic Paediatric Service, Hospital Robert Debré, 48 Bd. Serurier, F-75019 Paris, France.

Intercalary Allograft Reconstruction

M. G. Rock

Mayo Clinic and Mayo Foundation, Orthopaedic Department, Rochester, Minnesota, U.S.A.

Segmental intercalary deficits occur in varied clinical conditions including traumatic loss, post resection for extensive osteomyelitis, and after tumor resection for diaphyseal or periarticular lesions. The options that exist for bone reconstruction include cortical cancellous autograft, vascularized bone transfer, allograft, bone transport, salvage procedures, such as the creation of one-bone forearm and tibiofibular synostosis for diaphyseal tibial lesions. If none of these options are a viable alternative and/or the technical expertise does not exist amputation may be necessary.

Cortical cancellous or cancellous autograft can successfully be used to address deficiencies of 6 cm or less [3, 5, 15]. Such reconstruction has the advantage of being osteoconductive and osteoinductive with immediate transfer of the tissue from donor site to intercalary deficiency allowing for a small percentage of osteoblasts to survive. The surviving cells are dependent on surrounding soft tissue for nutrition and, therefore, the success of such a reconstruction is contingent on a viable envelope of soft tissue. The autograft so applied is replaced with creeping substitution allowing the graft to become fully incorporated into the host. The mechanical strength of nonvascularized cortical autografts may last up to one year during which incorporation should have been complete and remodeling initiated to successfully offset the stresses applied to the graft. Although favored for small intercalary deficits autograft procurement is associated with not uncommon complications. These include: significant increase in the operative time, perioperative bleeding necessitating transfusions and all the attendant risks with homologous blood product transfusions, fracture, nerve injury, infection, hernia, and persistent pain at the operative site.

With the advent of microvascular surgical technique vascularized bone transfer, either transposition or free grafts have become very popular to address deficiencies exceeding the indications for nonvascularized autografts [4, 15, 16, 17]. It has all the advantages of autograft tissue mentioned above but also heals without creeping substitution, it retains structural quality and integrity and if vascularity is maintained the segment hypertrophies according to Wolf's law (Fig. 1a–d). Additional advantages include the ability to span up to 24 cm of deficiency and include composite tissue transfer overlying muscle and skin. The maintenance of blood supply renders unimpaired microcirculation to the bone preserving both the periosteal and medullary blood flow. There are three principal sources of vascularized bone grafts which include the fibula with or without overlying soleus and skin, the iliac crest with or without overlying skin and subcutaneous tissue and rib (Table 1). The selection of one of these three sources is dependent on the length and shape of the defect, the need for composite tissue or an articulating surface as with distal radial deficiency being compensated with the proximal

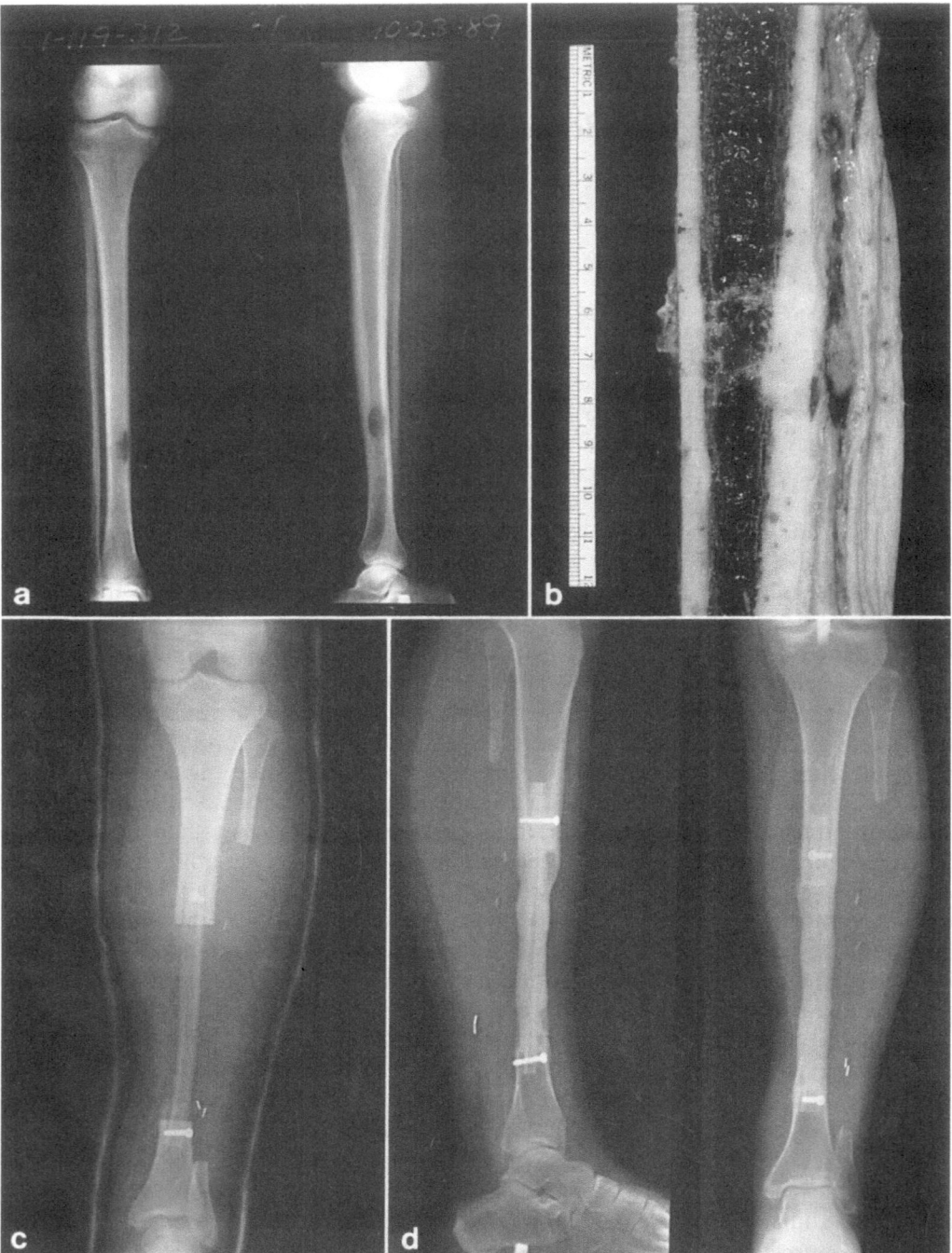

Fig. 1. a Forty-eight year old female with a low grade central osteosarcoma of the distal tibia as demonstrated on the AP and lateral radiograph; **b** Resected specimen after preoperative chemotherapy; **c** Immediate postoperative appearance of transposition of ipsilateral vascularized fibular graft; **d** Two and one-half years after the reconstruction showing significant hypertrophy of the transposed fibula and union at both proximal and distal juncture sites

Table 1. Vascularized bone graft donor sites

Site	Length	Shape	Structure	Artery
Fibula	22–26	straight	corticocancellous	peroneal
Rib	30	curved	membranous	posterior intercostal
Iliac crest	10	slight curve	corticocancellous	deep circumflex

fibula. An extensive recent review of our experience with vascularized fibula for intercalary deficiencies has been performed [6]. The intercalary deficits were due to tumor, osteomyelitis, trauma, and congenital anomalies. For the entire series the rate of union after the primary procedures was 61 percent with an additional 20 percent being salvaged with autogenous cortical cancellous grafting at one of the juncture sites. The success of the operation was largely dependent on the presence of infection in the wound prior to the vascularized bone transfer. The overall failure rate and persistent nonunion in the defects with previous infection were 25 percent versus 15 percent in those patients being treated for underlying tumor, traumatic or congenital anomaly defects. The overall 81 percent union rate and the incidence of failure appear to reflect the magnitude of the operations, the underlying conditions for which the operation is being performed and are commensurate with other large series in the literature. Recipient complications included 12 stress fractures of the transferred fibula, all of which were treated successfully either with immobilization or open reduction and grafting. The most devastating complication at the recipient site was that of infection. This occurred in 13 percent of the patients, all of whom had had either prior management of extensive osteomyelitis or tumor resection and reconstruction. Approximately half of these patients were ultimately rendered amputation for uncontrollable infection. Complications at the donor site included stress fracture of the ipsilateral tibia, contracture of the long flexor tendon of the great toe, compartment syndrome in the lower limb, particularly in those with combined tissue transfer and transient peroneal palsy. The latter occurred in five patients all of whom ultimately went on to have total return of function. The overall function of the donor limb was not significantly effected with full capability of performing day to day activities.

Vascularized tissue transfer continues to be a very viable alternative when addressing intercalary deficiencies exceeding 6 cm in wounds rendered dysvascular by previous trauma, osteomyelitis and tumor resection with adjuvant radiation and chemotherapy. If vascular supply is maintained the transferred graft resembles normal bone and maintains its strength, stiffness and torsional capability better than nonvascularized autograft tissue.

Limitations of vascularized fibular transfer include the presence of suitable tissue to transfer which sometimes can be compromised with ipsilateral contiguous bone involvement with tumor, infection or trauma. Additionally, defects in a large weightbearing bone such as the tibia or femur would demand extensive hypertrophy of the transferred fibula to allow continued weight bearing with or without repetitive stress fractures (Fig. 2). The majority of the failures based on anatomic site occurred in the femur (24 percent), and in the tibia (18 percent). It is likely optimistic to assume that a vascularized fibular graft by itself can compensate for a large metadiaphyseal defect of the distal femur or proximal tibia which is the preferred site of aggressive bone tumors and/or osteomyelitis. In such circumstances, larger structurally competent grafts or bone transport may be

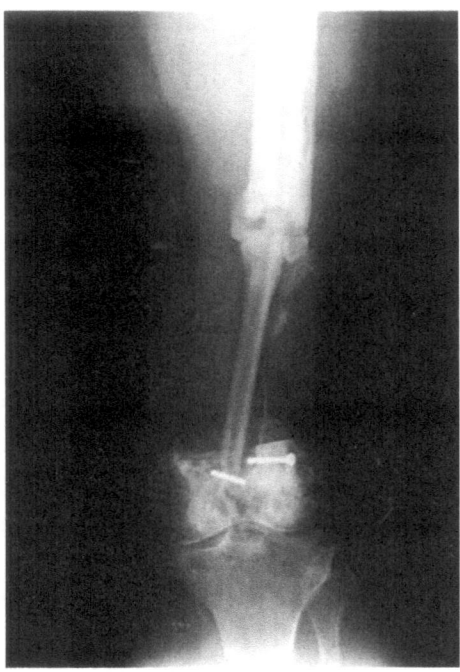

Fig. 2. Unsuccessful attempt at distal femoral inter-calary resection and reconstruction utilizing a vas-cularized fibula graft. Even with hypertrophy a transferred vascular fibula would not be able to sustain the mechanical stresses applied to this ana-tomical area and therefore an intercalary allograft of similar dimensions to that of the resected specimen would have been a more appropriate option for reconstruction

more appropriate. We have had no experience with bone transport in the presence of aggressive bone and/or soft tissue tumors. The need for continued postoperative chemotherapy and in some rare circumstances, radiotherapy, would likely preclude its use in malignant conditions. There are very few benign processes of bone for which diaphyseal and/or extra-articular resection arthrodesis would be necessary. For situ-ations in which vascularized tissue transfer is not going to address mechanical needs, most orthopedic oncologists have relied on the use of intercalary allografts which provide immediate structural stability and allow for the ultimate biologic incorporation. Additionally, given the comparable size of the allograft to the resected segment, fixation is more effectively achieved than in nonvascularized or vascularized autografts. This allows for earlier reconstitution of motion at the contiguous joint. Additional advan-tages of allografts include no host morbidity, unlimited segmental length, and being able to fashion the allograft to precisely offset the intercalary deficiency. One significant advantage using allograft is the incorporation of antibiotic impregnated cement within the medullary cavity which markedly increases the strength of the reconstruction, does not influence the incorporation at the host allograft juncture sites, and allows elution of antibiotics into the surrounding tissues for the first two to four weeks after recon-struction.

When compared to other forms of allograft reconstruction, intercalary diaphyseal reconstruction has been one of the more successful. In Mankin's series [12] 88 percent were considered either excellent or good which is similar to an 85 percent success rate noted in an experience among tertiary institutions in the United States [9, 10, 11, 13]. Similarly, in a recent review by Hernigou [7], 79 percent of his 14 patients with fresh frozen and irradiated intercalary allografts could be considered good or excellent. Additionally, Mnaymneh and Malinin [13] have reported 89 percent success in a group of 28 patients receiving intercalary allografts. Long term survivors have also been reported by Muscolo [14] with follow-ups ranging from 22 to 36 years. When intercalary allografts are used to gain arthrodesis principally at the knee and the shoulder the success rates drop off precipitously. This may be a product of the lack of a viable soft tissue envelope around the reconstruction site which facilitates union and minimizes the contamination of the graft with superficial infections or wound dehiscence. In Mankin's [12] series alloarthrodesis success occurred in 59 percent of patients. In the combined experience of other tertiary institutions in North America, an allograft arthrodesis has been successful in approximately 72 percent of cases [7, 10, 11, 13].

Despite the many successful reports of diaphyseal allograft reconstruction there have been reports of significant complications including infection, nonunion, graft resorption and fracture. In Hernigou's [7] review of 14 patients there was a 15 percent infection and 25 percent nonunion rate. Additionally in a review of 23 intercalary allografts and 2 alloarthrodeses of the knee, Loty [10] found infection in 8 percent, nonunion in 20 percent, resorption in 8 percent, fracture in 8 percent, with a total complication rate of 40 percent. Makley [11] has had a similar experience with 46 percent of patients having an overall event-free postoperative course. In his series he had five diaphyseal intercalary reconstructions and 8 alloarthrodeses. Complications in the diaphyseal reconstructions included infection in one and persistent pain in an additional patient. For the alloarthrodesis population there was one peroneal palsy, three wound breakdowns, 3 cases with persistent pain and one fracture. At the ten juncture sites of the five patients undergoing diaphyseal intercalary reconstruction, three proved to have nonunions whereas in the 16 juncture sites among 8 alloarthrodesis patients 4 went on to a nonunion and one to a partial union.

In his review of 31 massive allograft transplantations in 1985, Dick [2] suggested that the success of the allograft was not dependent upon the use of chemotherapy alone but is multifactorial. In his review of intercalary resection, Mnaymneh [13] suggested that patients receiving chemotherapy and having intercalary reconstructions had an overall success rate of 77 percent versus 89 percent of those who did not receive chemotherapy perioperatively. Other authors have reported that the success of intercalary allografts correlated with multiple factors such as graft fixation, age of the patient, size of the graft, natural history of high grade tumor, the presence or absence of chemotherapy, anatomical site, and whether the reconstruction is done diaphyseal or for attempted arthrodesis at the knee or the shoulder [1].

Given what appears to be a rather inordinate high complication rate with intercalary allografts and specifically alloresection and arthrodesis, we proceeded to perform a multivariate analysis to identify factors with a negative influence on intercalary allograft incorporation and longevity [8]. Thirty-one patients received segmental allografts for intercalary (11) or arthrodesis (20) reconstruction after resection of malignant bone tumors at the Mayo Clinic. There were 15 females, 16 males with the average age of 28 years. The average follow-up among the patients was 52 months. All tumors were either malignant conditions of bone or contiguous soft tissue that necessitated removal of large segments of bone. There were 17 osteosarcomas, 9 chondrosarcomas, 2 leiomyosarcomas, one liposarcoma, one malignant fibrohistiocystoma, and one fibrosarcoma. Anatomic localization included six humeral lesions, 15 femoral, 9 tibial and one iliac wing. The segmental length for allograft reconstruction averaged 16 cm. Neoadjuvant chemotherapy was administered to 12 patients and adjuvant chemotherapy to 4.

Of the 31 patients, 29 were available for extensive evaluation of functional results and a thorough multivariate analysis of the tumor or allograft related complications. Two patients were not included in the analysis, one due to an early infection and an arterial occlusion necessitating perioperative removal of the allograft and one additional patient who died within two months of the reconstruction from disseminated disease. The functional results included three excellent (10 percent), 15 good (52 percent) and 11 poor (38 percent) cases. Among the failures six had infection and five had local recurrence. When the tumor-related failures were excluded, overall acceptable results of segmental allografts was 75 percent. The overall survival rate in this patient population was 81 percent with 71 percent being disease-free. There were five local recurrences with three of these patients ultimately dying from metastasis. Four of the five patients who had local recurrences had amputation with two concurrently having infection within the allograft.

Allograft complications occurred in 14 of 31 patients (45 percent). Seven patients (23 percent) developed infection, 6 delayed or nonunion necessitating grafting in 5 patients (16 percent), one (3 percent) had graft resorption and one (3 percent) had fixation failure. We attempted to correlate the allograft-related complications with various possible prognostic factors using a multivariate analysis including allograft length, fixation method, the incorporation of vascularized fibula grafts, operative method in terms of arthrodesis or intercalary, perioperative chemotherapy, age and anatomical location. There was no statistical evidence to support that length of resection, fixation technique, the presence of vascularized fibula, and/or the use of perioperative chemotherapy had any effect on allograft success. Kattaprum et al. [9] reported no correlation between age, sex, location, previous treatment, diagnosis or complication on the surgical outcome of intercalary allografts. In our study we had a different observation in terms of age. Of the 13 patients under the age of 20, 31 percent had complications whereas of the 17 patients over 20 years of age, 59 percent had complications. Additionally, complications were statistically more likely to occur in alloarthrodeses than in diaphyseal intercalary resections. The infection rate was 6 of 20 patients undergoing resection arthrodesis versus 1 of 11 in the intercalary diaphysis. Additionally, of statistical significance was the association between complications and a poor functional outcome. Of 21 patients experiencing at least one complication, only 38 percent had excellent or good ultimate functional results. The 10 patients who experienced no complications postoperatively universally had excellent or good results.

The anticipated five year survival of allograft reconstruction at our institution was 68 percent. Most of the complications occurred within the first year and with the exclusion of infection, which inevitably necessitated the removal of the allograft and some other form of reconstruction or amputation, all other complications could be successfully managed without removal of the allograft. The allograft related complication rate was 46 percent which is comparable to that of the series mentioned previously. In our series and in that of Dick [2] and Czitrom [1] there did not appear to be any adverse effect of neo- or adjuvant chemotherapy. This may be a product of the chemotherapy being given to younger patients who, in our series and in those mentioned, appear to have a better overall functional result in spite of the need for chemotherapy.

We have learned from reviewing the experience of others as well as our own that intercalary allograft reconstruction can be a viable option in the treatment of intercalary diaphyseal or resection arthrodesis cases. In spite of the relatively high incidence of complications in the early postoperative course, segmental intercalary allografts or arthrodesis have predictably good long-term results. Methods to reduce complications, specifically infection, include the transposition of viable muscle over the reconstructive site and avoidance of placing the allograft in a subcutaneous location. Six of our seven cases of infection occurred in attempts at alloarthrodesis at the knee and at the shoulder without associated attempts at transposing local or possibly even free soft tissue

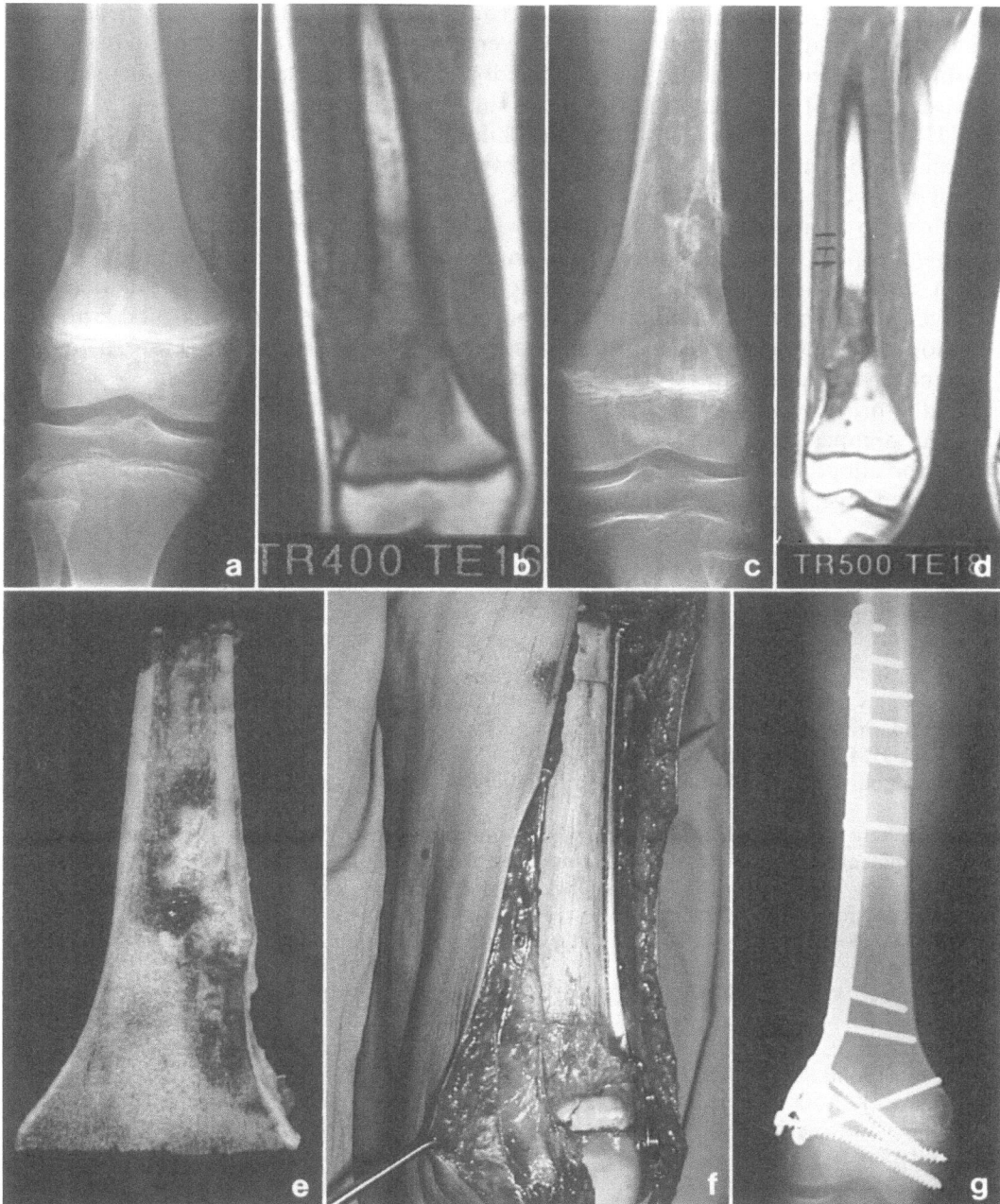

Fig. 3. a An 11-year-old girl appeared in our clinic with a classic high-grade osteosarcoma involving the distal aspect of the femur; **b** MRI at the time of presentation reveals a sizable soft tissue extension laterally with central edema of the femoral canal down to abutting of the epiphyseal growth plate; **c** After neoadjuvant chemotherapy the AP radiograph reveals maturation of the tumor and less local response; **d** MRI taken at the time of definitive surgical excision reveals considerable decrease in the soft tissue mass, loss of the edema extending down to the distal femur with the tumor being that much more encapsulated and defined; **e** Resected specimen showing the tumor 2 cm from the resection margin; **f** Intraoperative photo showing the diaphyseal intercalary allograft in place with the juncture site at the epiphyseal plate and approximated within the diaphysis of the femur being securely fixed with a condylar plate; **g** Postoperative x-ray revealing the intercalary allograft in place with excellent reconstitution of length and orientation of the limb

transfers over the reconstruction. It is now routine practice to transpose the medial and lateral head of the gastrocnemius muscle over alloarthrodesis at the knee and in similar fashion, transfer the ipsilateral latissimus dorsi by itself or associated myocutaneous transfer to overly the allograft arthrodesis site of the shoulder.

Historically most skeletally immature children with sarcomas were routinely treated by amputation, in part because of the inability to compensate for continued longitudinal growth of the long bone. With effective neoadjuvant chemotherapy allowing for predictable necrosis of the tumor, diaphyseal intercalary resections at or above the epiphyseal plate are becoming more popular trying to preserve the ipsilateral contiguous joint function (Fig. 3a–g). As such, intercalary resection and reconstruction with allogeneic tissue will assume greater importance among the options available to the orthopedic oncologist. This in large part is due to the increased success rate seen among intercalary resections and reconstructions than osteoarticular allografts or custom metallic prostheses. The results of previous series and ours would suggest that with careful preoperative planning and with the inclusion of effective soft tissue coverage over the allograft, a successful result can be anticipated. Perioperative chemotherapy in the younger patient has not precluded union at the two host allograft juncture sites.

References

1. Czitrom A, Campannacci R, et al (1989) Segmental allograft reconstruction concomitant with neoadjuvant chemotherapy. Presented at the Fifth International Symposium of Limb Salvage, San Malo, France
2. Dick HM, Malinin TI, Mnaymneh WA (1985) Massive allograft implantation following radical resection of high grade tumors requiring adjuvant chemotherapy treatment. Clin Orthop 197: 88
3. Enneking WF, Eady JL, Burchardt H (1980) Autogenous cortical bone grafts in the reconstruction of segmental skeletal defects. J Bone Joint Surg 62A: 1039–1058
4. Goldberg VM, Shaffer JW, Field G, Davy DT (1987) Biology of vascularized bone grafts. Orthop Clin N Amer 18: 197–205
5. Goldberg VM, Stevenson S (1987) Natural history of autografts and allografts. Clin Orthop 225: 7–16
6. Han CF, Wood MB, Bishop At, Cooney WP III (1992) Vascularized bone transfer. J Bone Joint Surg 74A: 1441–1449
7. Hemigou P, Delepine G, et al (1993) Massive allograft sterilized by irradiation. Clinical result. J Bone Joint Surg 75B: 904–912
8. Kang YK, Rock MG, et al (1992) Segmental allograft following radical resection of malignant bone tumors. Presented at the Minnesota Orthopedic Society Meeting, 1992. Clin Orthop Rel Res (submitted)
9. Kattaprum SV, Phillips WC, Mankin HJ (1989) Intercalary bone allograft: Radiographic evaluation. Radiology 170: 137
10. Loty B, et al (1990) Bone and allograft sterilized by irradiation; Biologic properties, procurement and results of 150 massive allografts. International Orthop 14: 237–242
11. Makley JT (1985) The use of allograft to reconstruct intercalary defects of long bones. Clin Orthop 197: 58–75
12. Mankin HJ, et al (1992) Current status of allografting for bone tumors. Orthopedics 15(10): 1147–1154
13. Mnaymneh W, Malinin T (1989) Massive allografts in surgery of bone tumors. Orthop Clin N Amer 20: 455–467
14. Musculo DL, et al (1992) Massive femoral allograft followed for 22 to 36 years. A report of six cases. J Bone Joint Surg 74B: 887–892

15. Shaffer JW, et al (1985) The fate of vascularized and nonvascularized autografts. Clin Orthop 197: 32–43
16. Weiland AJ (1981) Current concepts review. Vascularized free bone transplants. J Bone Joint Surg 63A: 166–169
17. Wood MB, Cooney WP, Irons GB (1984) Posttraumatic lower extremity reconstruction by vascularized bone graft transfer. Orthopedics 7: 255–262

Author's address: Michael G. Rock, M.D., Orthopedic Department, Mayo Clinic, 200 First Street SW, Rochester, MN 55905, U.S.A.

Spine and Trauma

Arthrodesis of the Spine with Bone Allografts

T. Malinin and M. D. Brown

Tissue Bank, Department of Orthopaedics and Rehabilitation, University of Miami-Jackson Memorial Medical Center, Miami, Florida, U.S.A.

Introduction

Arthrodesis of the spine is performed to stabilize the spinal column. The spinal column becomes unstable when it can no longer maintain normal anatomic alignment of adjacent vertebrae with their neural arches, intervertebral discs, facet joints and ligaments. Spinal instability results most frequently from severe degenerative disease involving intervertebral discs and posterior elements and it can also be caused by trauma, infections and tumors [13, 30].

One of the earliest uses of bone grafting was in the spines afflicted with tuberculosis [1]. Bone grafts stabilize the motion segments of the spine by creating a bone mass posteriorly and laterally, by obliterating intervertebral spaces, by providing structural support anteriorly, or by replacing vertebral bodies and the intervertebral discs. Bone grafts can also be used to maintain the increased diameter of the neural arch in laminoplasties.

Frequently bone grafting is performed concomitantly with the application of metallic internal fixation devices. The latter were initially developed for the correction of extensive spinal deformities, Harrington rods being the first universally accepted devices used for this purpose [20]. At first it was thought metallic rods would permanently stabilize the spine without arthrodesis, but this turned out not to be the case. When stainless steel rods were used alone they usually broke with time and the hooks became loose. Titanium instrumentation developed subsequently by Dwyer and later modified by Zielke likewise failed to provide permanent stability of the spine [15, 16]. Therefore supplementation of instrumentation with posterior or anterior fusions of the spine became a practice.

Introduction of segmental spinal instrumentation (SSI), a term generally used to describe metal implants attached to several contiguous vertebrae, also did not obviate the need for supplementary spine fusions.

Bone Grafts

Autologous Bone

Albee, as early as 1911, fused the spines of children with Pott's disease with tibia strut autografts [1]. Tibial bone is still used occasionally, as is the fibula, but corticocancellous bone from the ilium is now the most commonly transplanted autograft.

When placed in a wound bed with good blood supply, autologous bone induces osteogenesis from surrounding mesenchymal cells and provides scaffolding for the ingrowth of new host bone. Whether or not autografts actively contribute cells which significantly influence new bone formation is still an unresolved question. Carefully performed rodent experiments indicate that they do not [25]. In humans, if contribution of viable cells from a bone autograft does occur, it is probably limited to the surface cells from the endosteum. The presence of periosteum is not essential for successful transplantation of autologous grafts.

Since bone autografts are biologically active, and survive manipulations to which they are subjected in the operating room, their performance in spine fusions is used as a standard against which the performance of all other grafts is judged [4, 6, 17, 31].

Incorporation of bone autografts is biologically similar to the healing of fractures. After the initial inflammatory cell response, primitive mesenchymal cells of the host are activated to differentiate into osteogenic cells. Cancellous bone is replaced in a uniform manner throughout its thickness. In cortical grafts the periphery becomes pitted and replaced with new bone rather uniformly, but the interior of the graft is replaced in an irregular fashion [17]. In practice, bone autografts have their limitations. In some instances the quantity of autologous bone that can be obtained is inadequate. In elderly or debilitated patients autologous cancellous bone is often osteopenic. Morbidity associated with excision of bone from the iliac crest is not inconsiderable. Complications encountered with autologous bone grafts in spinal fusions include pseudarthrosis, graft collapse, resorption and occasionally bone mass overgrowth [30].

Allogeneic Banked Bone

The creation of numerous tissue banks during the last decade has virtually assured an unlimited availability of a wide variety of bone allografts employed for the fusions of the spine. Increase in bone banking activities has also resulted in the employment of widely divergent methods of allograft acquisition, processing and preservation. These can be roughly divided into methods which rely on strict aseptic surgical techniques employed during allograft excision and processing and those which rely on secondary sterilization by either chemical or physical means.

Clinical results reported thus far suggest that for spinal arthrodesis, aseptically processed bone approximates the behavior of the autografts the closest [28, 29, 46, 48]. Ethylene oxide sterilized bone allografts receive mixed reviews. On one hand Prolo et al. report good results in achieving arthrodesis of the spine with ethylene oxide sterilized bone allografts [37, 38]. On the other hand several other authors record poor results with these preparations. Herron and Newman reported a high incidence (76%) of pseudarthrosis in patients receiving ethylene oxide sterilized freeze-dried bone allografts, and stated that the use of these allografts in the fusion of the thoracic and lumbar spine cannot be recommended [21]. The studies by Jorgenson et al. support the same conclusion [22]. Since doses of ionizing radiation required to sterilize bone allografts significantly reduce or altogether abolish their osteogenicity, the use of irradiated bone allografts for arthrodesis of the spine likewise cannot be recommended [21, 22].

Cervical Spine

Anterior fusion of the cervical spine is a frequently performed operation. The preference for either the Smith-Robinson or Cloward technique varies with the times and with individual surgeons [8, 40]. Either technique produces satisfactory arthrodesis at single or multiple levels. However, the motion of cervical spine segments adjacent to the level of anterior interbody fusion increases after the fusion. The larger the number of the vertebral bodies fused, the greater is the motion of the adjacent segments. This causes not uncommonly observed degenerative changes in the intervertebral spaces below and above the fusion levels. The motion of the cervical spine does not decrease after cervical laminoplasty [34, 42]. Therefore transformation of stress to adjacent normal spinal segments does not occur. This is one of the reasons for the recent popularity of lamino-plasties which employ allografts.

In the cervical spine, aseptically excised and processed allografts, when placed in an interbody position, produce fusion rates identical or very similar to those obtained with autografts [6, 10, 17, 39, 43] (Fig. 1). The accumulated experience with freeze-dried or frozen dowel shaped or tricortical iliac crest allografts shows certain advantages offered by these grafts over autografts obtained from the ilium. Dowel shaped bone allografts are prepared from the femoral head, femoral condyles or tibial plateaus. Cancellous bone from these locations is compact, but the anatomical sites themselves preclude their use as autogenous grafts. Compact allograft bone avoids the problem of graft collapse which can occur with osteopenic iliac bone grafts [6, 10]. When tricortical iliac allografts are prepared from carefully selected donors osteopenic bone is likewise avoided.

Freeze-dried fibular allograft segments have also been used in the anterior interbody fusions at one, two and three levels in patients with cervical spine myelopathy. With the use of these grafts, a 92% union rate is obtained by six months after surgery [19].

The replacement of vertebral bodies destroyed by tumors, trauma and infections is accomplished through an interior approach. In these circumstances the use of allografts becomes very attractive, as these are readily available in appropriate sizes and shapes. When compared with methylmethacrylate, bone grafts provide reliable constructs which achieve spinal stability [51]. To replace spine bone loss from tumors, allografts of the

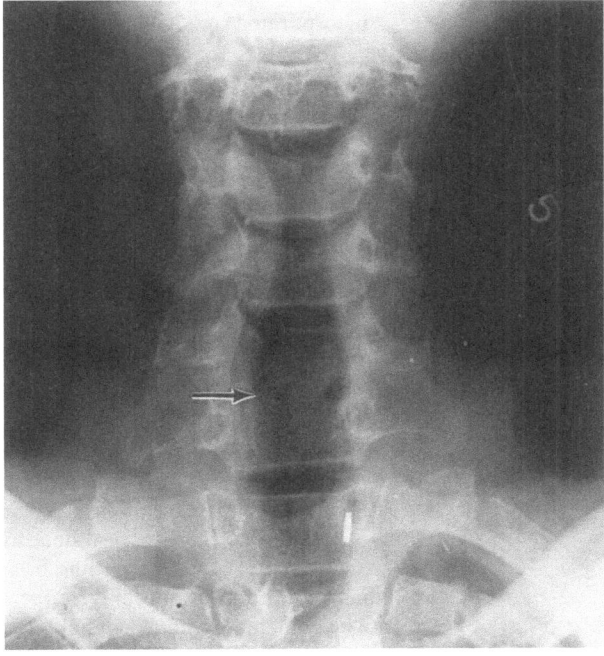

Fig. 1. 56 year old male with fracture dislocation of C-6. Roentgenogram taken 14 months after insertion of a frozen femoral head cadaver bone allograft following a decompression laminectomy. The allograft (arrow) is incorporated into the host bone

tibia, femur diaphyses or ilium blocks can be used. Fibular strut allografts as well as notched cortical allografts have also been employed with success for the replacement of vertebral bodies after partial or complete corpectomies [19, 41].

The only negative results with allografts as compared to autografts in anterior cervical spine fusions were reported by Zdbelick and Ducker [52]. In this report a higher rate of non-unions and graft collapse occurred in two level, but not one level fusions These authors did not state how the allografts were prepared in their series.

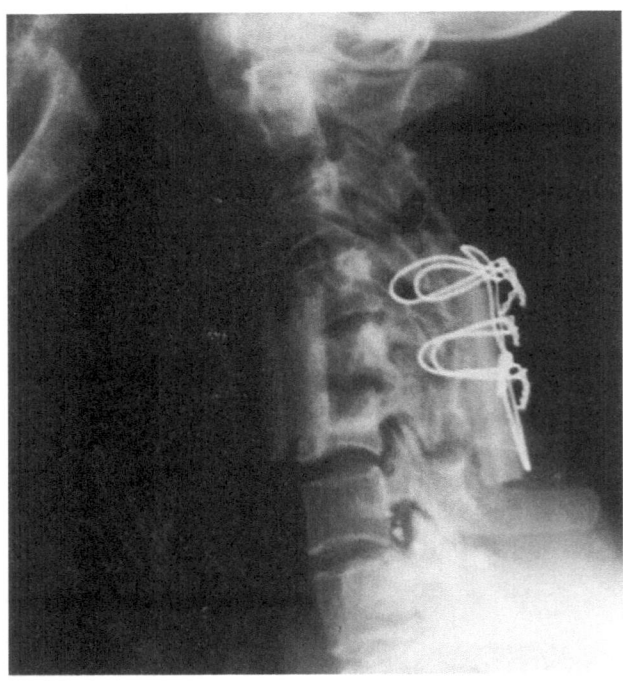

Fig. 2. Autologous fibula allograft was used anteriorly, and a cortical plate allograft posteriorly to stabilize the cervical spine in a patient with C-5 vertebral body destruction secondary to an infected anterior interbody autograft. Both bone grafts incorporated successfully

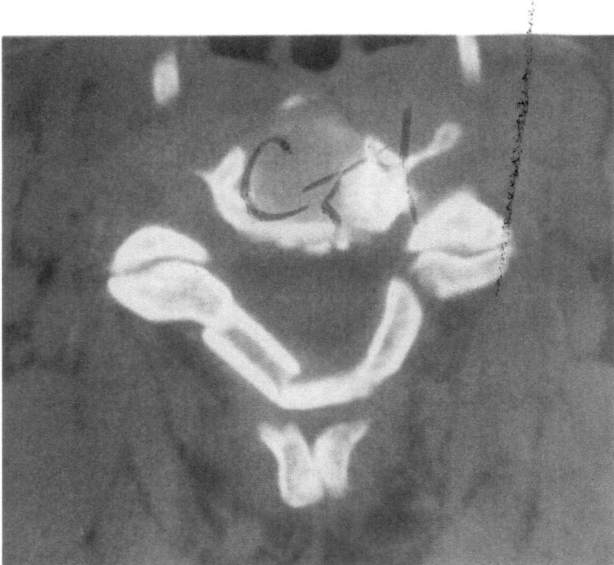

Fig. 3. This CT scan shows a 42 year old male with severe cervical stenosis and myelopathy. Lamina has been cut on both sides and hinged open. The fibular allograft which holds the lamina open is seen clearly

In posterior cervical fusions the indications for the use of allografts are not as clear as in anterior interbody fusions. In several instances failures of cortical allografts in posterior cervical spine fusions has been recorded, but the validity of the statement that bone allografts under tension will always be absorbed has been questioned [44, 50]. An example of an allograft in the posterior cervical fusion which performed well is shown in Fig. 2. Both the allografts from the rib and the fibula have performed well in posterior cervical laminoplasties (Fig. 3).

Arthrodesis of the Thoracic and Lumbar Spine in the Presence of Spinal Instrumentation

Arthrodesis of the thoracic and lumbar spine is most commonly performed for scoliosis or for unstable spinal fracture dislocations requiring open reduction and internal fixation. Instrumentation is also used for correction of severe spinal instability resulting from tumors or infections [18]. Instrument fixation used to realign the thoracic and lumbar spine must be supplemented with a bone fusion. Otherwise the fixation devices will usually fatigue and break. The posterior fusion technique used in conjunction with spinal instrumentation must include the destruction of the articular cartilage of the facet joints, adequate debridement of soft tissue attachments and decortication of host bone surfaces.

Several studies on autograft versus allograft bone in the surgery of idiopathic adolescent scoliosis report solid fusions with allografts. Dodd et al. compared two groups of patients, each receiving either frozen cortico-cancellous bone allograft or autograft from the iliac crest. There was no difference between the two groups in a blind radiographic assessment of bone graft mass or in the maintenance of the curve correction [14]. Aurori et al. reported similar findings, while McCarthy and co-workers observed that rates of complications and fusions were comparable with or better than those obtained with autologous bone graft [31, 32]. Freeze-dried cancellous bone allografts were also found safe and effective substitutes for autologous bone grafts in patients with cerebral palsy undergoing posterior spinal fusions [33]. On the other hand, Stricker and Sher demonstrated the efficiency of freeze-dried cortical bone allografts in effecting fusion in patients with idiopathic and other types of scoliosis [46]. Allograft bone clearly produces adequate fusion mass and stabilizes the spine in patients with idiopathic scoliosis. However, the type of the graft may not be as important as the fusion technique itself [23]. Strict adherence to facet obliteration, decortication and stable instrumentation are probably the most important factors in preventing pseudarthrosis.

The data accumulated thus far shows little difference between the allogeneic and autologous bone in posterior spinal fusions in patients with idiopathic adolescent and cerebral palsy scoliosis. In these patients the use of bone allografts markedly reduces the operative time and blood loss, and eliminates morbidity associated with the taking of autografts. Therefore, even in the presence of an adequate iliac crest, the use of aseptically excised and processed banked allograft bone is indicated for grafting in adolescent scoliosis surgery [14].

Posterolateral Lumbar Fusion

Unlike in idiopathic scoliosis, autograft remains the graft of choice in posterolateral fusions of the lumbar spine in adults, as most authors report significantly lower fusion rates with allografts as compared with autografts in these fusions [2, 35]. In patients with degenerative disease of the lumbar spine, allografts should be used as augmenting bone grafts, because with few exceptions neither freeze-dried nor frozen allograft bone alone perform as well as autograft.

The experience with posterolateral laminar or intertransverse fusions in the lumbar spine emphasizes that performance of bone grafts will depend on the environment into which they are placed. Mechanical factors such as motion at the specific intervertebral segment and the loading characteristics at that segment as well as the blood supply vary between cervical, thoracic and lumbar spines. Thus the performance of bone allografts in the cervical spine or the thoracolumbar spine in adolescents cannot be extrapolated to the lumbar spine in adults [5].

At this point it appears that current observations and conclusions regarding bone allografts in the posterolateral lumbar spine are accurate. While bone allografts perform well in some segments and locations in the spinal column, there is little data to suggest that allografts alone will act as efficiently as autografts in posterolateral fusions in the lumbar spine. Therefore, in these circumstances, the use of the allografts should be confined to patients with insufficient own bone, and then the fusion site should be supplemented with any available autogenous bone.

Posterior Lumbar Interbody Fusion (PLIF)

Posterior lumbar interbody fusion was originally described by Cloward, and subsequently modified by several surgeons [9, 26]. The placement of four thin iliac crest grafts into the intervertebral space is difficult, but the success of graft incorporation depends on the good alignment and the close match of these grafts. Cloward has used allografts for this procedure almost from its inception and reported good results with the same in 623 posterior lumbar interbody fusions [11]. However, he cautions, the graft must be placed in the prepared interspace so that the cortical surface of the graft lies in a vertical plane and the cancellous bone is in contact with the vertebral bodies. Subsequently posterior lumbar interbody fusions utilizing two larger grafts rather than four thin ones have been performed with success equal to that obtained by Cloward. The fusion rates with this procedure have been roughly the same regardless of whether the patients' own bone or allografts were used. Stefee combined posterior interbody fusions with segmental instrumentation and devised rectangular cancellous block grafts which are placed in the intervertebral body position [45]. He claims a predictable fusion outcome utilizing this technique.

Anterior Lumbar Interbody Fusion (ALIF)

Since the original description of anterior lumbar interbody fusion in 1933, different success rates have been described with this procedure. Allografts and autografts have been used interchangeably with equal success, although Crock, who described the use of ALIF for internal disc derangement favors autografts [12, 27].

Few spinal fusion operations theoretically appear as ideal and as unpredictable and difficult as the anterior lumbar interbody fusion, hence there are a number of discrepancies in reports dealing with it. Watkins et al. in a review of 82 patients with ALIF's recorded a 60% union rate for autografts and 64% for iliac crest block allografts, and noted that the fusion rate did not increase with additional postoperative time [48]

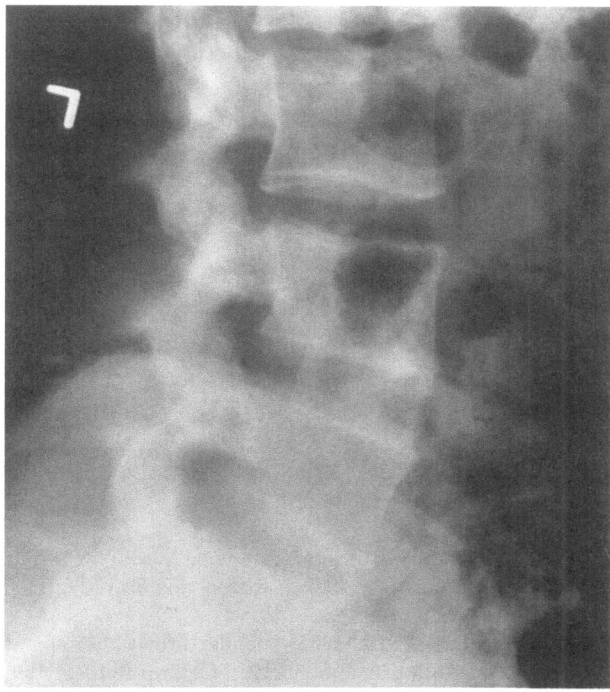

Fig. 4. Anterior interbody fusion with a freeze-dried iliac crest block four years postoperatively

(Fig. 4). On the other hand, Kozak et al. recorded a 97% fusion rate with composite allografts consisting of femoral rings and crushed cancellous bone [24]. However with the use of cortical bone allografts prepared from fibulas the fusion rate was only 58% [49].

Discussion

The ready availability of bone allografts has led to several advances in the reconstructive surgery of the axial skeleton. Correction and prevention of deformity as well as the replacement of bone loss can be accomplished with the aid of these grafts. However, surgeons contemplating transplanting allogeneic, preserved bone must be aware of the advantages and disadvantages of these transplants.

Despite long-standing interest by orthopaedic and neurologic surgeons in the replacement of the diseased segments of the spine and arthrodesis of the spine with bone from other individuals, systematic gathering of information of these efforts is relatively recent. By now we have accumulated sufficient clinical experience which suggests that there is an indication for allografting in spinal surgery. Understanding the biological behavior of bone transplants and the dependence of their success on osteoinduction is of paramount importance. Clearly allografts subjected to treatments which diminish or abolish their osteoinductive capacity will not function as well as their counterparts in which such activity is preserved. Curiously, in spinal surgery, allografts function well in some anatomical sites and not in others. This too must be borne in mind in determining whether to use or not to use an allograft.

The attention to details in the studies which report and analyze the results obtained with allografts is of paramount importance. This is particularly true when dealing with the preparation of allografts. Treatment of the allografts with various chemicals may influence their osteogenic activity, but reports giving the results with allografts rarely describe in detail the methods of their preparation. This omission makes the analysis of data difficult.

The attainment of a solid bone fusion is multifactorial. There is a race between bone resorption and new bone formation in creating a fusion mass which can withstand mechanical loads. Standard methods of bone allograft preparation are now widely accepted. However, the behavior of bone grafts cannot always be predicted. At this point in time we can recommend the use of bone allografts in spinal surgery where its effectiveness has been clearly established. Hopefully future clinical investigation and laboratory research will result in bone grafting material and methodology which will fulfill all of the demands of reconstructive surgery of the spine.

References

1. Albee IH (1911) Transplantation of a portion of the tibia into the spine for Pott's disease. JAMA 57: 885–887
2. An HS, Lynch K, Toth J (1995) Prospective comparison of autograft vs. allograft for adult posterolateral lumbar spine fusion: differences among freeze-dried, frozen and mixed grafts. J Spinal Disorders 8: 131–135
3. Aurori BF, Weirman RJ, Lowell MA, Nadel CI, Parsons JR (1985) Pseudarthrosis after spinal fusion for scoliosis: A comparison of autogeneic and allogeneic bone. Clin Orthop Rel Res 199: 155–158
4. Bassett CAL (1972) Clinical implications of cell function in bone grafting. Clin Orthop Rel Res 87: 49–59
5. Boden S (1994) Point of view. Spine 18: 2053
6. Brown MD, Malinin TI, Davis PB (1976) A roentgenographic evaluation of frozen allografts versus allografts in anterior cervical spine fusions. Clin Orthop Rel Res 119: 231–236
7. Bright RW, Smarsh JD, Gambill VM (1983) Sterilization of human bone by irradiation. In: Friedlaender GE, et al (eds) Osteochondral allografts. Boston, Toronto: Little, Brown & Co, pp 223–232
8. Cloward RB (1952) The treatment of ruptured intervertebral disc by vertebral body fusion. Ann Surg 136: 967–971
9. Cloward RB (1953) The treatment of ruptured lumbar intervertebral disc by vertebral body fusion I. Indications, operative technique, aftercare. J Neurosurg 10: 154–167
10. Cloward RB (1962) The anterior approach for removal of ruptured cervical discs. J Neurosurg 15: 602–617
11. Cloward RB (1963) Lesions of intervertebral disks and their treatment by interbody fusion methods. Clin Orthop Rel Res 27: 51–77
12. Crock HV (1982) Anterior lumbar interbody fusion. Clin Orthop Rel Res 165: 157–163
13. DePalma AF, Rothman RH (1970) Intervertebral disc. Philadelphia: W.B. Saunders
14. Dodd CAF, Fergusson CM, Freedman L, Houghton GR, Thomas D (1988) Allograft versus autograft bone in scoliosis surgery. JBJS 70B: 431–434
15. Dunn HK (1983) Spinal instrumentation. In: Evart CM (ed) AAOS Instructional Course Lectures, vol 32. St. Louis: S.V. Mosby, pp 209–218
16. Dwyer AF, Schafer MF (1974) Anterior approach to scoliosis. JBJS 56B: 218–224
17. Enneking WF, Morris JL (1972) Human autologous bone transplants. Clin Orthop Rel Res 87: 28–35
18. Fountain SS (1979) A single stage combined surgical approach for vertebral resections. JBJS 61A: 1011–1017
19. Grossman W, Peppleman WC, Baum JA, Kraus DP (1992) The use of freeze-dried fibular allografts in anterior cervical fusion. Spine 17: 565–569
20. Harrington PJ, Dickson JH (1973) An eleven year clinical investigation of Harrington instrumentation. Clin Orthop Rel Res 93: 113–130

21. Herron LD, Newman MH (1989) The failure of ethylene-oxide gas sterilized freeze-dried bone graft for thoracic and lumbar fusion. Spine 14: 496–500

22. Jorgenson SS, Lowe TG, France J, Sabin J (1994) A prospective analysis of autograft versus allograft in posterolateral lumbar fusion in the same patient. Spine 19: 2048–2052

23. Knapp RD Jr, Jones ET (1987) Use of cortical cancellous allograft in posterior spinal fusion. Clin Orthop Rel Res 229: 99–105

24. Kozak JA, Heilman AE, O'Brien JP (1994) Anterior lumbar fusion options. Technique and graft material. Clin Orthop Rel Res 300: 45–51

25. LaCroix P (1951) Organization of bones. London: J & A Churchill

26. Lin PM, Cantilli RA, Joyce MF (1983) Posterior lumbar interbody fusion. Clin Orthop Rel Res 180: 154–168

27. Loguidice VA, Johnson RG, Guyer RD, Stith WJ, Ohmneiss DD, Hochschuler SH, Rashbaum RF (1988) Anterior lumbar interbody fusion. Spine 13: 366–369

28. Malinin TI, Rosomoff HL, Sutton CH (1977) Human cadaver femoral head homografts for anterior cervical spine fusions. Surg Neurol 7: 249–251

29. Malinin TI, Brown MD (1981) Bone grafts in spinal surgery. Clin Orthop Rel Res 154: 68–73

30. Malinin TI, Eismont FJ, Brown MD (1986) Materials used in spine stabilization. In: Dunster M, et al (eds) The unstable spine. Philadelphia: W.B. Saunders pp 25–43

31. Marx RE, Snyder RM, Kline SN (1979) Cellular survival of marrow during placement of marrow cancellous bone graft. J Oral Surg 37: 712–715

32. McCarthy RE, Peek RD, Morrissy RT, Hough AJ Jr (1986) JBJS 68-A: 370–375

33. Montgomery OM, Aromson DD, Lee CL, LaMont RL (1990) Posterior spinal fusion: Allograft versus autograft bone. J Spinal Disorders 3: 370–375

34. Naito M, Ogata K, Kurose S, Oyama M (1994) Canal-expansive laminoplasty in 83 patients with cervical myelopathy. A comparative study of three different procedures. Int Orthop 18: 347–351

35. Nasca RJ, Whelchel JD (1987) Use of cryopreserved bone in spinal surgery. Spine 3: 222–227

36. Nishizawa K (1995) Problems of interbody fusion with bank bone allografts. Abstracts, 14th Annual Meeting Japan Society of Bone, Joint and Soft Tissue Transplantation, Kyoto, Japan p 28

37. Prolo DJ, Pedrotti PW, White, DH (1980) Ethylene oxide sterilization of bone, dura mater and fascia lata for human transplantation. Neurosurgery 6: 529–539

38. Prolo DJ, Oaklund SA (1983) Sterilization of bone by chemicals. In: Friedlaender GE, et al (eds) Osteochondral allografts. Boston, Toronto: Little, Brown & Co., pp 233–238

39. Rish BI, McFadden, Penix JP (1976) Anterior cervical spine fusions using homologous bone grafts: A comparative study. Surg. Neurol 5: 119–121

40. Robinson RA, Walker AE, Fezlic DC, Weikling DK (1962) The results of anterior interbody fusion of the cervical spine. JBJS 44A: 1569–1586

41. Rossier AB, Hussey RW, Kenzoza JE (1977) Anterior fibular interbody fusion in the treatment of cervical spinal cord injuries. Surg Neurol 7: 55–60

42. Sato T (1962) Radiological follow-up in the cervical spine after surgery. J Japanese Orthop Assoc 66: 607–620

43. Schneider JR, Bright RW (1976) Anterior cervical fusion using preserved bone allografts. Transpl Proc 8 [Suppl 1]: 73–76

44. Stabler CL, Eismont F, Brown MD, Green BA, Malinin TI (1985) Failure of posterior cervical fusion using cadaveric bone graft in children. JBJS 67A: 370–375

45. Stefee AD, Sitkowski DJ (1988) Posterior lumbar interbody fusion and plates. Clin Orthop Rel Res 227: 99–102

46. Stricker SJ, Sher JS (1996) Freeze-dried cortical allograft in posterior spinal arthrodesis. Orthopaedics (In press)

47. Urist MR, Hernandez A (1974) Excitation transfer in bone. Archives of Surgery 109: 486–494

48. Watkins RG, Springer D, Wiltse L, Champoux J, Schilz J, Hodge B (1985) Anterior interbody fusion of the lumbar spine—a review. Orth Trans 9: 430

49. Wetzel FT, Hoffman MA, Arcieri RR (1993) Freeze-dried fibular allograft in anterior spinal surgery: cervical and lumbar applications. Yale J Biol & Med 66: 263–275

50. White AA 3rd, Panjabi MM (1984) The role of stabilization in the treatment of the cervical spine injuries. Spine 9: 512–522

51. Whitehill R, Barry JC (1985) The evolution of stability in cervical spinal constructs using either autologous bone graft or methylmethacrylate cement. A follow-up report on a canine in vivo model. Spine 10: 32–41
52. Zdeblick TA, Ducker TB (1991) The use of freeze-dried allograft bone for anterior cervical fusion. Spine 16: 726–729

Authors' address: Theodore Malinin, M.D. and M.D. Brown, M.D., Ph.D., Department of Orthopaedics and Rehabilitation, P.O. Box 016960 (R-12), Miami, Florida 33101, U.S.A.

Allografts for Spinal Surgery

A. Nather and J. Thambiah

National University Hospital Bone Bank, Department of Orthopaedic Surgery, National University Hospital, Singapore

Introduction

With the official setting up of the National University Hospital Bone Bank in October 1988 [13, 14, 15, 18], the use of bone and ligament allografts has increased tremendously. It is therefore not surprising that bone allografts are increasingly being used for spinal surgery.

Background

Legal Status

Bone transplantation is legal in Singapore. It does not follow the Human Organ Transplant Act of 1987 [20]. Instead, the procurement of musculoskeletal tissues follows the Medical (Therapy, Education and Research) Act of 1972 [25] whereby consent is needed from the next of kin or relative.

Development of The National University Hospital Bone Bank

The National University Hospital (NUH) Bone Bank was established in October 1988 [13, 14, 15, 18] by the first author with a research grant from the National University of Singapore. Two electrical freezers were commissioned for storage of bones and ligaments at $-80°C$. This being the only bone bank in the country, the bank provided allografts not only to National University Hospital but also to all hospitals in Singapore [13, 14, 15, 18].

Because of the increasing demand for both deep frozen and lyophilised allografts, the bank received a further grant from the National University of Singapore and an additional grant from the Totalisator Board to upgrade the bank to a national bone bank status [18, 19]. It is now equipped with four electrical freezers and two lyophiliser units, each unit including a shaker bath, a lyophiliser, a laminar flow cabinet, a bench saw and an impulse autosealer. Lyophilised bones have been produced and used since July 1994 [18, 19].

NUH Bone Bank Protocol

The bank has its own protocol taking into acount the guidelines set up by the American Association of Tissue Banks [24], European Association of Tissue Banks [5] European Association of Musculoskeletal Transplantation [23] and the American Red Cross Tissue Services [22].

All donors were screened by detailed medical history, detailed medical examination and laboratory test for Aids, Hepatitis B and C, Syphilis and culture and sensitivity tests for aerobic and anaerobic microgranisms [13, 14, 15, 17].

Procurement

Small bones were procured from living donors using the sterile double jar technique. To date 166 femoral heads and bone slices from 77 total knee replacement operations have been retrieved.

Long bones were procured from deceased donors using the sterile triple wrap technique. So far, 31 femora, 34 tibiae, 20 fibulae, 35 patella ligaments, 15 humeri, 7 radii, 7 ulnae, 8 iliac crests, 5 tibialis posterior and tibialis anterior tendons, 4 pieces of fascia lata, and 15 menisci have been procured from 20 deceased donors. The first cadaveric procurement was performed in September 1989.

Documentation

Detailed documentation was carried out for both donors and recipients, all data being computerised.

Processing

NUH Protocol favored the use of allograft-prosthetic composites for joint reconstruction [13, 14, 15, 18]. Most long bones were gamma irradiated at a dosage of 25 KiloGrays at the Cobalt 60 Plant in the Malaysian Institute of Nuclear Technology (MINT) in Bangi, Selangor under the direction of Dr Norimah Yusof, Head, Isotope and Radiation in Biology and Agriculture [18, 19]. This joint collaboration between NUH Bone Bank and MINT was started in September 1992 under the auspices of the International Atomic Energy Agency. The bones were packed in dry ice and air flown to MINT for irradiation and then flown back the same day within 10 hours for re-storage in the freezer.

All morsellised bones were lyophilised [18, 19]. The processing included cutting the bones into various shapes and sizes, percolation with normal saline, pasteurisation, lyophilisation, triple packing in special polyethylene bags and gamma irradiation at 25 KiloGrays. The irradiation of the morsellised bones was performed by Dr Liew Soo Chin of the Physics Department of the National University of Singapore using Gamma Chamber 4000 A [18, 19].

Transplantation

The first bone transplantation was performed in June 1989. Since then, 144 allograft transplantations have been performed in various hospitals in Singapore including 82 at the National University Hospital and 35 at the Singapore General Hospital. These included 50 cases for spinal surgery, 26 cases for hip surgery, 7 cases for massive allograft reconstruction for tumors and 33 anterior cruciate ligament reconstruction.

Transplantations in Spinal Surgery

Bone grafting (autografts) has a major role in orthopaedic surgery and is frequently used in spinal surgery [3]. It is therefore not surprising that allograft tissues are also increasingly used in spinal surgery [1, 2, 3, 4, 6, 7, 8, 9, 10, 11, 21].

Allografts have been used in spinal surgery for anterior cervical fusion [4, 8, 9, 11, 21, 27], posterolateral spinal fusion in adults [6, 10, 11, 16, 19, 26], posterior spinal fusion in children [16, 19], posterior lumbar interbody fusion [2], anterior lumbar interbody fusion [7], and massive anterior spinal reconstruction.

Spinal Surgery in Singapore

Between January 1991 and September 1994, spinal surgery using allografts was carried out in 50 patients in Singapore [19], 39 cases were performed for posterolateral fusion in adults, 4 cases for posterior spinal fusion in children and 7 cases for massive anterior spinal reconstruction.

Posterolateral Spinal Fusion in Adults

Study Population

Posterolateral fusion using allografts was carried out in 39 patients in the Division of Spinal Surgery, National University Hospital between January 1991 and October 1993 [16, 19]. The patients age ranged from 19 to 85 years, the average age was 47 years. There were 23 males and 16 females. The duration of follow-up ranged from 12 months to 41 months with an average of 18 months.

Indications

The indications for operation were shown in Table 1 [16, 19]. Most patients were elderly with degenerative stenosis or degenerative spondylolisthesis and spinal instability. Two patients with osteoporotic burst fractures presented with neurological compression.

Operative Technique

A mid line incision was made to expose the spinous processes at the affected level. Where indicated, spinal decompression was first performed. The spinous processes were removed and the bone from the laminectomy was preserved as autograft to be used together with allograft bone. At the start of the operation, the allografts to be used were carefully prepared. The femoral heads or bone slices from total knee replacements were thawed in normal saline containing Ampicillin and Cloxacillin. The articular cartilage was meticulously removed from all allografts. The allograft bones were then ground into small pieces using a sterile bone mill.

Table 1. Indications for posterolateral fusion

Indications	No. Patients
Degenerative Stenosis	8
Degenerative Spondylolisthesis	8
Spondylolysis	6
Spondylolytic Spondylolisthesis	5
Burst Fracture	6
Fracture – Dislocation	2
Osteoporotic Burst Fracture	2
Secondaries with Cord Compression	1
Traumatic Spondylolisthesis	1
Total	39

The most crucial step in the operation was the meticulous preparation of the fusion bed [11, 16, 19]. Facet joints, laminae and transverse processes including the ala of the sacrum in relevant cases were completely exposed and thoroughly rawed. After preparation of the fusion bed, instrumentation was performed and the bone graft consisting of a 50% mixture of allograft and autograft was properly packed into the fusion bed. Where laminectomy was performed, there was no need to procure autograft. Bone from the removed spinous processes and from the laminectomy was enough to provide a 50% mix with allograft bone. Where decompression was not performed, procurement of bone autograft was necessary to provide live bone to the mixture and give it osteogenic potential.

Instrumentation

Except in one case where there was severe osteoporosis, instrumentation was performed in all cases. Hartshill instrumentation was used in 30 cases, Cottrel Dubousset instrumentation in 17 cases and Stefee plating in 1 case.

Results

No infection was encountered. There were 4 cases of implant failure, all involving Hartshill instrumentation. Allografts are useful particularly in elderly patients where the iliac crest bone is porotic and fatty [16, 19].

Posterior Spinal Fusion in Children

Allografts were used in 2 cases with congenital scoliosis and in 1 case of neurofibromatosis with kyphoscoliosis. In-situ fusion was achieved in all 3 cases. Allografts were also used in a 10 year old chinese male who was operated on for a double-curve scoliosis from T4 to L4 using a Harrington rod and autograft in October 1991 and who presented with a pseudoarthrosis in April 1993 [16, 19]. In this case autograft was procured from both iliac crests in the first operation.

Table 2. Anterior spine fusion

Case	Sex/Age	Indication	Bone Used	Length	Instrumentation
1.	F/79	Osteoporotic Burst L1	Femur (DF)*	5 cm	Not used
2.	F/67	Osteoporotic Burst L1	Tibia (DF)*	8 cm	Isola
3.	F/75	Osteoporotic Burst T12, L1	Tibia (DF)*	10 cm	Kaneda
4.	F/77	Osteoporotic Burst L1	Femur (FD)**	6 cm	Kaneda
5.	F/44	Ca Breast T11, T12, L1	Femur (DF)*	2 cm	DCP
6.	M/27	Mediastinal Germ Cell Tumour T9	Humerus (DF)*	6 cm	Kaneda
7.	M/60	Ca colon T12	Femur (DF)*	6 cm	Isola

  * Deep Frozen
**Freeze-Dried

Allografts are essential in very young children where donor bone is not available since the iliac crest is mainly cartilaginous [16, 19].

Massive Anterior Spinal Reconstruction

Massive allografts were used for anterior vertebral column reconstruction in 7 cases as shown in Table 2. The two main indications were osteoporotic burst fracture with neurological compression and metastatic disease with cord compression [16, 19].

Instrumentation

The Kaneda device was used in 3 cases (Cases 3, 4 and 6). In Case 5 where a 12 centimeter defect was too long to be bridged by the Kaneda device, a Dynamic Compression Plate was used to stabilize the long allograft. Isola instrumentation was used in Case 2 (see Figs. 1 and 2) and Case 7 where a combined anterior and posterior approach was employed. No instrumentation was performed in Case 1.

Choice of Allograft

Two factors should be considered in choosing the allograft, namely the size of the allograft and the type of allograft. With regards to the size of allograft needed, the diameter of the diaphyseal allograft used should match the diameter of the vertebral column to be reconstructed. For reconstruction of the thoraco-lumbar spine, the femur and in some cases the tibia was the ideal choice [19]. For upper thoracic spine reconstruction, the humerus was the allograft of choice [19].

In young patients subjected to greater biomechanical loading, the stronger deep frozen gamma irradiated allografts should be used. However, in elderly patients where the bones are porotic and the functional demands are not great, lyophilised allografts are preferred. It is easier to use lyophilised allografts because one does not have to prepare the graft beforehand. Lyophilised grafts of the femur, tibia and humerus are available in ready made lengths (4, 6, 8, 10, 12 and 14 centimeters) in triple packs which have been

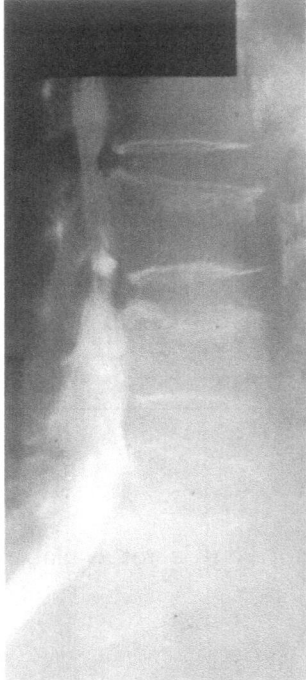
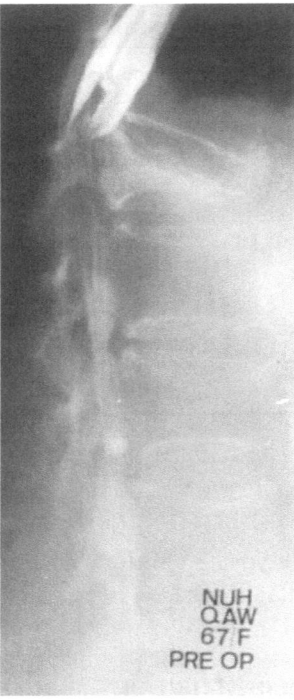

Fig. 1. Myelogram of a 67 year old Chinese female showing partial block at L1, L2 level from an osteoporotic burst fracture L1 with neurological deficit

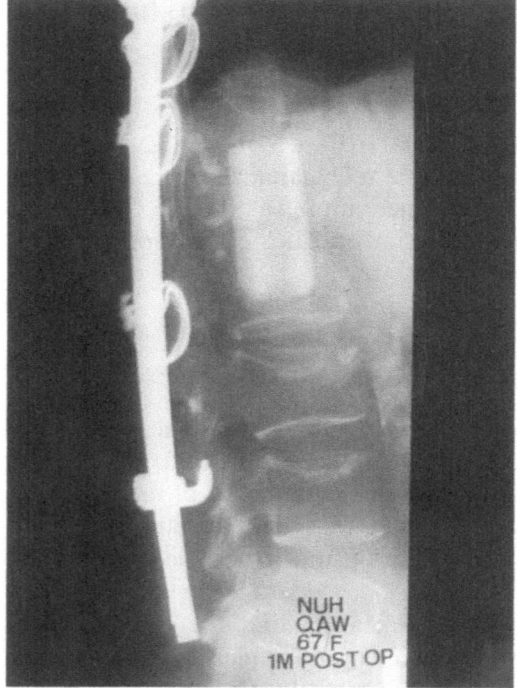

Fig. 2. Showing reconstruction anteriorly using a 6 cm deep-frozen femoral allograft with Isola instrumentation posteriorly

gamma irradiated and stored at room temperature [18, 19]. In all cases, deep-frozen allografts were used except in Case 4 (Table 2) where the readily available freeze-dried femoral shaft was preferred [19].

Allograft—Autograft Composite

Recently, the medullary canal of cylindrical allografts was packed with autografts obtained either from the rib removed during the approach or with autografts taken from the iliac crest. This ensures better graft healing and is recommended for all future cases.

Discussion

In spinal surgery, allografts are used to serve two functions namely to act as a buttress and to enhance fusion [3]. The need to buttress occurs every time the anterior column is compromised [3]. Buttressing is the primary function in anterior bone grafting procedures as in anterior cervical fusions, anterior lumbar interbody fusions and anterior thoracic fusions. In these cases, an additional aim is to achieve fusion of the segments involved. In anterior spinal surgery, the allografts are inserted into well vascularized beds in the vertebral bodies. Cortico-cancellous buttressing allografts with good osteoconductive properties are rapidly incorporated giving a high clinical success rate after anterior cervical fusions [4, 8, 9, 21, 27]. The osteoconductive function is also responsible for the clinical success reported with xenografts such as Kiel bone [27]. In our experience, healing has occurred in all 7 cases where massive anterior allografts have been used.

In posterior spinal surgery, the fuction of the graft is to induce fusion [3]. Morsellised allografts are used for this purpose. However, because allografts lack osteogenic and osteoinductive properties, they should only be used for augmenting the quantity of graft in mixtures with autograft bone [3, 16, 19]. In children, under some circumstances they can be used alone [3]. For posterior spinal fusion deep frozen allografts gave better results than freeze-dried allografts [9]. Because of their osteoinduction properties, demineralized bone allografts are becoming more widely used in spinal surgery, particularly for posterior spinal fusion [3].

Acknowledgements

The authors would like to thank the National University of Singapore and the Totalisator Board for funding this project, Mr. S.C. Yong and A. Mathiyalagan for the technical assistance rendered, Mr. B.K. Tan and Mr. S.S. Moorthy for the excellent photographs taken and Ms. J. Baharim for typing the manuscript.

References

1. Cloward RB (1980) Gas sterilised cadaver bone grafts for spinal fusion operations. Spine 5: 4–10
2. Cloward RB (1985) Posterior lumbar fusion updated. Clin Orthop 93: 16–19
3. Czitrom AA (1994) Biology of bone grafting and principles of bone banking. In: Weinstein SL (ed) The pediatric spine: Principles and practice. New York: Raven Press, pp 1285–1298
4. Frothingham RE, Solomon A (1988) The use of allografts in anterior cervical interbody fusion. J Miss Med Assoc 29: 71–74

5. General Standards for Tissue Banking (1995) European Association of Tissue Banks. Austria, Gutezeichen
6. Herron LD, Newman MH (1989) The failure of ethylene oxide gas-sterilised freeze-dried bone grafts for thoracic and lumbar spinal fusion. Spine 14: 496–500
7. Loguidice VA, Johnson RG, Guyer ED (1988) Anterior lumbar interbody fusion. Spine 13: 366–369
8. Malinin TI, Rosomoff HL, Sutton CH (1977) Human cadaver femoral head homografts for anterior cervical fusion. Surg Neurol 7: 249–251
9. Malinin TI, Brown MD (1981) Bone allografts in spinal surgery. Clin Orthop 154: 68–73
10. Montgomery DM, Aronson DD, Lee CL, La Mont RL (1990) Posterior spinal fusion: Allograft versus autograft bone. J Spinal Dis 3: 370–375
11. Nasca RJ, Whelchel JD (1987) Use of cyropreserved bone in spinal surgery. Spine 12: 222–227
12. Nather A (1990) Healing of large diaphyseal allograft transplants. An experimental study. Proceedings 2nd Conference of International Society for Fracture Repair, 6–7 September, Mayo Clinic, USA, pp 90
13. Nather A (1991) Organisation, operational aspects and clinical experience of National University of Singapore Bone Bank. Ann Acad Med Singapore 20: 453–457
14. Nather A (1991) The present status of bone banking in Singapore. In: Itoman M (ed) Musculo-skeletal tissue banking and grafting. Tokyo: Walsh Japan Co, pp 41–45
15. Nather A (1992) Bone banking and transplantation in developing countries. Trans Proc 24: 1944–1945
16. Nather A, Thambiah J, Lee ST (1992) Spinal fusion using allografts. Proceedings 7th International Conference on Biomedical Engineering, 2–4 December, Singapore, pp 249–251
17. Nather A (1992) Value of screening procedures in femoral head procurement for allograft transplantation. The NUS bone bank experience. J ASEAN Orthop Assoc 6: 39–42
18. Nather A, Thambiah J, Yong SC (1994), Singapore National Bone Bank: 6 years of experience. Proceedings 3rd European Conference on Tissue Banking and Clinical Application of Grafts, 4–7 October, Vienna, pp 17
19. Nather A, Thambiah J, Yong SC (1994) Allografts for spinal surgery. Proceedings 8th International Conference on Biomedical Engineering, 7–9 December, pp 173–176
20. Republic of Singapore Government Gazette Acts Supplement: The Human Organ Transplant Act 1987; 15: 411–421
21. Rish BL, Mc Fadden JT, Penix JO (1976) Anterior cervical fusion using homologous bone grafts. A comparative study. Surg Neurol 5: 119–121
22. Standards of the American Red Cross Tissue Services Sixth Edition (May 1994) KD Campagnari, JPO' Maley (eds). Washington: American Red Cross
23. Standards for tissue banking and current developments (1994) European Association of Musculo Skeletal Transplantation
24. Technical manual for tissue banking (1992) McLean, VA, American Association of Tissue Banks
25. The statutes of the Republic of Singapore Medical (Therapy, Education and Research) Act (Chapter 175): Act 23 of 1972; 12: 1–6
26. Urist MR, Dawson E (1981) Intertransverse fusion with the aid of chemosterilized autolyzed antigen—extracted allogeneic (AAA) bone. Clin Orthop 154: 97–113
27. Vich JMO (1985) Anterior cervical interbody fusion with threaded cylindrical bone. J Neurosurg 63: 750–753

Authors' address: A. Nather and J. Thambiah, National University Hospital Bone Rank, Department of Orthopaedic Surgery, National University Hospital, Singapore.

The Use of Bone Allografts in Spine Surgery Indications and Results

O. Schwarzenbach, P. Heini, U. Berlemann, and E. Gautier

Department of Orthopaedic Surgery, University of Bern, Inselspital, Switzerland

Introduction

For several decades, bone allografts have been widely used in orthopaedic surgery, with the main application being in the reconstruction of large skeletal defects [4].

In the field of spine surgery, the main use of bone allografts is for spinal fusions, specifically for the treatment of cervical and thoraco-lumbar degenerative spine disease and spinal deformities. There are few reports in the literature describing the application of bone allografts in trauma and tumor surgery of the spine or of its use in the management of infective lesions of the spine [12, 15, 16, 26].

Indications and Results of Bone Allografts in Spine Surgery

Cervical Spine

In anterior cervical spine fusions, bone allografts have been used for many years with good results. Several authors have compared the clinical and radiological results of allogeneic and autogenous bone grafts for cervical spine fusions. Brown et al. have compared fresh autograft with frozen ($-20°$C) allograft iliac crest bone for anterior cervical spine fusion in 63 and 76 spinal levels respectively [3]. There were no differences in clinical results and fusion rates between the groups with autografts (97%) and allografts (94%). Brown noted a higher incidence of allograft collapse, particularly in those patients undergoing multilevel fusions. Overall there was a 28% incidence of graft collapse when allograft was used compared with 14% when autograft was employed. A 30% collapse rate had also been described by Zdeblick and Ducker while using freeze-dried allogeneic tricortical iliac crest grafts [30]. In their study, the fusion rate in allografts was clearly lower in two-level fusions when compared with autografts (38% vs 83%), but the overall clinical results at 2 year follow-up were identical between the two groups. Similarly, no significant difference in the clinical and radiographic results using freeze-dried allografts versus autografts had been noted in an earlier study by Rish et al. [24].

Allografts from donor sites other than iliac crest have been used by Malinin et al. and Grossman et al. [13, 20]. Freeze-dried grafts from femoral heads or freeze-dried fibular grafts have been implanted successfully with comparable results to the previously mentioned studies. Specifically, fibular grafts have demonstrated good compressive strength and, in the patient population followed by Grossmann et al., allograft collapse did not occur [13, 29].

It has been suggested that in multilevel fusions, additional plate fixation might further decrease the incidence of allograft collapse, but this has not been investigated thus far. In a recent study at our clinic in which iliac crest autografts were augmented with plate fixation in anterior cervical spine fusions, we noted no graft collapse at all.

The donor site is a potential source of a number of complications, although these are generally of a minor nature. In a review of 1,244 cases, Whitecloud reported a complication rate of 20% at the donor site, whereas there was only a 0.2% complication rate occurring from the neck incision [28]. Considering the high incidence of donor site morbidity of iliac crest autografts in anterior cervical spine fusion, and the good results and minimal risks of using allografts in this operative technique, we conclude that the application of allograft bone for anterior cervical fusion is a safe and efficacious method.

According to the literature, the preoperative preparation of the graft seems to play a minor role for the clinical outcome. It seems that freeze-dried fibular and iliac crest allografts are favoured today. The storage of these grafts needs no special equipment and the antigenicity of freeze-dried allografts is very low [8].

In children with cervical instability due to a congenital anomaly or secondary to trauma, the results of spinal fusion with cadaveric bone grafts have not been satisfactory. In a study by Stabler et al., bone allografts were felt to be contraindicated in posterior cervical fusion in children [27].

Lumbar Spine

Degenerative disc disease in the lumbar spine may be treated by posterior, posterolateral or interbody fusion. The interbody fusion may be performed through an anterior approach (ALIF) or through a posterior approach (PLIF). In the operative treatment of degenerative disease of the lumbar spine, allogeneic bone graft is preferred in lumbar interbody fusions since the fusion rate is as high as with autogenous bone. Table 1 represents an overview of some reports combining PLIF and ALIF with allograft bone. Most surgeons use freeze-dried or ethylene-oxide sterilized bone without additional

Table 1. Result of spine fusions using allograft bone

Author		Graft	Fusion rate autografts	Fusion rate allografts
Cloward [6]	1985	Gas-sterilized PLIF		87–92%
Ma [19]	1985	Gas-sterilized PLIF		74%
Rish [25]	1989	Bank bone PLIF	84.3%	86.3%
Collis [7]	1985	Bank bone PLIF		94%
Loguidice [18]	1988	Cadaveric bone ALIF	75%	75%
Kozak [17]	1994	Femur allograft ALIF		97%

spinal instrumentation. Loguidice et al. and Rish have noted that the fusion rate depends on the lumbar level and number of levels fused [18, 25]. The 85% fusion rate of one level fusions drops to 50% in three level fusions [18]. The lumbo-sacral junction L5/S1 has a significantly higher fusion rate than the lumbar segments L4/L5 and L3/L4. Addition of spinal instrumentation clearly enhances the fusion rate [11].

The biomechanical properties of allograft bone has been of concern in lumbar interbody fusions. In an experimental study, Brantigan has shown that a large amount of processed allogeneic bone did not have adequate strength to withstand the expected mechanical loads in interbody lumbar fusion [2]. This is mainly true for iliac crest allografts and other cancellous bone blocks. Only fibular strut and femoral cortical ring allografts manifold exceed the load demands of approximately 2400 N during daily activities. Published results of studies in which allografts were used to achieve posterior or posterolateral fusion in the degenerative lumbar spine are mixed. The applied load on the fusion mass in extension may have a negative effect on the rate of healing. Additionally, the host environment in the posterolateral and lateral gutter is biologically less conducive to the formation of the fusion mass than the intervertebral space after complete discectomy. Herron reported a 76% pseudarthrosis rate with ethylene-oxide sterilized allogeneic bone. Nasca and Whelchel however described a fusion rate of 87% using cryopreserved allografts [14, 23]. It seemed that gas sterilization of the graft bone led to deterioration in graft incorporation [6, 14].

At our center, allograft bone for lumbar fusions is not used routinely. Only when the patient's bone stock is of very low quality, i.e. mainly in osteoporotic elderly people, do we add milled fresh frozen ($-70°C$) allogeneic femoral heads to the autogeneic bone harvested from the spinal decompression or the posterior iliac crest.

Another application of allograft bone in the lumbar spine is shown in Fig. 1. We routinely use allograft bone for the transpedicular filling of compression or burst fractures of the spine that have been reduced and stabilized by the internal fixator system.

Deformities

The use of allogeneic bone grafts as supplements in spinal fusion for scoliosis can offer several advantages over autogenous iliac grafts. The total operative time and blood loss can be decreased and possible complications related to the donor site can be avoided. These complications can include hematoma, infection, dysesthesia, pain in the hip or leg, gait disturbance, retroperitoneal hematoma, osteomyelitis, and wound dehiscence or unsightly scar if a separate incision is used.

Table 2 shows some results of different studies that compared the application of allogeneic bone in spinal fusion for scoliosis to the fusion with autogeneic bone. Operative time and blood loss have always been reduced if allograft had been used for fusion. The donor site morbidity, which may have a very high incidence with autograft harvesting is not an issue when allograft is used. The fusion rate is comparable between the allograft and autograft groups. In patients with neuromuscular scoliosis, the fusion rate was as high when using allografts as when using autografts. In these patients in whom iliac crest bone stock may be deficient, allogeneic bone provides the only available bone source. The infection rate with allograft fusions has not been increased. Because the transmission of infectious disease by bone grafts can be decreased by graft pretreatment, the use of processed allogeneic bone should be recommended in this young patient population.

Between 1988–1993 we operated on 31 patients with neuromuscular scoliosis at our center. In this patient group, we routinely used allograft bone for the posterior spinal

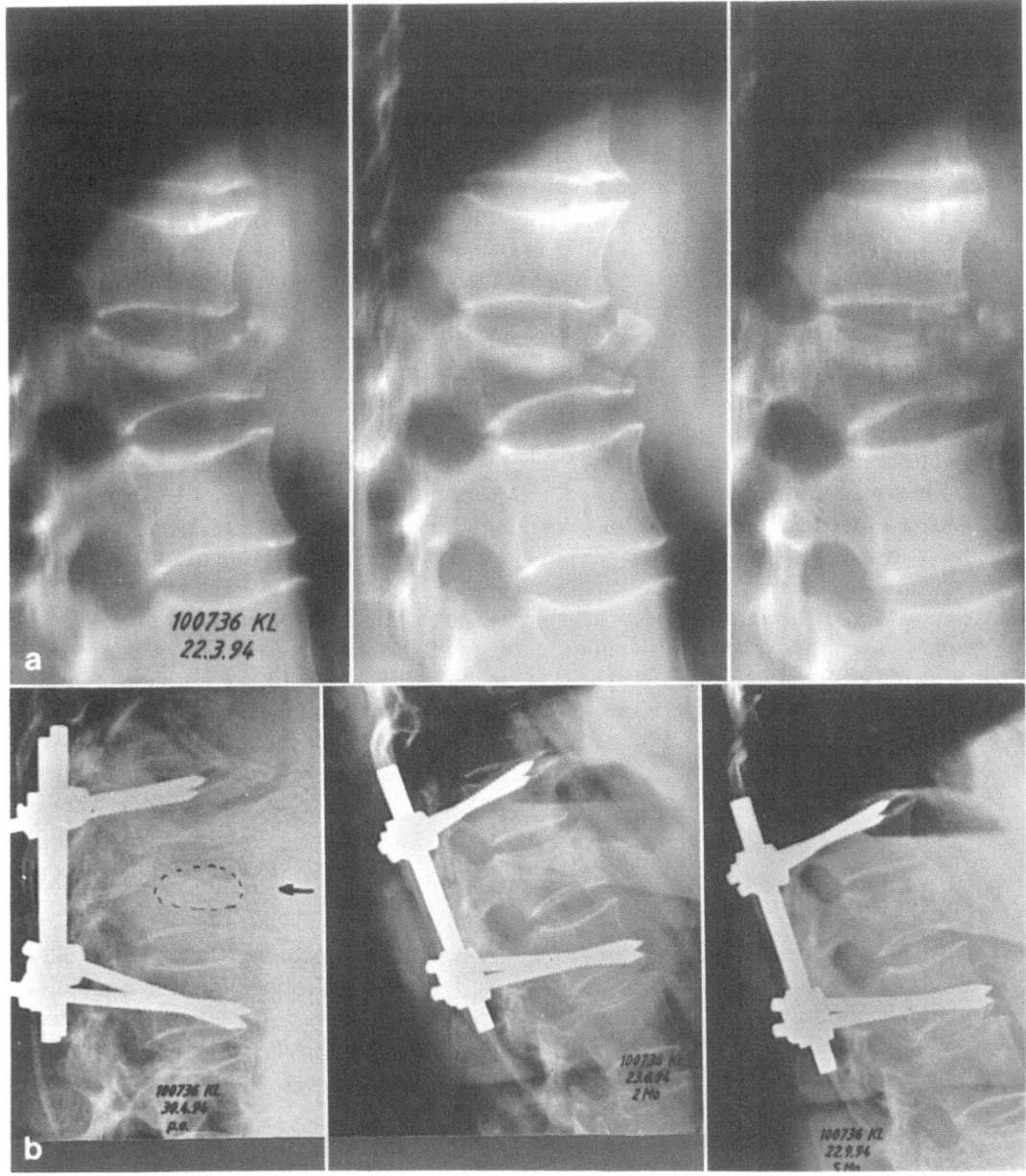

Fig. 1a. Incomplete burst fracture of 12th thoracic vertebral body in a 59 year old woman. Lateral tomogram. **b.** Follow-up after operative fracture treatment with internal fixator and transpedicular allogeneic bone grafting of fractured vertebral body (circle = allograft bone)

fusion. These patients were evaluated clinically and radiologically after a mean follow-up time of 3.4 years (range 10 months – 6.5 years). All patients except one had been stabilized by posterior instrumentation alone using the technique of Luque sublaminar wiring combined with pedicle screws placed in the S1 pedicles. The mean preoperative Cobb angle was 67°. Postoperatively, this had been corrected to 28°. There were no major preoperative or postoperative complications except one deep wound infection

Table 2. Allografts versus autografts in scoliosis surgery

Author	Diagnosis	Graft	No. of patients	Blood loss	Operation time	Infection	Non-union	Loss of correction	Donor site compl.
Fabry [1991]	Idiopathic scoliosis	Autograft	83			None	1/83	9%	20%
		Allograft (d.f.)	99	Ns decrease	Significant decrease		1/99	7%	None
Montgomery [1990]	Neuromusc. scoliosis	Autograft	18			1 superf.	1/18 (6%)	46%	?
		Allografts (f.dr.)	12	Significant decrease	Significant decrease	2 (1 late)	None	38%	None
Dodd [1988]	Idiopathic scoliosis	Autograft	20			None	None	9%	40%
		Allograft (d.f.)	20	Ns decrease	Significant decrease	None	None	4%	None
McCarthy [1986]	Neuromusc./ paralytic	Allografts (d.f.)	32	—	—	3 (2 deep)	None	11%	
Aurori [1983]	Idiopathic scoliosis	Autograft	114			1	5/114		
		Allograft (d.f.)	94	Significant decrease	Significant decrease	3	5/94		

d.f. = deep-frozen
f.dr. = freeze-dried

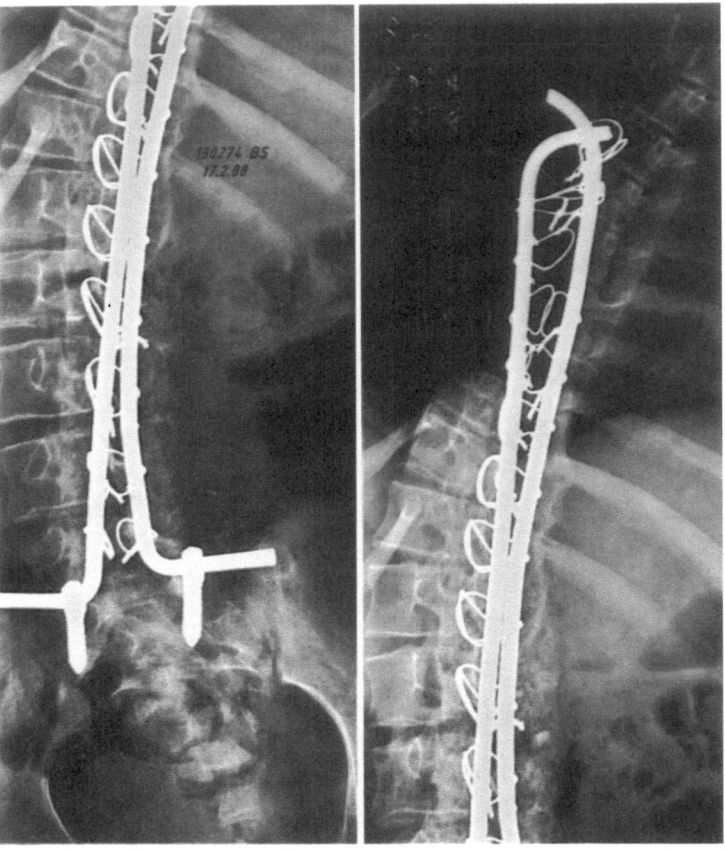

Fig. 2. One year follow-up after instrumentation and fusion of a neuromuscular scoliosis. Solid posterolateral allograft bone fusion mass

that healed after revision surgery. During the follow-up period we have seen 2 implant failures with breakage of the rods or wires. In these patients we suspect a vertebral non-union. None of them have required revision thus far. Figure 2 shows the 2 year result of a posterior instrumentation and fusion with allograft bone in a patient with neuromuscular scoliosis.

Conclusion

Bone autograft remains the most effective grafting material because it provides the three elements required for bone regeneration: osteoconduction, osteoinduction and osteogenic cells. However, autogenous grafting is associated with some shortcomings and complications, including limited quantities of bone for harvesting and donor-site morbidity. Therefore, alternative grafting substitutes such as bone allografts, ceramics, demineralized bone matrix etc. have been used. Based on the literature reviews, we conclude that bone allografts are a good, reliable and inexpensive alternative to bone autografts in the treatment of different spinal diseases requiring spine fusion. The advantage of the bone allograft is the easy availability without any donor site morbidity and everlasting quantity. If the donor selection and graft procurement have been done following the modern standardized rules of tissue banking, the risk of transmitting a disease is very low [5].

In the cervical spine the most common application is in anterior interbody fusion. The main problem here is the increasing probability of graft collapse correlating with the number of levels fused. This problem could possibly be solved with the addition of plate fixation.

In degenerative disease of the lumbar spine, bone allografts are widely used for anterior or posterior lumbar interbody fusions. Because of the higher biomechanical loads of the lumbar spine compared to the cervical spine, the risk of graft collapse in this region is even higher. The choice of a mechanically strong graft, like the cortical femoral ring, seems to be advisable when attempting to eliminate this problem. The biomechanical properties of commercially procured and prepared bone allografts should be controlled and declared.

In young patients with spinal deformities, bone allografts have also been widely used with good results. In these situations, the spinal instrumentation together with a thorough decortication of the dorsal spine elements enhances the bone healing.

Acknowledgement

Linguistic help by David L. Kramer, M.D., Brookline MA, U.S.A.

References

1. Aurori BF, Weierman RJ, Lowell HA, Nadel CI, Parsons JR (1985) Pseudarthrosis after spinal fusion for scoliosis. Clin Orthop 199: 153–158
2. Brantigan JW, Cunningham BW, Warden K, McAfee PC, Steffee AD (1993) Compression strength of donor bone for posterior lumbar interbody fusion. Spine 18: 1213–1221
3. Brown MD, Malinin TI, Davis PB (1976) A roentgenographic evaluation of frozen allografts versus autografts in anterior cervical spine fusions. Clin Orthop 119: 231–236
4. deBoer H (1989) Early research on bone transplantation. In: Aebi M, Regazzoni P (eds) Bone transplantation. Berlin Heidelberg: Springer, pp 7–19
5. Buck BE, Malinin TI, Brown MD (1989) Bone transplantation and human immunodeficiency virus: An estimate of risk of Acquired Immunodeficiency Syndrome (AIDS). Clin Orthop 240: 129–136
6. Cloward RB (1985) Posterior lumbar interbody fusion updated. Clin Orthop 193: 16–19
7. Collis JS (1985) Total disc replacement: A modified posterior lumbar interbody fusion. Clin Orthop 193: 64–67
8. Czitrom AA (1989) Bone transplantation, passenger cells and the major histocompatibility complex. In: Aebi M, Regazzoni P (eds) Bone transplantation. Berlin Heidelberg: Springer, pp 103–110
9. Dodd CAF, Fergusson CM, Freedman L, Houghton GR, Thomas D (1988) Allograft versus autograft bone in scoliosis surgery. J Bone Joint Surg 70-B: 431–434
10. Fabry G (1991) Allograft versus autograft bone in idiopathic scoliosis surgery: A multivariate statistical analysis. J Pediatr Orthop 11: 465–468
11. Gill K, O'Brien JP (1993) Observation of resorption of the posterior lateral bone graft in combined anterior and posterior lumbar fusion. Spine 18: 1885–1889
12. Griss P, Pfeiffer M (1991) Vertebral body replacement with homologous femoral head transplants. Int Orthop (SICOT) 15: 65–69
13. Grossman W, Peppelman WC, Baum JA, Kraus DR (1992) The use of freeze-dried fibular allograft in anterior cervical fusion. Spine 17: 565–569
14. Herron LD, Newman MH (1989) The failure of ethylene oxide gas-sterilized freeze-dried bone graft for thoracic and lumbar spinal fusion. Spine 14: 496–500

15. Kemp HBS, Jackson JW, Cook JDJ, Cook J (1973) Anterior fusion of the spine for infective lesions in adults. J Bone Joint Surg 55-B: 715–734
16. Knapp DR, Jones ET (1988) Use of cortical cancellous allograft for posterior spinal fusion. Clin Orthop 229: 99–106
17. Kozak JA, Heilman AE, O'Brien JP (1994) Anterior lumbar fusion options. Technique and graft materials. Clin Orthop 300: 45–51
18. Loguidice VA, Johnson RG, Guyer RD, Stith WJ, Ohnmesis DD, Hochschuler StH, Rashbaum RF (1988) Anterior lumbar interbody fusion. Spine 13: 366–369
19. Ma GWC (1985) Posterior lumbar interbody fusion with specialized instruments. Clin Orthop 193: 57–61
20. Malinin TI, Rosomoff HI, Sutton CH (1977) Human cadaver femoral head homografts for anterior cervical spine fusions. Surg Neurol 7: 249–251
21. McCarthy RE, Peek RD, Morrissy RT, Hough AJ (1986) Allograft bone in spinal fusion for paralytic scoliosis. J Bone Joint Surg 68-A: 370–375
22. Montgomery DM, Aronson DD, Lee CL, La Mont RL (1990) Posterior spinal fusion: Allograft versus autograft bone. J Spinal Disord 3: 370–375
23. Nasca RJ, Whelchel JD (1987) Use of cryopreserved bone in spinal surgery. Spine 12: 222–227
24. Rish BL, McFadden, JT, Penix JO (1976) Anterior cervical fusion using homologous bone grafts: a comparative study. Surg Neurol 5: 119–121
25. Rish BL (1989) A critique of posterior lumbar interbody fusion: 12 years' experience with 250 patients. Surg Neurol 31: 281–289
26. Roy-Camille R, Saillant G, Mazel Ch, Lapresle Ph (1986) Utilisation des tetes femorales de banque dans les reconstructions apres corporectomies dorsales et lombaires. Rev Chir Orthop [Suppl II] 73: 168–170
27. Stabler CL, Eismont, FJ, Brown MD, Green BA, Malinin TI (1985) Failure of posterior cervical fusions using cadaveric bone graft in children. J Bone Joint Surg 67A: 370–375
28. Whitecloud TS III (1978): Complication of anterior cervical fusion. In: American Academy of Orthopaedic Surgeons: Instructional Course Lectures, Vol 27. St. Louis: CV Mosby, pp 223–227
29. Wittenberg RH, Moeller J, Shea M, White III AA, Hayes WC (1990) Compressive strength of autologous and allogenous bone grafts for thoracolumbar and cervical spine fusion. Spine 15: 1073–1078
30. Zdeblick TA, Ducker TB (1991) The use of freeze-dried allograft bone for anterior cervical fusions. Spine 16: 726–729

Authors' addresses: Othmar Schwarzenbach, M.D., Paul Heini, M.D., Ulrich Berlemann M.D., Emmanuel Gautier, M.D., University of Bern, Department of Orthopaedic Surgery, Inselspital, CH-3010 Bern, Switzerland.

The Role of Massive Bone Allografts in Traumatic Bone Loss

M. Salai, Y. Amit, S. Velkkes, and H. Horosowski

The Orthopaedic Wing, Chaim Sheba Medical Center, Tel Hashomer Hospital, Israel

Summary

Traumatic bone loss is often the result of injuries such as: missiles (either high or low velocity) or motor vehicle accidents (MVA).

These types of injuries are often associated with major bone loss, soft tissue damage, and frequently also injury to the neurovascular bundle.

Early reconstruction of the bone deficits by massive bone allografts, offers immediate stabilization by a bony scaffold, allowing early rehabilitation and resumption of function.

The indications, prerequisites, technique and illustrative cases are presented and discussed.

Introduction

The increasing numbers of traumatic bone loss poses major difficulties and challenges to the orthopedic surgeon. Traumatic bone loss is characterized by high energy dicipated into the tissues which causes major soft tissue damage as well as severe comminution of bone [1, 2, 3, 4, 12]. Often, these injuries are associated with damage to the adjacent neurovascular bundles threatening the viability of the limb [7, 8].

Since most of these injuries are "open" Gustilo 3-A/B, infection is a major threat to the success of treatment [5, 11].

Classically, these injuries were treated in the past by primary amputation, and more recently, by external fixation along with delayed bony reconstruction [10]. Traditionally, the wounds were left open until the risk of infection had subsided. Nevertheless, a high percentage of cases resulted in amputation regardless of which method was used especially when a neurovascular injury was encountered [6, 9].

With the development of rapid evacuation modalities from the scene of injury, wide spectrum antibiotic therapy, advanced vascular and microsurgical repair techniques, improved external fixation systems, and increased experience of trauma surgeons, it became logical to replace the bone loss as soon as possible. This is now feasible because major trauma centers have access to tissue banks set up for other fields of reconstructive orthopedic surgery.

These advances enabled us to treat selected cases of traumatic bone loss by early evacuation, meticulous debridement, and replacement of the bone defect with a massive bone allograft as a primary modality of treatment.

Material and Methods

Between 1973–1993 we have treated 19 patients who suffered major traumatic bone loss. There were 16 males and three females. The cause of injury was missiles in 13 patients and motor vehicle accident (MVA) in the other 6. The major bone loss was in the tibia in 11 patients, proximal ulna in 4, distal femur in 3, and distal humerus in one. All the patients were evacuated and reached the operating room in less than 10 hours after injury. Antibiotic therapy was initiated less than 4 hours after injury and all patients were operated on by the same senior surgical team. Six patients had additional vascular injury which needed vascular reconstruction. Eight patients had additional nerve injuries. Bone allograft of different sizes was used in all patients. The allografts were fresh, irradiated (by 3 Megarads of Gamma irradiation) and frozen to −80 degrees centigrade.

The size of the allografts ranged from 4–22 cm. Three patients received osteo-articular allografts. (The articular surface was preserved with 10% DMSO solution). All patients received wide spectrum antibiotics for six weeks or longer if there was any specific infecting organism.

Results

Only one leg was amputated among this group of patients. Three patients developed chronic osteomyelitis in whom the infection subsided eventually in two. The third patient has a draining sinus and refused any surgical intervention. Seven patients needed additional surgical procedures: bone grafting in four patients, split thickness skin graft in two, and vascularised musculocutaneous free flap in one. Three patients are walking with the help of a cane. Seventeen patients resumed their work following their treatment, and nine returned to full pre-injury sports activities. From the patients' perspective, despite the prolonged need for rehabilitation (6–18 months), the end result of their physical status is preferrable for amputation.

Illustrative Cases

Case 1 S.A. A 20 year old soldier sustained a high velocity missile injury to his leg. On admission, no pulses were palpable in his foot and the radiographs (Fig. 1) showed a severely comminuted fracture of the middle third of the tibia. At surgery, vascular repair followed reconstruction by a massive bone allograft and intramedullary nail (Fig. 2). The nail was removed later with excellent functional result 20 years following his injury. Case 2 J.K. A 41 year old male was involved in a road accident in which he sustained other major injuries and a severely open comminuted fracture of the proximal ulna (Fig. 3).

At surgery, reconstruction of, the humero-ulnar joint was not feasible. Osteoarticular allograft replacement of the whole proximal ulna was performed (Fig. 4). At 3 1/2 years following injury he has a functional stable elbow with a range of movement of −20 to 100 degrees.

Discussion

Amputation is often the best surgical solution in critically injured limbs, especially when a major bone defect and neurovascular impairment co-exist [7, 9]. However, even in

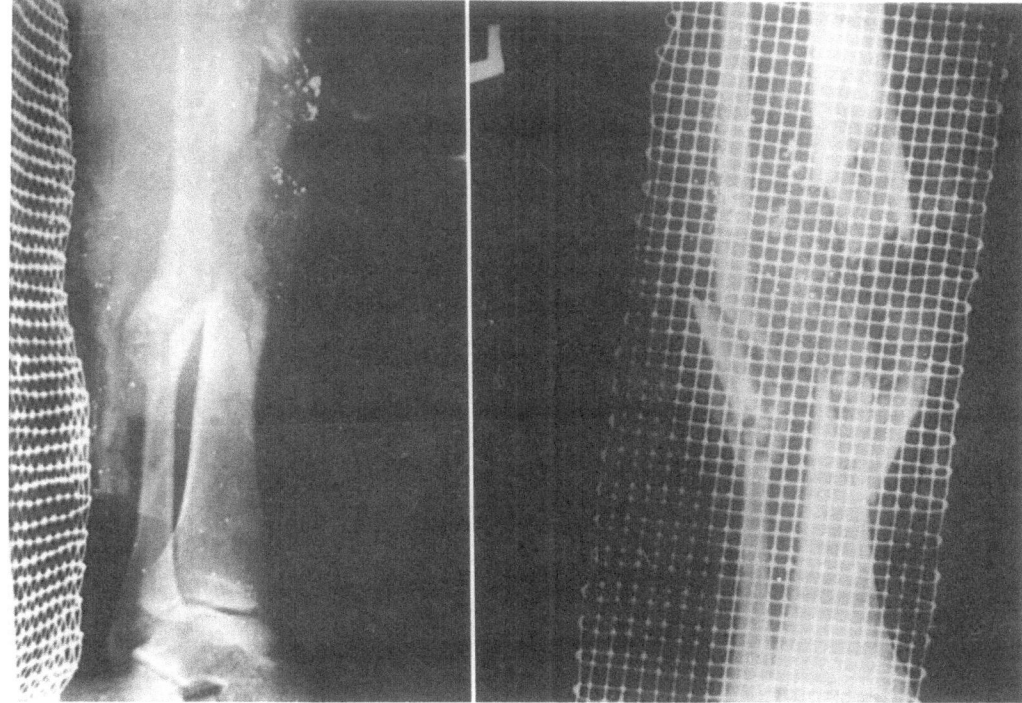

Fig. 1. Case No. 1: Radiograph of the leg on admission. Severe comminution of the middle third of the tibia is demonstrated

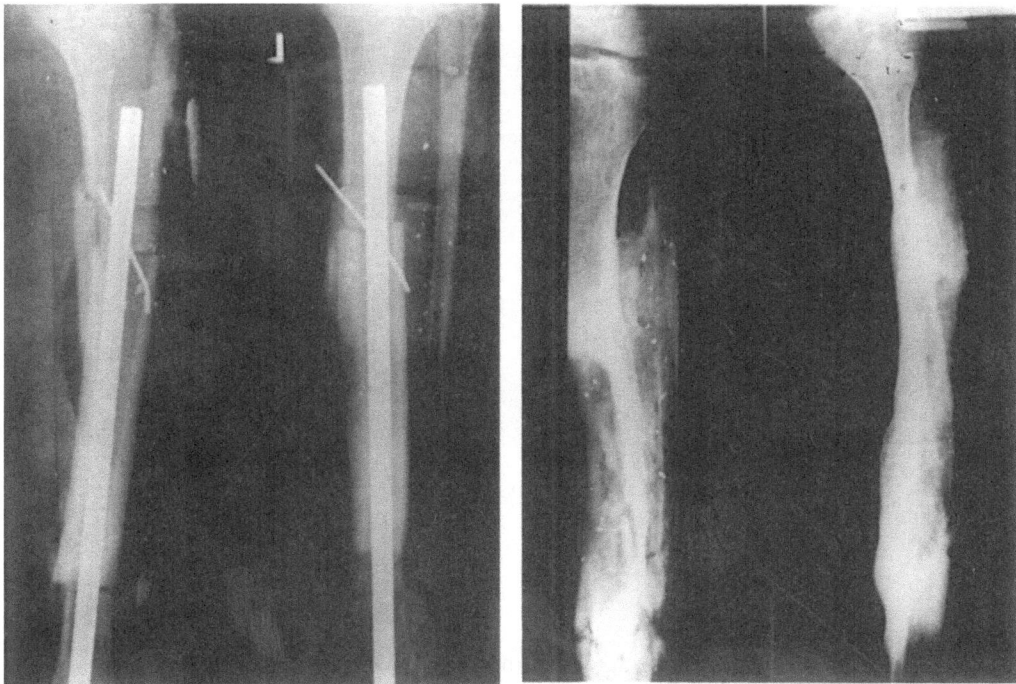

Fig. 2. Case No. 1: Massive bone allograft used to reconstruct the defect in early postoperative stage and 15 years later after reconstruction

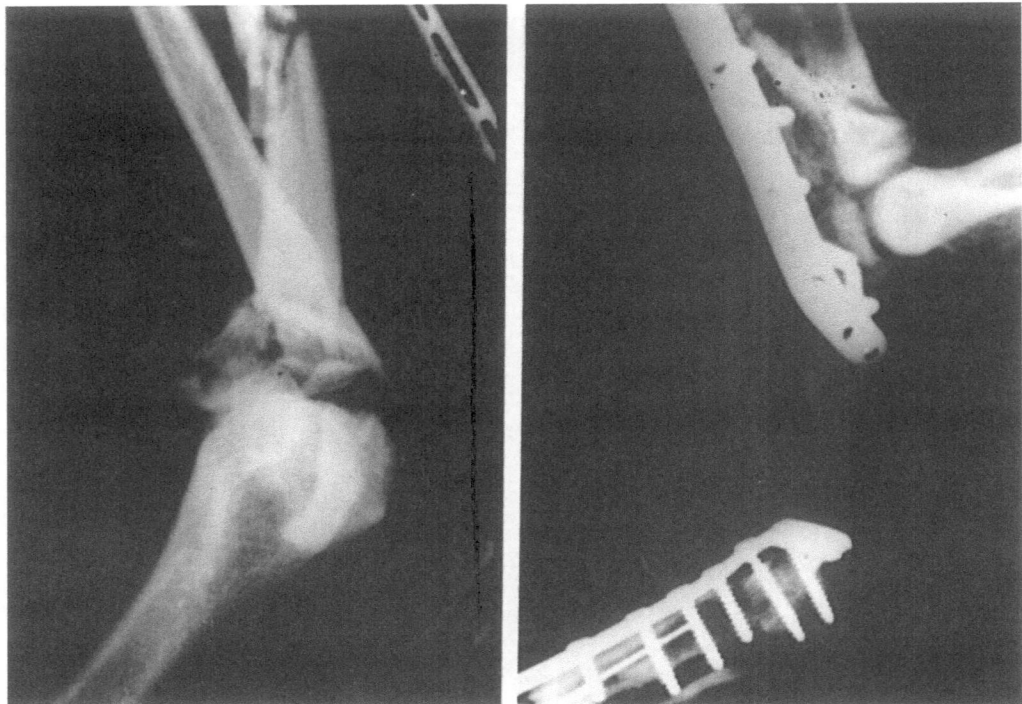

Fig. 3. Case No. 2: Radiograph of the elbow on admission: severe comminution of the proximal ulna is demonstrated

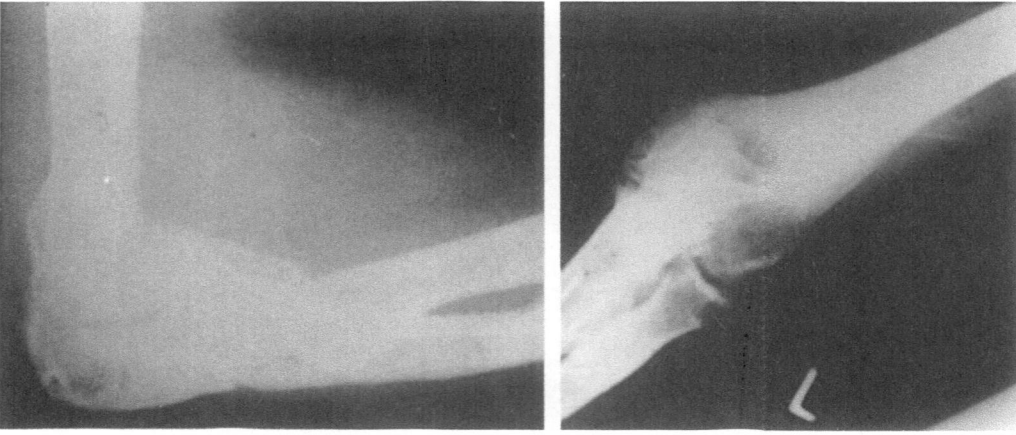

Fig. 4. Case No. 2: Reconstruction at 3 1/2 years follow-up showing good incorporation of the osteoarticular allograft of the proximal ulna

such devastating conditions, under certain circumstances limb salvage is possible. Vascular impairment, soft tissue damage and major bone loss are the main factors that jeopardize the viability of the injured limb [12]. The following factors are prerequisites for successful limb salvage:

a) Means for rapid evacuation, within 6–8 hours of injury, to a level 1 trauma center which has all the necessary facilities for the treatment of such cases. This should often be accomplished by helicopters.

b) Availability of specially trained and experienced trauma orthopedic surgeons able to perform a meticulous debridement of the wounds and knowledgeable in allograft reconstruction of bone defects.

c) Availability of early wide spectrum intravenous antibiotic therapy to be initiated at the scene of injury.

d) Collaboration of experienced surgeons in subspecialities such as: vascular, plastic and microvascular surgery.

e) Access to a regional bone or tissue bank which can supply at short notice all the donor tissue necessary for such cases including various osteoarticular allografts.

In our experience massive bone allografts united with the host bone even though the preliminary conditions were unfavorable for bone remodeling. The rate of non-union necessitating bone grafting was low.

In conclusion, bone allografts should be added to the armamentarium of methods employed in the treatment of traumatic bone loss.

References

1. Amato JJ (1971) High velocity arterial injury: a study of the mechanism of injury. J Trauma 11: 142–146
2. Celavland M, Manning J (1951) Care of battle casualties and injuries involving bone and joints. J Bone Joint Surg 33A: 517–523
3. De Muth WE Jr (1966) Bullet velocity and designs as determinants of wounding capability: an experimental study. J Trauma 6: 226–228
4. Hennessy M, Banks HH (1976) Extremity gunshot wounds and gunshot fractures in civilian practice. Clin Orthop 114: 296–303
5. Patzakis MJ, Harvey JP (1974) The role of antibiotics in the management of open fractures. J Bone Joint Surg 56A: 532–537
6. Robins W, Kuswetter W (1982) Fracture typing of human bone by assault missile trauma. Acta Chir Scand [Suppl] 508: 233–227
7. Russotti GM, Sim FH (1985) Missile wounds of the extremities: a current concept review. Orthopedics 8: 1106–1110
8. Rybeck B, Janzon B (1985) Absorption of missile energy in soft tissue. Acta Chir Scand 142: 201–205
9. Salai M (1990) Massive bone allograft: a salvage procedure for complex bone loss due to high-velocity missiles—A long-term follow-up. Mil Med 155, 7: 316–318
10. Standford JP, Evans JR (1957) An experiment evaluation of usefulness of antibiotic agents in the early management of contaminated traumatic soft tissue wounds. Surg Gynecol Obst 105: 5–10
11. Thoresby FP, Darlow HH (1967) The mechanism of primary infection of bullet wounds. Br J Surg 54: 359–363
12. Ziperman HH (1961) The management of soft tissue missile wounds in war and peace. J Trauma 1: 361–366

Authors' address: M. Salai, Y. Amit, S. Velkkes and H. Horosowski, The Orthopedic Wing, Chaim Sheba Medical Center, Tel Hashomer Hospital, 52621 Israel.

Tendon, Meniscus and Osteochondral Grafts

Clinical Applications of Tendon Allografts

A. Lechat[1] and M. Martens[2]

[1] Orthopaedic Surgery-Traumatology, Keerbergen, Belgium
[2] Orthopaedic Surgery-Traumatology, University Hospital Antwerp, Edegem, Belgium

Ligament injuries are common and potentially disabling. The healing of certain ligaments remains unpredictable for reasons that are still poorly understood. In recent years there has been an increase in the number of reconstructive procedures performed for different kinds of acute or chronic ligament injuries. For these reconstructive procedures many surgeons still use an autograft. The use of autografts bears some limitations. It is a mutilating surgery where one structure is sacrificed to replace another. This aspect not only limits the choice of tendon removal but also the amount of available graft material. It leads to extensive surgery, it is time consuming and may have adverse effects and complications due to the resection of a tendon or part of a tendon. These complications, such as a muscle hernia after MacIntosh ligametoplasty, rupture of the patellar tendon [27] or tendonitis after Jones or Imbert plasty are inherent to the applied techniques. Consequently, various types of artificial ligaments and heterologous bioprostheses have been developed. Clinical trials of these materials have proved that they can provide neither a long-standing prosthetic substitute nor an innocuous scaffold which will induce thick fibrous tissue [12]. Problems relate to a lack of bone ingrowth at the osseous tunnels and also to biocompatibility, deformity and fatigue characteristics of the artificial ligament. In our center we revised several artificial ligaments that failed.

The use of tendon allografts for surgical procedures has been documented by experimental and clinical studies but is not yet fully accepted nor commonly used by orthopaedic surgeons. We wanted to find out whether tendon allografts are suitable for surgical use.

When we started using tendon allografts in 1986 there was not much literature available on results of this procedure. So far we have only used tendons procured from multi-organ donors. Achilles tendon and tensor fascia lata were removed with a bone block and split in two. Patellar tendon was removed with bone blocks from the tibial tuberosity and patella with the attached quadriceps tendon and also split. Tibialis anterior, peroneal tendons, foot extensors and flexors were also removed. The donor selection was done by the transplant coordinator according to AATB criteria. The tendons were procured under strict aseptic conditions in the operating room. After taking cultures the tendons were double packaged in sterile plastic containers, sealed and labeled. They were stored in a deep-freezer at $-80°C$. Initially, the tendons were only rinsed in physiological solution before storage. We did not add antibiotics in order to be able to clinically evaluate the patient after transplantation (intra-articular antibiotics can cause chemical synovitis which would have been difficult to differentiate from a rejection reaction causing an effusion). More recently, due to awareness of the possibly longer window period for HIV, we immerse the tendons in 70% Hibitane Alcohol for 30 minutes. They are then rinsed and stored. This procedure does not seem to cause any clinical problem. It is not known whether the alcohol penetrates to the center of the tendons.

We looked into the possible use of freeze-dried tendons. These are easier to store and handle, safer regarding the transmission of disease, and superior in terms of reducing the immunogenicity of the tissues [4]. In 1978 Neviaser et al. [9] reported the successful use of freeze-dried allogeneic tendon to repair massive chronic ruptures of the rotator cuff at the shoulder. Bright and Green [1] also reported in 1981 on the clinical use of freeze-dried fascia lata allografts in various types of orthopaedic reconstructions. Shino [13] on the other hand, stated in 1986 that he prefers non-lyphilized tendons because he fears that freeze-drying might reduce the mechanical strength of the tissues.

We investigated fresh, frozen and freeze-dried tendons by microscopy. In comparison to the frozen tendons the freeze-dried tendons, after 4 hours of rehydration, showed massive destruction. This indicated that freeze-dried tendons may be biomechanically inferior to frozen tendons and therefore not good enough for clinical use. We investigated the reason for the microscopic findings with the hypothesis that freeze-drying perhaps breaks the cross-links between the alpha-chains of the collagen. In collaboration with the Department of Rheumatology of the Leuven University (Prof. Dequecker) identical portions of fresh, frozen and rehydrated freeze-dried tendons were disolved and fractionated into tropocollagen bundles. Chromatography was performed and the results showed no difference between the three groups, indicating that freeze-drying as such does not destroy the cross-links and does not damage the collagen. It is not known if irradiation damages cross-links of collagen, further experiments with irradiated freeze-dried tendons will resolve this question.

In collaboration with the Biomechanical Engineering Department (Prof. R. Van Audekercke) of our university and the UCL Tissue Bank (Dr. Chr. Delloye) biomechanical tests were performed on 30 pairs of patellar tendons. We compared the strength to failure of frozen and freeze-dried tendons. Two techniques of freeze-drying were used. We also compared left to right. The tendons were tested with an Instron testing system with a deformation rate of 1000 mm/min. Results are shown in Table 1. There was no difference in strength between frozen and freeze-dried tendons, and the technique of freeze-drying had no effect on the biomechanical characteristics of the tendons. There was no significant difference between left to right in the control group.

It is surprising that freeze-drying does not affect the biomechanical properties of tendon allografts. It is possible that if this experiment was repeated on freeze-dried "irradiated" tendons, a difference might be found. So far our studies have suggested that freeze-dried tendons are as good and as strong as frozen tendons and probably safer because they are sterilized and therefore carry a diminished risk for infectious contamination.

Another important aspect of the use of tendon allografts is the immunological response. Numerous studies have examined the biology of tendon allografts in various clinical and experimental settings [3, 5, 8, 11, 13]. It has been shown that collagen of the extracellular matrix of connective tissue can be weakly antigenic. It is generally accepted that the immune response is mainly directed toward the cellular components of the transplanted tendon [3, 4, 5, 6, 8, 13]. Studies have shown that tendon allografts possess major histocompatibility antigens which are expressed on the surface of cells of tendon tissue [8]. Destruction of the cellular elements of bone and tendon resulted in improved acceptance when these tissue allografts were placed into a mismatched host [3, 4, 5, 6, 8, 13]. Freeze-drying and deep-freezing have been shown to render connective

Table 1. Comparison of strength to failure of freeze-dried and frozen patellar tendons

Group 1:	
Freeze dried	Frozen $-80°C$
n = 14 pairs	
$3299 \pm 1110\,N$	$3244 \pm 1153\,N$
$\Delta = 55.21$	$p = 0.45$
No significant difference	
Group 2:	
N_2 boiling point (195,8°C)	Frozen $-80°C$
n = 11 pairs	
$3936 \pm 957\,N$	$4069 \pm 953\,N$
$\Delta = 133\,N$	$p = 0.37$
No significant difference.	
Group 3:	
Control left	Right
n = 5 pairs	
$3877 \pm 628\,N$	$3839 \pm 910\,N$
$\Delta = 37.4\,N$	$p = 0.47$
No significant difference.	

tissue allografts less antigenic [3, 4, 5, 6, 8]. It is probable that such preservation techniques kill the cells within the tissue thus altering their immunogenicity.

In 1988 a prospective study regarding the immunological response to tendon allografts was conducted in collaboration with the HLA laboratory of the blood transfusion center (Dr. M.P. Emonds). At the time when the study was performed 113 tendons had been inserted in 111 patients. The tendons were procured from multi-organ donors, and stored at $-80°C$ for at least 3 months prior to transplantation. 75 patients were evaluated. 2 patients had operations on both knees for chronic instability.

All patients were HLA typed before surgery. HLA-antibody screening was performed on the patients' sera in a standard microlymphocytotoxity test on a selected frozen lymphocyte panel, before and at least once between 2 and 6 months post-transplantation. 48 HLA Class I antigen specificities were included. Two techniques were used to detect the HLA-antibodies. One was the standard National Institute of Health (NIH) test on total peripheral blood lymphocytes in Terasaki trays. The second test was the more sensitive two-color fluorescence test on labeled B lymphocytes. As all tendons came from HLA-typed multi-organ donors whose spleen cells had been frozen, HLA crossmaches were performed retrospectively. Pre-transplantation HLA-antibody screenings were negative in all patients. Post-transplantation we found HLA-antibody (with low PRA in the beginning) detectable with the standard NIH test in 47% of the patients. With the more sensitive B cell test cytotoxicity was present in 75% of the patients. Shortly after transplantation the antibodies showed a narrow specificity (but positive on the tendon donor lymphocytes).

HLA crossmatches on frozen tendon-donor spleen lymphocytes were performed retrospectively on all patients with HLA-antibodies and a few negative controls. All patients with HLA-antibody also had positive crossmatches. Negative controls were not reactive with their tendon donor lymphocytes. This proved the donor specificity of the antibodies formed. Clinically we did not see any synovitis or any other rejection reaction.

We concluded that tendon allograft implantation can induce an immunological response on a subclinical level. This sensitization is important if the patient is on a waiting list for organ transplantation. In such patients the surgeon is advised to use a freeze-dried tendon in order not to compromise the patients' chance for an organ transplantation. So far we have mainly used tendon allografts for the reconstruction of an ACL with chronic instability of the knee. From 1986 till now over 600 patients had reconstructions carried out in two centres. Criteria for surgery were frequent giving way in daily life in the not very sports active patients. Active young athletes were advised to have reconstructive surgery if they had a strong wish to continue vigorous sports including jumping, sudden turning or body contact. In most patients an intra-articular reconstruction was performed using either half of a patellar tendon, half of an Achilles tendon, half of a tensor fascia lata or a tibialis anterior. Initially an open procedure was performed in most patients. The tendon was fixed at the tibia osseous tunnel by means of the bone block attached to the tendon. The tendon was passed through the tibial and femoral tunnels by means of a Chinese finger. A bone plug was then inserted at the femoral tunnel. With the rest of the tendon an extra-articular augmentation was done and it was fixed at the tubercle of Gerdi with a staple. More recently the procedure has been carried out arthroscopically.

The possibilities for using tendon allografts are increasing steadily. PCL ruptures (acute and chronic) are treated with very satisfactory results with Achilles tendon allograft transplantation combined with L.A.D. augmentation. Severe lesions of the lateral collateral ligament and the lateral capsular structures of the knee are treated primarily by an allograft since suturing is often not possible or not efficient to secure knee stability.

We have used tendon allografts in about 30 patients with chronic lateral ankle instability. We used a modified Chrisman Snook procedure. Instead of using the patients' own peroneus brevis tendon, which has to be split, we used a peroneal tendon allograft. This shortened the procedure, the patient needed a much smaller incision, and recovered more quickly than after the use of an autograft. (Fig. 1; Fig. 2).

We have used extensor tendons to repair the Achilles tendon after a third rupture. Many other conditions can be treated by using an allograft rather then an autograft or a synthetic graft. We have used extensor tendons from the foot of a multi-organ donor to replace flexor or extensor tendons at the hand. We mainly use foot tendons because it is very difficult to get permission to remove tendons from the hand. The family of the donor usually gives permission to procure on the condition that nothing can be seen after the procedure. This cannot be guaranteed if the hands, that are usually very visible, are operated on. In one patient, in whom we reconstructed 5 flexor tendons, (Fig. 3) we had the chance to have a second look 3 months later (Fig. 4), since the patient developed some adhesions at the level of the anastomosis at the forearm. We took some biopsies, that showed no necrosis at all. There was no abnormal infiltration. The tendon, macroscopically and microscopically, looked like a normal tendon. Our surgeons have used several tendon allografts for hand surgery recently, both in primary reconstruction or after the implantation of Silicone rods for 6 weeks, without experiencing any problems.

Frozen or freeze-dried fascia lata can be used for duraplasty by the neurosurgeons or they can be used to close large inguinal or abdominal herniations. The advantage over Marlex meshes is that these tissues quickly revascularize and behave as normal biological tissues. There is less chance for infection, which always exists if you implant a foreign material and you can do a reintervention through the graft after some time without any problem.

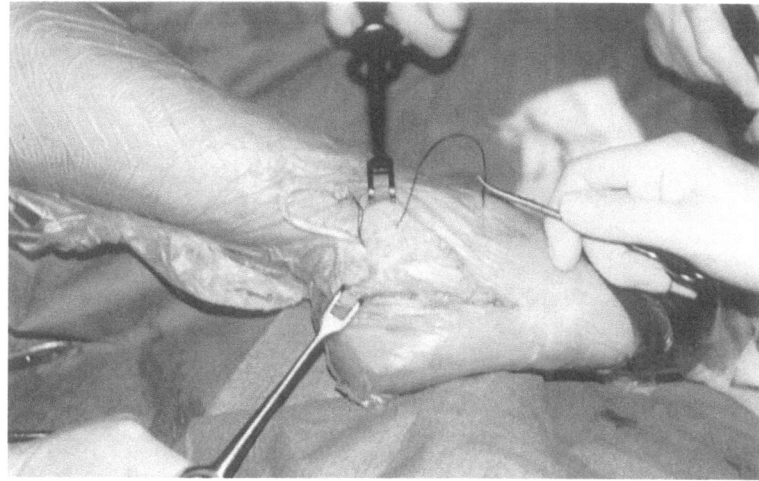

Fig. 1

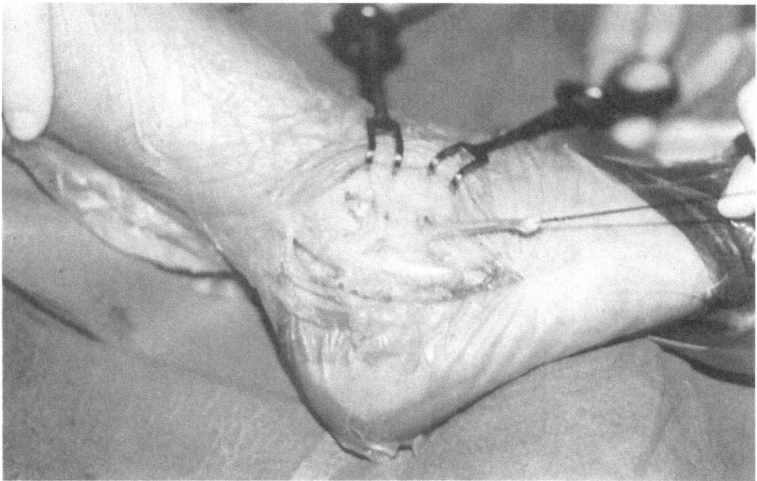

Fig. 2

Figs. 1 and 2. Peroneal tendon allograft used for reconstruction of chronic lateral ankle instability

Soft tissue allografts can also be used to provide stability about the hip joint when the abductor musculature is deficient or inadequate. A variety of ligamentous and tendinous repairs are possible for conditions such as sternoclavicular separation, acromioclavicular separation, hallux valgus, atlanto-axial subluxation from juvenile rheumatoid arthritis, quadriceps, patellar and Achilles tendon ruptures and other defects.

In conclusion we can state that an allograft is a valuable and suitable alternative to an autograft. Although both have mechanical characteristics that do not meet those of the original structure one may recognize some obvious advantages with regard to the use of an allograft. We are using biological material achieving the same end result as with an autograft but by a far less mutilating procedure, with shortened and limited surgery avoiding certain complications that are inherent to the use of an autograft. We must pay

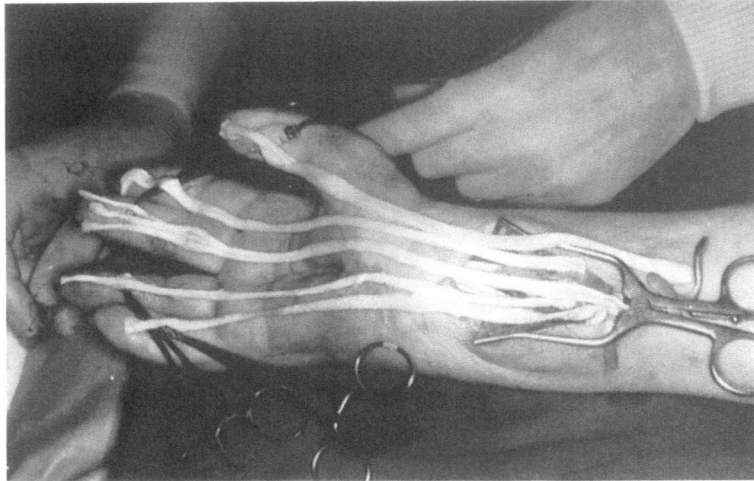

Fig. 3. Extensor tendons from the foot used to reconstruct the flexor tendons of the hand

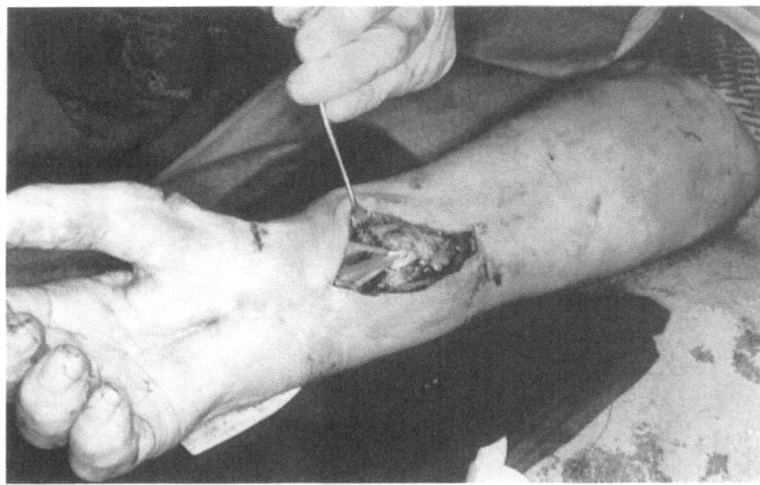

Fig. 4. Reintervention 3 months post-transplantation. The tendons look like normal tendons

attention to find a safe solution with regard to the immunological response and disease transmission including possible transfer of hepatitis, HIV etc.

The principal disadvantage of allografts is that they are in short supply. If it becomes possible to obtain large numbers of tendon allografts under ideal sterile conditions, and to process them in a way that allows storage for long periods, their application would be considerably broadened.

References

1. Bright RW, Green WT (1981) Freeze-dried fascia lata allograft: a review of 47 cases. J Pediatric Orthop 1: 13–22
2. Bonamo JJ, Krinick RM, Sporn AA (1984) Rupture of the patellar ligament after use of its central third for anterior cruciate reconstruction. A report of two cases. J Bone Joint Surg 66-A: 1294–1297

3. Cameron RR, Conrad RN, Sell KW, Latham WD (1971) Freeze-dried composite tendon allografts: an experimental study. Plast Reconstr Surg 47: 39–46

4. Friedlaender GE, Strong DM, Sell KW (1976) Studies on the antigenicity of bone. Freeze-dried and deep-frozen bone allografts in rabbits. J Bone Joint Surg 58-A: 854–858

5. Graham WC, Smith DA, McGuire MP (1955) The use of frozen stored tendons for grafting. An experimental study. Proceedings of the Orthopaedic Research Society. J Bone Joint Surg 37-A: 624

6. Gresham RB (1964) Freeze-drying human tissue for clinical use. Cryobiology 1: 150–156

7. McCarroll JR (1983) Fracture of the patella during a golf swing following a reconstruction of the anterior cruciate ligament. A case report. Am J Sports Med 11: 26–27

8. Minami A, Ishii S, Ogino T, Oikawa T, Kobayashi H (1982) Effect of the immunological antigenicity of the allogeneic tendons on tendon grafting. Hand 14: 111–119

9. Neviaser SJ, Neviaser RJ, Neviaser TJ (1978) The repair of chronic massive ruptures of the rotator cuff of the shoulder by use of a freeze-dried rotator cuff. J Bone Joint Surg (Am) 60-A: 681–684

10. Noyes FR, Grood ES (1976) The strength of the anterior cruciate ligament in humans and rhesus monkeys: age-related and species-related chanes. J Bone Joint Surg (Am) 58-A: 1074–1082

11. Peacock EE Jr, Petty J (1959) Morphology of homologous and heterologous tendon grafts. Surg Gynecol Obstet 109: 735–742

12. Rushton N, Dandy DJ, Naylor CPE (1983) The clinical arthroscopic and histological findings after replacement of the cruciate ligament with carbon fiber. J Bone Joint Surg 65-B: 309

13. Shino K, Kawasaki T, Hirose H, Gotoh I, Inoue M, Ono K (1984) Replacement of the anterior cruciate ligament by an allogeneic tendon graft. An experimental study in the dog. J Bone Joint Surg 66-B (5): 672–681

Authors' addresses: Dr. Ann Lechat, Orthopaedic Surgery—Traumatology, Haachtsebaan 150A, B-3140 Keerbergen, Belgium; Prof. Mark Martens, Orthopaedic Surgery—Traumatology, University Hospital Antwerp, Wilrijkstraat 1,B-2650 Edegem, Belgium.

The Use of Fresh Frozen Soft Tissue Allografts in Knee Ligament Surgery

D. L. Johnson[1] and C. D. Harner[2]

[1]Division of Orthopaedics Chief: Section of Sports Medicine, University of Kentucky, Lexington, Kentucky, U.S.A
[2]Department of Orthopaedics, Chief, Division of Sports Medicine, University of Pittsburgh, Pittsburgh, U.S.A

The use of soft tissue allografts in knee ligament reconstruction has an important role in the surgical treatment of patients in the field of sports medicine. Currently, the most common uses for soft tissue allografts involve isolated anterior cruciate ligament (ACL) and posterior cruciate ligament (PCL) reconstruction, revision ACL and PCL reconstruction, medial collateral ligament augmentation, lateral collateral ligament augmentation, and combined ligamentous injuries of the knee. This chapter will highlight the current basic science, clinical knowledge, and controversies regarding the use of fresh frozen allograft tissues. In addition, we report the results of our early clinical experience using fresh frozen soft tissue allografts in knee ligament reconstruction. We will be focussing our attention on fresh frozen allografts as this has been our preferred allograft of choice since 1985. The use of freeze-dried allografts will only be mentioned briefly in this chapter.

Patient Selection

Selecting to use a soft tissue allograft is often patient specific. Thus the surgeon has carefully considered the advantages and disadvantages of using a soft tissue allograft for that particular individual. The principal advantage of a soft tissue allograft is that it obviates the need to harvest autogenous tissue from the patient. Weakening of the donor muscle groups can occur by violating the normal extensor mechanism or harvesting the hamstring tendon. Other advantages include improved cosmesis, decreased tourniquet/operative time, ability to "customize" the size of the allograft to that individual patient's requirement (increased graft selection), and decreased postoperative pain. Another relative advantage includes the individual who may be at risk of developing a "stiff knee" postoperatively. The greatest potential disadvantage is the remote possibility of transmission of the human immunodeficiency virus (HIV) and other diseases to the recipient. Additional concerns include the delayed biologic incorporation of allograft tissue compared to autogenous tissue, possible effects of increased laxity compared to autogenous grafts, and the unknown long-term results (five to ten years) which are currently being defined.

The primary advantage of allograft tissue in knee ligament surgery is the situation when autogenous tissue is not available or is undesirable. This includes the patient on whom autogenous tissue has been used for a previous reconstruction which has failed and who now requires revision surgery. When performing multiple ligament reconstruction (i.e., surgery in the dislocated knee), allograft tissue is particularly advantageous because there frequently is insufficient autogenous tissue available to replace all of the torn and irreparable structures. In other select cases, the patient's own autogenous tissue is undesirable for one reason or another. For example, a patient who sustains a PCL tear secondary to a "dashboard" injury in an automobile accident may have traumatic injury to the extensor tendon mechanism. Other examples include patients with a history of patello femoral pain, dysfunction, or malalignment. In individuals with a "small" patellar tendon, allograft reconstruction may be preferable to autogenous reconstruction. In addition, older patients with symptomatic ACL deficiency who have failed non-operative management and have early evidence of patello-femoral degenerative joint disease, harvesting of the central-third patellar tendon may exacerbate the patello-femoral symptoms postoperatively.

Allograft Tissue Availability, Procurement, and Storage

There are two basic types of allograft tissue. One is composed of soft tissue alone; others contain a bony block on one or both ends. Currently, the majority of allograft reconstructions are performed with bone-patellar tendon-bone (BPTB) or bone Achilles tendon grafts. Other allograft tissues which have been used for knee ligament reconstruction include the fascia lata, semitendinosus, gracilis, flexor tendons of the hand, anterior or posterior tibialis tendons, peroneal tendons, and ACL allografts. Allograft tissue with attached bone is advantageous over soft tissue allograft because of the ability of the surgeon to provide increased fixation strength at the time of reconstruction.

Several steps are taken to minimize the risk of disease transmission when using soft tissue allografts. Unequivocally, the most important of these is meticulous donor screening. The American Association of Tissue Banks has developed criteria to minimize the risk of transmission of neoplastic and infectious diseases [1]. Current exclusion criteria include men who have had sex with another man since 1977, persons immigrating from countries where heterosexual transmission of HIV is believed to be common (Central Africa and Haiti), hemophiliacs who have received clotting factors, men and women who have engaged in prostitution since 1977, and sexual partners of any of the above people mentioned. Tissue is not recovered from potential donors whose medical history reveals ongoing infections, positive blood cultures, history of neoplasms, positive serologic screens, autoimmune diseases, or trauma to, or previous surgery in, the sites where tissue recovery is planned. It is the responsibility of the surgeon who elects to use allograft tissue to confirm that their local tissue bank which provides the allograft tissue is strictly adhering to the standards set by the American Association of Tissue Banks. At the current time there is no regulatory body which maintains quality control over local tissue banks in the United States. This will undoubtedly change in the near future.

Tissue retrieval is an obvious key step in maintaining graft sterility. Standard operating room techniques in sterile tissue handling and transportation ensure that the risk of any bacterial contamination is minimized. In addition to taking precautions of not using tissue from an infected donor, most tissue banks perform secondary sterilization to ensure allograft sterility. Methods of secondary sterilization include exposure to ethylene oxide and gamma irradiation. Unfortunately, these secondary sterilization processes lead to other problems. The use of allografts exposed to ethylene oxide has been associated with serious adverse reactions demonstrated in the basic science laboratory as well as the clinical situation [9, 23]. Currently, the use of ethylene oxide as a form of "secondary sterilization" for ligaments is contraindicated in humans. The current recommendation of the American Association of Tissue Banks for secondary sterilization of allografts by irradiation is between 1.5 to 2.5 Mrads, which decreases the tissues' viral biologic burden. Unfortunately, the irradiation dose needed to kill the hepatitis viruses and HIV has not been adequately investigated. Fideler et al. has recently shown that a minimum of 3.0 Mrads may be required to completely eliminate the possibility of HIV transmission [2]. This increase in requirement of irradiation to eliminate the potential of disease transmission may have an untoward outcome as the use of the irradiation has been shown to have a dose dependent affect on the material properties of soft tissue allografts [3]. How this ultimately affects graft healing, incorporation, mechanical properties, and clinical outcome remains to be determined. Once the allograft is secondarily sterilized it is frozen at $-80°$ Celsius in storage until use in the operating theater. An alternative method of preservation/storage is "freeze-drying". Advantages include "off the shelf" storage eliminating the need for a dedicated allograft freezer. Disadvantages include a magnified negative biomechanical effect when secondarily sterilized with irradiation. Both deep freezing and freeze-drying decrease immunogenicity by killing nucleated cells (white blood cells and osteocytes, osteoblasts, and osteoclasts) which are stimulators for the recipient's immune system.

Graft Preparation/Operative Techniques

Once allograft tissue has been selected for a patient's knee ligament reconstruction, the surgeon should confirm with the tissue bank to determine tissue availability. The tissue is transferred to the hospital on dry ice and then stored in a dedicated bone freezer at $-80°$ Celius until surgery. At the time of surgery, we have found that three basins with normal saline antibiotic solution are required to thaw and rinse the graft. The graft should be thawed at temperatures well below $40°C$ to prevent denaturing of the collagen and weakening of the graft.

Once the graft is thawed, it needs to be sized and shaped for implantation. Surgeons should customize the graft (size and shape) to the particular needs of the patient. For example, in a patient undergoing revision ligament surgery with a previous large tibial tunnel, it is beneficial to shape the bony portion of the allograft to form a customized fit within the previous tibial tunnel to enhance graft fixation [10]. It is important to be meticulous when preparing the graft to avoid damage of the collagen fiber insertion into the bone. It is beyond the scope of this chapter to completely review the operative techniques used for each type of ligament reconstruction as these have been previously published [18]. The authors' allograft of choice for primary/revision ACL reconstruction and lateral collateral ligament augmentation is patellar tendon [12]. For PCL reconstruction and medial collateral ligament augmentation, we prefer Achilles tendon bone allograft [13].

Results: Animal and Human

Basic science studies using different animal models have verified that incorporation of allograft tissue parallels that of autogenous tissue: necrosis, revascularization, cellular repopulation, new matrix and collagen formation, and remodelling. Except for initial cell viability, incorporation of allograft tissue proceeds along a course similar to that of autografts. Differences may exist in the timing of certain stages and the source of repopulating cells. Jackson et al. have shown in a goat model that autograft tissue has a more robust biologic response than that of allograft tissue [7]. He noted that allografts had lower strength and cross-sectional area than did autografts 6 months after implantation. Additionally, he performed electron microscopy on the specimens and found that allografts retained the larger diameter collagen fibers longer, suggesting a more sluggish biologic replacement. While it has been shown during the incorporation process of autogenous and allograft tissue that the graft tissue may lose a significant amount of its original ultimate strength, there appears to be no significant difference in ultimate strength between allograft and autograft tissue once the incorporation and remodelling process has been completed. Unfortunately, it remains unclear in the current literature when the allograft tissue has maximally incorporated and remodeled.

There is still a considerable amount of controversy surrounding the cellular repopulation of allograft tissue [8, 20]. While most authors have agreed about the cellular repopulation of the "superficial" portion of the allograft, considerable differences have been reported in cellular repopulation of the "deep" portions of the allograft. It has been shown that in the initially acellular graft a synovial covering develops within two months after surgery. The cellularity increases from the periphery and spreads centrally over the ensuring months. The vascularity is increased within the first few months of the allograft reconstruction and does not subside until between nine and fifteen months postoperatively. Some studies have suggested that it may take 18 to 24 months before a normal orientation of collagen bundles and normal cellular patterns are evident in allograft tissue, twice the time it takes for autograft incorporation. The comparison of biopsies taken from ACL allograft ligaments ranging from 3 to 36 months after implantation is exceedingly difficult because of the differences in the location and depth of where the biopsy was taken. Additionally, electron microscopy has shown differences in fibril diameter distribution in the proximal, middle, and distal normal ACL [11]. In summary, it appears from the literature that allograft viability is not uniform and varies from patient to patient. In certain patients it appears that larger allografts may remain relatively acellular within the central portion of the allograft, possibly predisposing to an increased risk of "stretching out" over time. Further research is required to confirm the vascularity, cellularity, and remodelling of allograft ligament reconstructions.

The immunogenicity of a potential allograft is of foremost concern as any allograft must not elicit a marked inflammatory response if it is to be revascularized and survive. We have performed extensive clinical studies on the immune response to fresh frozen non-irradiated allograft tissue in ACL reconstruction [24]. The details of this research will not be covered except to mention that 45% of the allograft recipients developed antibodies to the donor tissue. Examination of the functional outcome of this unique study population may provide a correlation between the humoral immune response and clinical success of fresh frozen ACL allograft reconstruction.

Clinical studies in humans with long term follow-up have begun to appear in the literature over the last few years. In comparing results of these studies it is necessary to compare allografts of the same type (patellar tendon versus Achilles tendon bone) which have undergone the same process of harvesting, secondary sterilization, and storage. Indelicato et al. reported two studies on ACL reconstruction using non-ethylene oxide sterilized allografts [5, 6]. In 1990, he published results comparing freeze dried and fresh frozen patellar tendon allografts. They found that the recipients of fresh frozen allografts did slightly better than those patients with freeze-dried allografts. More recently they have published a prospective study using fresh frozen allograft tissue. At an early follow-up period of two years or more, results using allografts were generally good, however, no comparison was made with autograft controls in the study group. Noyes et al. have published extensively on the use of allograft tissue for the treatment of the acute, chronic, and "failed" ACL deficient knee [14–16]. While their results tended to show improvement in the objective and subjective parameters studied, they still recommended autogenous tissue as a primary graft choice. One must be careful with these authors' conclusions however, because they do not include an autograft control group in their studies. Shino et al. have published extensively on the clinical use of allograft tissue in knee ligament reconstruction [20–22]. Their results which reflect an average follow up period of 5 years after surgery were good. However, they also did not compare the results to patients receiving autogenous tissue.

Over the last ten years at the University of Pittsburgh we have had extensive experience using fresh frozen allograft tissue in the treatment of the ligament deficient knee. Our patients which have undergone primary ACL, revision ACL, PCL, and multiple ligament reconstruction have achieved significant improvements in subjective, objective and functional measures compared to their pre-operative status at a minimal follow-up period of two years. A detailed evaluation of thirty-three patients after primary ACL allograft reconstruction showed that greater than 70% of the patients were able to return to their pre-injury level of sports activity and demonstrated less than three millimeters of increased laxity in their reconstructed knee compared with their intact side when tested with a knee arthrometer [17]. Four patients were found to have greater than 5 mm side to side difference on knee arthrometer testing. A critical review of 18 patients who underwent isolated PCL reconstruction using fresh frozen Achilles tendon bone allograft with an average follow up of 2.5 years demonstrated improvements in subjective and objective criteria in all patients [13]. Over 50% were able to return to their pre-injury sports with over 80% of the patients being able to return to the pre-injury frequency level of activity. The corrected knee arthrometer score was less than 5 mm for 73% of the patients and less than 10 mm in all patients. We recently reported our results of using fresh frozen allograft tissue in the knee which had failed a previous primary intra-articular reconstruction [10]. The anterior-posterior displacement was improved in all patients. 64% of the patients had less than a 5 mm side to side difference on arthrometric testing. 76% of the patients were found to be completely satisfied with the results and would undergo revision surgery again. Of 21 patients who underwent arthroscopically assisted reconstruction for the multiply ligament injured knee, no patients reported limitations with activities of daily living; 40% of the patients were able to return to their pre-injury level of activity. All patients had full return of extension and only 2 demonstrated greater than 25 degrees loss of flexion. Lachman translation was less than 5 mm in all subjects and the posterior drawer was less than 10 mm in 92% of the subjects.

There are only a few studies in the literature which attempt to compare the use of allograft and autograft tissue in the ligament deficient knee. Noyes et al. and Indelicato et al. have made general comparisons to autograft tissue in reporting the results of ACL allograft ligament reconstruction. Unfortunately, there was no specific group mentioned with which to compare the allograft tissue in their published articles. We have recently reported our 3 to 5 year results comparing autograft versus non- irradiated fresh frozen allograft in primary ACL reconstruction [4]. Using a matched pair analysis to eliminate as many confounding variables as possible and to permit direct comparison between allograft and autograft tissue, we found no significant differences in clinical outcome. Unfortunately, because of the complicated issues surrounding the use of allograft tissue, it will be exceedingly difficult in the future to conduct a truly prospective study on comparing the use of allograft versus autograft tissue in the treatment of the ligament deficient knee.

Conclusions/Future Directions

The use of soft tissue allografts for ligament reconstruction has increased dramatically over recent years. This has been brought about by our increased knowledge gained from the basic science laboratory and clinical studies. The potential advantage of using allograft instead of autograft which include decreased surgical morbidity, decreased surgical time, increased graft selection, decreased postoperative pain, and increased flexibility when autogenous tissue is inadequate, must be weighed against the known potential disadvantages. Fresh frozen allografts appear to perform slightly better than freeze-dried grafts in humans, even though preceeding animal studies do not demonstrate a significant difference. Secondary sterilization with ethylene oxide cannot be recommended for use in humans. Patients must be adequately informed of the experimental nature of the use of allografts for ligament reconstruction, with the potential for allograft failure and/or rejection. There are many questions which remain to be answered concerning the use of soft tissue allograft reconstruction in the ligament deficient knee. We believe that allograft use at the present time should be performed at centers with adequate clinical and technical support for graft storage and implantation under the specific guidelines of the American Association of Tissue Banks and under protocols where adequate clinical follow up can be obtained. Postoperative care and follow up must respect the particular characteristics of allograft maturation and ligament reconstruction. Current specific indications include the multiply ligament injured knee, selective cases of ACL and PCL reconstruction, failed primary autograft, and patients over 40 years of age with low demand but significant instability.

There are many areas of future research which need to be addressed involving the use of soft tissue allografts. The role of the immunologic response in the success or failure of allograft use in knee ligament surgery has yet to be determined. Animal models have been used in an attempt to define the difference between the biology of allograft and autograft incorporation, however, they only indirectly assess the role of the immune response in healing. Clinically, only two studies have attempted to assess directly the immune response in human allograft ACL reconstruction. Thompson et al. found evidence of a humoral immune response in 45% of cases that have undergone ACL reconstruction using non-irradiated fresh frozen allograft tissue. Rodrigo et al. found that 3 of 18 patients developed an anti-human lymphocyte antibody reaction 3 to 12 months after undergoing ACL reconstruction using freeze-dried, ethylene oxide treated, patellar tendon allografts [19]. These studies seem to suggest that an immunological reaction is present but it is unknown whether this response is detrimental with the potential for bone tunnel resorption and ligament failure. Until the existence and degree of the cellular and molecular mechanism of the immune response is better defined, the exact effect of the immunological response in allograft surgery remains undetermined.

Other research investigations should include longer follow up of irradiated fresh frozen allografts in vivo, as well as further studies on the efficacy of Achilles tendon bone allograft and other allograft sources. Viscoelastic and age related biomechanical properties of fresh, fresh frozen, and irradiated allograft tissue need to be further evaluated with animal and human tissue. Finally, the risk of HIV transmission has to be minimized while producing the fewest adverse reactions upon the allografts biomechanical and clinical performance. Although the above future research is clearly needed, there are sufficient animal and clinical data to support the selective use of fresh frozen allograft tissue for ligament reconstruction. Clinically, the demand for patellar tendon allografts may already exceed the supply. It is important for the surgeon who chooses to use an allograft that one be familiar with the American Association of Tissue Banks recommendations. One must be confident that the tissue bank is following these recommendations. The surgeon may even wish to set his own set of criteria for donor selection. Patients should be fully informed about the risk and benefits of allografts. Surgeons selecting these techniques should be concerned about the type and quality of tissue used, and the way in which it is harvested and procured. With this knowledge, allografts have significantly increased the treatment options available for the treatment of the ligament deficient knee.

References

1. American Association of Tissue Banks (1989) Standards for tissue banking. McLean VA. American Association of Tissue Banks
2. Fideler BM, Vangness Jr CT, Moore T, et al (1994) Effects of gamma irradiation on the human immunodeficiency virus. J Bone Joint Surg 76A: 1032–1035
3. Gibbons MJ, Butler DL, Grood ES, et al (1991) Effects of gamma irradiation on the initial mechanical and material properties of goat bone-patellar tendon-bone allografts. J Orthop Res 9: 209–218
4. Harner CD, Irrgang JJ, Johnson DL, et al (1994–1995) Three to five year outcome of anterior cruciate ligament reconstruction using allograft versus autograft tissue: A matched pair analysis. Orthop Trans 18(4): 987
5. Indelicato PA, Bittar ES, Prevot TJ, et al (1990) Clinical comparison of freeze dried and fresh frozen patellar tendon allografts for anterior cruciate ligament reconstruction of the knee. Am J Sports Med 18: 335–342
6. Indelicato PA, Linton RC, Huegel M (1992) The results of fresh-frozen patellar tendon allografts for chronic anterior cruciate ligament deficiency of the knee. Am J Sports Med 20: 118–121
7. Jackson DW, Grood ES, Goldstein J, et al (1991) Anterior cruciate ligament reconstruction using patella tendon autograft and allograft—an experimental study in goats. Trans Orthop Res Soc 16: 208
8. Jackson DW, Simon TM, Kurzweil PR, et al (1994) Survival of cells after intra-articular transplantation of fresh allografts of the patellar and anterior cruciate ligaments. J Bone Joint Surg (Am) 74: 112–118
9. Jackson DW, Windler GE, Simon TM (1990) Intra-articular reaction associated with the use of freeze-dried, ethylene oxide-sterilized bone-patella tendon-bone allografts in the reconstruction of the anterior cruciate ligament. Am J Sports Med 18(1): 1–11
10. Johnson DL, Swenson TM, Irrgang JJ, et al (1996) Revision ACL reconstruction using fresh frozen allograft tissue: The Pittsburg Experience. Clin Orthop Rel Res (In press)
11. Marks PH, Harner CD, Livesay GA, et al (1994) Quantative electron microscopy of the human cruciate and meniscofemoral ligaments. Trans ORS 19(2): 604
12. Miller MD, Harner CD (1993) The use of allograft: Techniques and results. Clin Sports Med 12(4): 757–771
13. Miller MD, Johnson DL, Harner CD, et al (1993) Posterior cruciate ligament injuries. Orthop Rev 22(1): 1201–1210
14. Noyes FR, Barber SD, Mangine RE (1990) Bone-patellar ligament-bone and fascia-lata allografts for reconstruction of the anterior cruciate ligament. J Bone Joint Surg 72A: 1125–1136
15. Noyes FR, Barber SD (1992) The effect of a ligament augmentation device on allograft reconstruction for chronic ruptures of the anterior cruciate ligament. J Bone Joint Surg 74A: 960–973
16. Noyes FR, Barber-Westin SD, Roberts CS (1994) Use of allografts after failed treatment of rupture of the anterior cruciate ligament. J Bone Joint Surg 76A: 1019–1031
17. Olson EJ, Harner CD, Fu FH, et al (1993) Clinical use of fresh frozen soft tissue allografts. Orthopaedics 15: 1225–1232

18. Paulos LE, Cooper JL (1993) Surgical technique for the use of allografts as an anterior cruciate ligament, posterior cruciate ligament, medial collateral ligament and lateral collateral ligament substitutes. Sports Med and Arthroscopy Rev 1(1): 92–102

19. Rodrigo JJ, Jackson DW, Simon TM, et al (1993) The immune response to freeze dried bone tendon bone allografts in humans. Am J Knee Surg 6(2): 47–53

20. Shino K, Inove M, Horibe S, et al (1988) Maturation of allograft tendons transplanted into knee. An arthroscopic and histological study. J Bone Joint Surg (Br) 70B: 556–560

21. Shino K, Inove M, Horibe S, et al (1990) Reconstruction of the anterior cruciate ligament using allogenic tendon. Long term follow-up. Am J Sports Med 18: 457–465

22. Shino, Nakata K, Horibe S, et al (1993) Quantitative evaluation after arthroscopic anterior cruciate ligament reconstruction. Allograft versus autograft. Am J Sports Med 21(4): 609–616

23. Silvaggio VJ, Fu FH, Georgescu HI, et al (1993) The induction of IL-I by freeze-dried ethylene oxide-treated bone-patellar tendon-bone allograft wear particles. Arthroscopy 9(1): 82–86

24. Thompson WD, Harner CD, Jamison JP, et al (1994) The immunologic response to fresh frozen bone-patellar tendon-bone allograft ACL reconstruction. Trans ORS 19(2): 624

Authors' addresses: Darren L. Johnson, M.D., University of Kentucky, Sports Medicine Center, 740 South Limestone, Kentucky Clinic, K429, Lexington, Kentucky 40536-0284, U.S.A.; Christopher D. Harner, M.D., Department of Orthopaedics, University of Pittsburgh, Pittsburgh, U.S.A.

Meniscal Allografts

E. M. Goble and S. M. Kane

Western Surgery Center, Logan, Utah, U.S.A.

Meniscal Function

Within the knee, the menisci perform vital biomechanical functions which contribute to the maintenance of articular cartilage and provide a protective barrier against degenerative joint disease. Removal or damage to all, or part of the meniscus has been generally felt to increase the likelihood of articular degeneration and the development of osteoarthritis [1]. Currently, it is felt that the function of the menisci include shock absorption, load transmission, secondary mechanical stability and possible joint lubrication and/or nutrition.

During the normal gait pattern, the articular surface of the knee bears between 4.5 and 6.2 times body weight with 72.2% of that load being transmitted to the medial tibial plateau [2, 3]. The menisci increase the contact area between long bones and consequently reduce the magnitude of compressive forces at the articular cartilage. Under static conditions, the load transmitted through the menisci in extension is 50% of the body weight which increases to 85% at 90° of knee flexion [4].

The anatomical configuration of the menisci which forms a semilunar, wedge-shaped structure, enhances tibial femoral joint stability by filling the void created by the incongruous femoral condyle and tibial plateau [5]. Through deepening of the tibial socket, mechanical tests suggest that the menisci provide secondary knee stability through enhancement of positional control and alignment of the knee [6]. Further studies imply that the soft viscoelastic meniscus has the ability to attenuate shock waves generated through the normal gait pattern, and through the intrinsic material properties of the meniscus, decrease stress loading of the articular cartilage [7, 8, 9]. Moreover, the menisci are felt to contribute to the nutritional environment of the knee as proposed by MacConaill [10]. Finally, the menisci may enhance lubrication of the joint through an influence toward even distribution of the synovial fluid within the knee.

Previous studies have shown that both menisci play a role in joint stability, albeit the medial meniscus contributes a greater percentage to the overall stability within the knee. For obvious reasons, therefore, the preservation of the menisci is desirable [11]. Furthermore, it is felt that the medial meniscus posterior horn, which is attached through the posterior oblique ligament, functions as a synergist to the anterior cruciate ligament and, therefore, loss of a major portion of the posterior horn of the medial meniscus significantly increases rotatory instability of the knee and may ultimately accelerate the development of osteoarthritis in the ACL deficient knee [12, 13].

Meniscectomy

Meniscal tears may create symptoms of pain and dysfunction within the knee and may predispose the knee to osteoarthritis and cartilage degeneration. While it is true that not all meniscal tears result in clinical symptoms, a torn meniscus may or may not retain its biomechanical function [14]. Currently the gold standard of care for meniscal pathology emphasizes that a meniscal tear be repaired when possible with certain tears being allowed to heal, particularly in younger individuals. However, partial and total meniscectomies are still at times necessary when repair or nonoperative treatment is not possible. Fairbank, in 1948, reported arthritic changes following complete meniscectomy which included joint space narrowing, flattening of the femoral condyle and spurring at the medial femoral condyle [15]. At that time Fairbak indicated that these changes were primarily due to the loss of load bearing capacity at the menisci and researchers have since demonstrated an increased incidence of degenerative changes after partial or total meniscectomy [16, 17, 18, 19]. Additionally, it appears that a lateral meniscectomy accelerates osteoarthrosis more readily than a medial meniscectomy. This is felt to be due in part to the fact that under normal physiological conditions the lateral meniscus carries most of the load in the lateral compartment while the medial compartment shares the load approximately equally between the meniscus and the exposed cartilage [20]. Furthermore, it has been shown that removal of the medial meniscus may cause a reduction in the contact area by up to 70%, and that the absence of a meniscus increases the pressure gradient considerably near the margin of the articular contact area [21]. It can be said that the single most predictive factor in the development of degenerative arthritis is the time since the meniscectomy was performed, and therefore, research into meniscal transplantation certainly warrants a well designed and closely scrutinized clinical investigation.

Literature Review

Animal studies have contributed greatly to our understanding of meniscal transplantation and the ability of a transplanted meniscus to survive within the knee. Milachowski et al. transplanted the medial meniscus in thirty sheep while altering the method of sterilization and preservation [13, 22]. In this paper it was shown that those sheep who had received lyophilized, gamma irradiated allografts had a healed meniscal rim at six weeks and were fully remodeled at 48 weeks, while those sheep receiving deep frozen specimens, were noted to have a healed meniscal rim at 48 weeks but showed little revascularization and disorganized remodeling over time. This led Milachowski to write in 1994: "The results seen in lyophilized transplants were less satisfactory due to a reduction in size" [23].

Arnoczky reported on fourteen canines who received cryopreserved meniscus transplants, with follow-up at six months following the operation. At six months, the allografts had healed at their periphery, with normal gross appearance and function. Histological studies further demonstrated an initial two week post-transplantation decrease in cellularity which subsequently increased along with metabolic activity at one month. At three-to-six months, the cellular metabolic activity within the graft returned to normal [24]. In additional studies, Arnoczky further evaluated the cellular repopulation of deep frozen meniscal autografts in the canine model, where it was shown that deep freezing the menisci killed all cells within the graft, but the periphery still had the ability to heal, and at three months the entire graft, except centrally, was repopulated with host cells. Examination under polarized microscopy at six months showed a disruption of the normal collagen orientation [25]. Host cell graft repopulation was confirmed by Jackson et al. [26] who showed that at four weeks post transplantation of fresh goat meniscal allografts, no donor DNA could be demonstrated within the graft and that the host DNA content approached or exceeded the amount present in the contralateral control meniscus. Revascularization within the transplanted meniscus has been evaluated as well and it has been shown that in the deep frozen transplanted menisci, revascularization tends to remain in a more physiological distribution in the outer one-third. Freeze drying of the allograft, however, resulted in a more extensive revascularization and remodeling which has been associated with graft shrinkage [27]. When comparing fresh frozen and cryopreserved meniscal allografts in goats, Jackson et al. [28] noted that six months post implantation, both types of grafts appeared to have a grossly normal architecture, with good peripheral healing, accompanied by revascularization and graft incorporation. It was, however, noted that a decrease in uronic acid and an increase in water content had occurred in both groups, which may suggest early meniscal degeneration. In more recent animal studies Mikic et al. [29] reported normal meniscal architecture eight-to-twelve months post fresh medial allograft transplantation in twenty canine knees. These menisci were also noted to have less cellularity upon microscopic evaluation than that which was found in control specimens.

Canhan [30] evaluated the effectiveness of a glutaraldehyde prepared allograft in five canine knees. This "bioprosthesis", when compared to autograft and tissue culture prepared allografts, showed less satisfactory postoperative attachment to the joint capsule and resulted in recurrent joint effusions postoperatively.

In terms of immunologic rejection of allografted menisci, to date no animal study has shown the presence of an immunological response to the allograft. Lanzer showed that allografted menisci in greyhound dogs showed no immunologically mediated rejection, either histologically or by way of laboratory criteria at three weeks, six and twelve months [31].

Clinical Trials

In 1984 and again in 1989, Milachowski reported the results from a group of fifteen patients who had undergone meniscal allograft transplantation. These allografts were implanted through the use of an arthrotomy, with ten of the fifteen grafts being freeze dried (lyophilized) and then irradiated, while five of the grafts were deep frozen. At the time of follow-up, which averaged thirteen months, thirteen of the fifteen patients were very satisfied with the result and only two patients reported occasional knee pain. A second look arthroscopic evaluation in nine patients revealed that only one had a non-healed meniscal rim. Milachowski's report in 1989 included seven additional patients and reported a disturbing trend for graft shrinkage which was more commonly found in the lyophilized, gamma irradiated group of allografts [22].

Since Milachowski's contribution to the clinical trials of meniscal allograft surgery, many physicians have implanted, and are currently following groups of patients who have undergone meniscal allograft transplantation. In 1987, Keene reported on the successful placement of a fresh meniscal allograft into the knee of a professional Australian football player who had previously undergone a total meniscectomy. At six months, the follow-up arthroscopic evaluation showed a normal appearing meniscus with some evidence of incomplete healing at the anterior and posterior horns [32].

Zukor et al., reported on a series of thirty-three fresh meniscal and osteochondral allografts, wherein the etiology of the meniscal deficient knee was traumatic. Follow-up at one year revealed that twenty-six patient (75%) where clinically successful with no failures attributable to meniscal pathology. Within this study ten patients underwent a second look arthroscopy, at which time all menisci were stable at their peripheral attachment with several small degenerative areas noted on the graft [33].

In 1993, Garrett reported on forty-three open allograft transplantations (16 fresh, 27 cryopreserved). Within this population, seven patients received isolated meniscal transplantations while 36 others received meniscal allografts in combination with either an ACL reconstruction or an osteotomy. At a two year minimum follow-up, twenty-eight of the patients underwent an arthroscopic reevaluation, which showed a well healed meniscal rim and no significant graft shrinkage in twenty patients. Fifteen other patients who did not undergo arthroscopic reevaluation remained asymptomatic. It is of note that in those patients in which clinical symptoms were less than satisfactory, it was felt that a preoperative grade four chondrosis had contributed to the deterioration of the clinical result [34].

Noyes in 1995, presented a series of ninety-six meniscal allografts (seventy-nine medial, seventeen lateral) in eighty-three patients. At a preoperative evaluation, all patients were noted to have had symptomatic arthritic degeneration at the meniscal deficient compartment. The meniscal allografts implanted in this study were deep frozen and received 2.5 Mrad of gamma irradiation prior to implantation through an arthroscopic procedure. Twenty-nine menisci (twenty-two medial, seven lateral) subsequently failed secondary to degeneration at the meniscus or because of a recurrence of a meniscal tear and were removed at a mean of fourteen months postoperatively. Sixty-seven menisci were, therefore, available for long term follow-up, of which sixty-two returned at a mean of thirty months postoperatively. Second look arthroscopic examinations were performed in thirty-five patients (56%) at a mean of sixteen months following the index procedure. At that time, 9% were classified as well healed, 31% were felt to have only partially healed and 58% were felt to have failed to exhibit adequate peripheral healing and 2% were unknown. This gave an overall healing rate, for the sixty-seven menisci which had survived at least two years postoperativly, of 13% healed, 45% partially healed, 40% failed and 2% unknown. It is of note that it was felt by the author that there remained a statistically significant relationship between the overall healing rate of the allograft and the preoperative arthrosis noted on MRI. Finally, ten of the thirty-five meniscal allograft patients viewed at follow-up, were noted to have small meniscal tears identifiable during the arthroscopy. These tears were noted to be typically located at the inner and middle one-third regions of the allograft, and six of these required partial resection with four being stable to probing and were left undisturbed [35].

Veltri reviewed his results of sixteen deep frozen or cryo preserved meniscal transplantations, in which eleven of the reported cases underwent either ACL or PCL reconstruction at the time of surgery. At follow-up, only two of fourteen patients complained of persistent joint line tenderness in the affected articular compartment. Seven of eleven patients at six months or greater follow-up, underwent an arthroscopic evaluation which revealed five menisci to have complete healing at the periphery. It was, however, noted at that time, that one of the well healed grafts had undergone a significant amount of degeneration in the mid portion of the meniscus. The remaining two patients showed evidence of impaired healing at the posterior horn attachment. Four patients were not arthroscopically examined while remaining clinically asymptomatic [36].

In Goble's series of forty-seven cryo-preserved meniscal allografts in forty-five patients, seventeen of eighteen (94%) patients who have reached two year follow-up reported a significant decrease in knee pain and improvement in function on a subjective evaluation. A second look arthroscopy was performed on thirteen patients (thirteen grafts) of which ten (71%) had a well healed and functional meniscus. Four of the grafts demonstrated a noticeable pattern of degenerative wear or peripheral detachment at the posterior horn. It was felt at that time that the failure of healing at the posterior horn was secondary to inadequate surgical technique in the early cases. Biopsy performed on eight of fourteen grafts revealed an average of 80% viable meniscal tissue. Only one graft was judged to be a failure which required meniscal resection. (Goble personal communication).

In a report obtained from Crylolife Incorporated (personal communication) cryo-preserved meniscal allografts implanted between November of 1989 and January of 1994, numbered 267, divided between nine surgical centers. The data compiled from the nine centers participating in this study, showed that 109 of the meniscal allografts had been secured through bone anchors while 114 were secured with suture fixation only (44 unreported). Thirty-two percent of the patients receiving meniscal allografts within this group of patients, an ACL reconstruction at the time of meniscal allograft surgery, while eighteen patients received a realignment osteotomy. The degree of preoperative degenerative joint disease present was reported in 221 of the 267 recipients with forty-five classified as a grade one osteoarthritis, while eighty-five were classified as grade two. Advanced arthritic knees having grade three changes, consisted of fifty-nine compartments with only thirty-two having been reported as severe arthritis (grade four). Second look arthroscopic procedures were performed on ninety of the meniscal allografts at an average postoperative period of 291 days. From these second look cases fixation was reported as firm in 41 (45%) cases, good in 19 (21%), incomplete in 5 (5%), and poor in 1 (1%). Findings in twenty-four patients were not reported. It was noted that no cases of poor fixation were found where meniscal attachment had been carried out through use of bone anchors. The integrity of the meniscal surface was defined in forty-three allografts, of which 33 (76%) were documented to have an abrasion free surface while 10 (23%) were considered only moderately abraded. Shrinkage was documented in twelve grafts and in five of the grafts, previously reported as inadequately fixed. There were forty-three reported complications of the 267 meniscal allografts, which included increased or continued compartmental pain, full or partial loss of graft function, failure of the graft to properly heal and progression of degenerative arthritis within the knee requiring a total knee replacement. When the complications were further classified into three categories which included cases requiring total removal, partial removal or non-removal failures, fifteen of the allografts required total removal. It is of interest that in thirteen of the fifteen cases where the meniscus required subsequent removal, grade three or greater degenerative joint disease was noted at the time of meniscal transplantation. Twenty-three transplanted menisci required partial removal at the time of second look with fifteen of those patients having been defined as high grade degenerative arthritis at the time of transplantation. Eight meniscal allografts were found to have significant meniscal tears at the time of arthroscopic reevaluation and required partial meniscectomy at that time.

Discussion

In light of the difficulty in locating, harvesting and distributing fresh donor allografts to a size matched recipient, as well as the real possibility of disease transmission through allograft implantation, fresh menisci, suitable for allograft implantation, have given way to bank preserved meniscal allografts. The manner in which the menisci are preserved and stored, and the subsequent clinical outcome thereof constitutes a major portion of what has been reported in the recent orthopedic literature. Currently, preservation of meniscal allografts is carried out in one of three different ways: deep freezing, freeze drying (lyophilization), and cryopreservation. Of these three processes, cryopreservation has been shown to be the only reproducible method in which a substantially viable cell population is maintained. While it is possible to confirm through literature review, the potential for good results with freeze dried (lyophilized), deep frozen, and cryopreserved meniscal allografts, Milachowski, Kohn, and other authors have reported a greater tendency towards shrinkage and inappropriate remodeling over time with the use of lyophilized meniscal allografts. Additionally, it cannot be overlooked, that gamma irradiation may possibly be a contributing factor to the comparative poor results of Milachowski's population. This argument seems to gather strength when one evaluates the data from Noyes's series which also showed a significant failure rate in deep frozen meniscal allografts which had also received gamma irradiation.

While it is hard to substantiate a long-term clinical difference between the results of deep frozen and cryopreserved allografts, the fact that most reports on fresh allograft transplantation are associated with comparatively good results, suggests that a viable meniscal chondrocyte population may have a beneficial effect on the long-term survival and function of the graft [37]. Finally, cryopreservation is not considered a process through which sterilization can be assured, and the remote risk of disease transmission through the usage of cryopreserved tissue is a matter of concern. It is for this reason that processes which effectively eliminate the risk of viral transmission (freeze drying, gamma irradiation) may continue to have an application in the transplantation of meniscal allografts [38].

Techniques

Surgical techniques for meniscal allograft transplantation include both open and arthroscopically assisted procedures. Most series to date, have reported the use of an arthrotomy for meniscal transplantation. Variations within the open surgical technique include both medial and lateral incisions, tibial tubercle osteotomy and collateral ligament releases, in order to allow easier access to the medial and lateral compartments. Recently advances within the realm of arthroscopic surgery have allowed for meniscal transplantation to be completed without the need for a formal arthrotomy. Many authors currently feel that transplantation performed arthroscopically is a much more desirable, yet significantly more difficult procedure. The obvious advantages of an arthroscopic allograft insertion include decreased morbidity, avoidance of collateral ligament disruption and facilitation of early rehabilitation. Early reports of problematic-healing at both the anterior and/or posterior horn attachments of the allograft meniscus, have been primarily seen with those procedures wherein the allograft was implanted through suture fixation only. This has given some credence to the possible advantages of fixation with circular donor bone plugs which are press fit or affixed into predrilled tunnels in the anterior and posterior horns of the recipient tibial plateau. Another method which has been advocated by certain authors, entails the use of a single anterior to posterior horn bone block which is press fit into a size matched trough within the recipient tibia. It should, however, be noted, that no direct inference of superiority can be gained by review of the literature as it pertains to the method of securing the allograft within the host knee.

Finally, it is the author's opinion that aside from the issue of graft preservation and sterilization, the most critical factor in the successful outcome of meniscal allograft transplantation lies within the ability of the surgeon to carry out the procedure in such a way as to assure that a well sized graft is securely and evenly affixed at it's periphery without damaging the meniscus. It must be stated that the meniscus is a relatively delicate structure, and the allograft can be easily lacerated or damaged by careless usage of suture needles or other instrumentation. Defects or lacerations within the meniscus that are iatrogenically created, can only lead to a less than optimal long term success rate for meniscal transplantation.

Indications for Meniscal Allograft Transplantation

The overall clinical success of meniscal transplantation depends largely upon appropriate patient selection. Secondary to the fact that this procedure is an evolving technique, the indications for transplantation must be considered strict. Further experience with tissue processing and surgical technique may subsequently allow for expansion of these criteria but the initial study subjects must be as homogenous and defined as possible.

Meniscal dysfunction results from either a disruption in the meniscal architecture or from a generalized degeneration at the cellular level. Mechanical changes result primarily from traumatic influences upon the meniscus which may result in meniscal tears or damage to the supporting structures of the knee. Consequently, the uninvolved soft tissue and bone in proximity to the injury are presumed to be essentially normal.

Conversely, conditions which result in the degradation of the cellular matrix of the meniscus often involve the surrounding tissue, cartilage and subchondral bone and, in this situation, the associated joint structures may also show microstructural derangement. This fact indicates that these tissues are abnormal. Degenerative joint disease of this type is a progressive and poorly understood process which often results in a meniscectomy but is not caused by the meniscectomy. As such, meniscal allograft reconstruction is contraindicated in these patients and should be considered only a useful procedure in those individuals who have lost their menisci through traumatic causes.

In identifying potential candidates, it is of paramount importance to focus on the goals of treatment. Several studies have demonstrated that patients who undergo meniscal allograft reconstruction may experience measurable relief of pain and corresponding increase in their functional level. (Wojtys, Goble, Garrett; Personal Communication). At this point, however, these benefits are only known from short term studies and obviously need a longer term follow-up

It has been shown that a meniscectomy may initiate a series of degenerative changes that have been well documented in the literature. Fairbank, in his classic article, clearly documents the progression of arthritis in meniscectomy knees and describes three stages of radiographic changes that consistently delineate the evolving pathology [18]. In this article, stage one is defined as the formation of an antero-posterior ridge projecting downwards from the margin of the femoral condyle over the meniscal site. Stage two, consists of a generalized flattening of the marginal half of the femoral articular surface, on the side of the meniscectomy, while stage three consists of narrowing of the joint space on the side of the meniscectomy with occasional associated varus valgus deformity of the knee. Theoretically, restoration of the normal meniscal anatomy should be able to decelerate or prevent further degenerative changes. However, up to this point no study has been able to demonstrate scientifically that a meniscal allograft implantation has had a significant impact on progressive joint destruction. Therefore, the indications for patient selection should focus on patients who have realistic expectations from the procedure. Most often they are defined as patients with significant knee pain and limitation of function who are skeletally mature but are still considered to be too young to be adequate candidates for total knee arthroplasty. Candidates must have demonstrable radiographic progression of their disease over a two year period, and should have exhausted all other options for medical management of their pain, including a thorough trial of conservative therapy and bracing techniques. The "compartment unloading braces" have been shown to decrease compression loads significantly in the affected compartment and are occasionally used with significant success. Several authors have suggested that advanced arthritis is an absolute contraindication to meniscal allograft transplantation, primarily because of questionable graft survival [34, 36, 37]. However, it has been shown in a limited fashion that transplanted menisci will heal and provide pain relief in properly selected grade three and four osteoarthritic patients. (Goble, Wojtys: Personal Communication) Therefore, it may be stated that, as experience with this technique improves, advanced arthritis may come to represent only a relative contraindication.

It should be noted that it is important to document the integrity of the ligamentous stabilizers of the knee, for it is often necessary to perform a ligamentous reconstruction prior to a meniscal transplantation in order to provide adequate soft tissue protection and balancing for the transplanted meniscus. Finally, the authors wish to state that secondary to the fact that those authors who are currently reporting failures within a population of meniscal allograft transplantations, have most commonly done so in patients with grade three or higher arthritic changes within the transplanted compartment, it may very well be, that after an adequate evaluation of the procedure has been completed, meniscal transplantation in earlier, nonsymptomatic, post-meniscectomy patients may be appropriate. At this point, however, one could only consider this to be experimental in nature. Secondarily, the possibility of disease transmission must be considered and completely explained to the patient and documented in a preoperative evaluation.

Summary

The use of meniscal allografts in the treatment of a meniscal deficient knee has progressed to a point where under well controlled situations, a good result in relief of pain may be expected short-term. Efficacy of the procedure on a long-term basis, however, remains unproven and mandates that meniscal allograft transplantation be considered an investigational procedure.

References

1. Mow VC, Ratcliff A, Chern KY, et al (1992) Knee meniscus basic and clinical foundations, edn 1. New York: Raven Press, pp 37–57
2. Rohrle H, Scholten R, et al (1984) J Biomech 17: 409–424
3. Hsu RWW, Himeno S, Coventry MB (1988) Transactions of 34th Annual Meeting of the Orthopedic Research Society, Vol 13. Parkridge, Illinois: Orthopedic Research Society, p 282
4. Ahmed AM, Burke DL (1983) J Biomech Eng 105: 216–225
5. Fu FH, Thompson WO (1992) Knee meniscus basic and clinical foundations, edn 1. New York: Raven Press, pp 75–89
6. Spilker RL, Donzeley, PS (1992) Knee meniscus basic and clinical foundations, edn 1. New York: Raven Press, pp 91–115

7. Kraus WR (1996) General Bone and Joint Surgery, pp 559–604
8. Kurosawa H, etc., et al (1980) Clin Orthop 149: 283–290
9. DeHaven KE (1990) The role of the meniscus. In: Ewing JW (ed) Articular cartilage and knee joint function: basic science and arthroscopy, edn 1. New York: Raven Press, pp 103–115
10. MacConaill (1932) The function of the interarticular fibrocartilage with special reference to the knee and inferior radial ulnar joints general anatomy. 66: 210–227
11. Deboer HH, Koudstal J (1991) The fate of meniscus cartilage after transplantation of cryopreserved nontissue antigen matched allograft. Clin Orthop 116: 145–151
12. Levy IM, Torzilli TA, Warren F (1982) The effect of medial meniscectomy on anterior posterior motion of the knee. J Bone Joint Surg 64A: 883–888
13. Milachowski KA, Weismeier K, Worth CJ, Kohn D (1988) Meniscus transplantation experimental study, clinical report arthroscopic findings. Surgery and Arthroscopy of the Knee, Second Congress of the European Society, edn 1. Berlin, Heidelberg: Springer, pp 380–388
14. Dehaven KE (1992) Meniscectomy Vs. repair: clinical experience. In: Mow VC, Arnoczky SP, Jackson DW (eds) Knee meniscus basic and clinical foundation, edn 1. New York: Raven Press, pp 131–139
15. Fairbank TJ (1984) Knee joint changes after meniscectomy. J Bone Joint Surg 30B: 664–670
16. O'Brien WR (1993) Degenerative arthritis of the knee following anterior cruciate ligament injury role of the meniscus. Sports Med Arthroscopy Rev 1: 114–118
17. Lynch MA, Henning CE, Glick KR (1983) Knee joint surface changes: long-term follow-up meniscus tear treatment and stable anterior cruciate ligament reconstruction. Clin Orthop 172: 148–153
18. Lynch MA, Henning CE (1988) Osteoarthritis in the ACL deficient knee. In: Feagin, JA, Jr (ed) The cruciate ligaments, edn 1. New York: Churchill, Livingston, pp 385–391
19. Johnson RJ, Kettlekamp DB, Clark W, Weaverton P (1974) Factors affecting late results after meniscectomy. General Bone Joint Surg 56A: 719–729
20. Walker BF, Erkman MJ (1975) The role of the menisci in forced transmission across the knee. Clin Orthop 109: 184–192
21. Ahmed AM (1992) The load bearing of the knee meniscus. In: Mow VC, Arnoczky SP, Jackson DW (eds) DDS: Knee meniscus basic and clinical foundations, edn 1. New York: Raven Press, pp 59–73
22. Milachowski KA, Weismeier K, Worth CJ, Kohn, D (1989) Homologous meniscus transplantation: Experimental and clinical results. Int Orthop 13: 1
23. Milachowski KA, Kohn D, Worth CJ (1984) Transplantation of allogenic menisci orthopade 1994 (APR) 23 (2): 160–163
24. Arnoczky SB, McDivot CA (1990) Meniscal replacement using cryo preserved allograft: Experimental study in the dog. Clin Orthop 252: 121
25. Arnoczky SB, O'Brien S, DeCarlo E, et al (1988) Cellular repopulation of deep frozen meniscal allograft: Experimental study in the dog. Transact Orthop Res Soc 34: 145
26. Jackson DW, Whelan J, Simon TM (1993) Cell survival after transplantation of fresh meniscal allograft, DNA probe analysis in a goat model. Am J Sports Med 21: 540–550
27. Arnoczsky SB, Milochowski KA (1990) Meniscal allografts: Where do we stand? In: Ewing JW (ed) Articular cartilage and the knee joint function: basic science and arthroscopy. New York: Raven Press, p 129
28. Jackson DW, McDivot CA, Simon TM, et al (1992) Meniscal transplantation using fresh and cryopreserved allograft, and Experimental study in goats. Am J Sports Med 20 (6): 646–656
29. Mikic ZD, Brankoy MZ, Tubic MV, et al (1993) Allograft meniscal transplantation in a dog. Acta Orthoscand 64 (3): 329–332
30. Canhan W, Stanish W (1986) A study of the biological behavior of the meniscus as a transplant in the medial compartment of dog knees. Am J Sports Med 14 (6): 376–379
31. Lanzer WA (1991) Allograft transposition of knee menisci: An animal study. Presented at Association of Bone and Joint Surgeons
32. Keene GCR, Paterson RS, Teague DC (1987) Advances in arthroscopic surgery. Clin Orthop 224: 64
33. Zucor DJ, Cameron JC, Brooks PJ, et al (1990) The fate of human meniscal autografts. In: Ewing, JW (ed) Articular cartilage and knee joint function: basic science and arthroscopy. New York: Raven Press, p 147

34. Garrett JC (1993) Meniscal transplantation: Review of forty-three cases with two-to-seven year follow-up. Sports Medicine and American Arthroscopic Review 1: 164–167
35. Noyes FR, Barber-Weston SD (1995) Irradiated meniscal allografts in the human knee: a two-to-five year follow-up study presented at the 1995 AAOS Orlando
36. Veltri DM, Warren RF, Wickiewicz TL, O'Brien SJ (1994) Current status of allograft. Meniscal Transplantation Clinical Ortho and Related Research 303: 44–45
37. Siegel MG, Roberts CS (1993) Meniscal allografts. Clin Sports Med 12 (1): 59–80
38. American Association of Tissue Banks (1987) Technical manual for surgical bone banking. McLean, VA: American Associations of Tissue Banks

Authors' address: E. Marlowe Goble, M.D. and Steven M. Kane, M.D., Western Surgery Center, 850 East 1200 North, Logan, Utah 84321-2800, U.S.A.

Meniscal Transplantation: The Hannover Experience

D. Kohn[1] and C. J. Wirth[2]

[1] Orthopädische Universitätsklinik Homburg (Saar) and
[2] Orthopädische Klinik der Medizinischen Hochschule Hannover, Hannover, Federal Republic of Germany

Not all damaged menisci can be treated by partial excision or by repair. The loss of a meniscus will be followed by the development of osteoarthrosis in the majority of cases [3, 4, 16, 20, 21, 23, 24, 28, 29]. Standard treatment options for symptomatic postmeniscectomy osteoarthrosis include osteotomy [15] and knee arthroplasty [34]. Both procedures give benefit only for a limited period of time and are therefore less well suited for the younger patient. Based on this dilemma the idea of meniscus replacement was established [2, 11]. Meniscus transplantation was the first and remains to be the most frequent type of meniscus replacement to date.

After removal of a meniscus from an otherwise intact knee, the patient will remain symptom-free for more than ten years in the majority of cases [33]. He will seek medical advice again, when unilateral osteoarthritis starts to evolve. If meniscectomy was performed in an anterior cruciate deficient knee, symptoms of knee instability will bring the patient to the orthopaedic surgeon earlier. The aims of treatment are to reduce pain, to stop the progress of degenerative arthritis and to enhance the stability of the involved knee.

The typical candidate for medial meniscus replacement is the young and active individual that has lost or has severly damaged the medial meniscus in an anterior cruciate ligament deficient knee. Reconstruction of the anterior cruciate ligament alone will not render an entirely stable knee. It was shown, that by adding a medial meniscal allograft to the ligament reconstruction better stability can be achieved [32].

Animal Experiments

Meniscus transplantation was investigated in an animal model in 1982 [34]. The medial meniscus was removed in 30 skeletally mature female Merino sheep. 15 animals received lyophilized gamma irradiated meniscus allografts and 15 received deep frozen meniscus allografts. Results in both groups were followed 6, 12, 24 and 48 weeks postoperatively by macroscopic, histological, microangiographic, biomechanical and scanning electron microscopy studies. Lyophilized menisci had completely healed after 48 weeks. The synovium remained hypertrophied and microangiography showed almost complete revascularization. Deep frozen menisci were also incorporated. After 48 weeks healing was complete, but revascularization was only slight and remodeling did not occur. The tensile strength of the deep frozen transplants corresponded to that of lyophilized transplants at 6 weeks, 12 weeks and 24 weeks. The deep frozen transplants were stronger after 48 weeks. The tensile strength of the genuine menisci was never achieved. In summary both types of allografts healed to the capsule, looked like menisci macroscopically, but remained mechanically inferior.

Clinical Series

In 1984 the first patient received a meniscus allograft at our institution. All patients entered in this study had ACL deficient, medial meniscus deficient knees with medial instability.

All operations were performed with a standardized technique using an anteromedial arthrotomy, replacement of the ACL by a bone-tendon-bone patellar tendon autograft, femoral detachment and reinsertion of the medial collateral ligament. The fixation of the posterior and the anterior horn of the meniscus allograft as well as the fixation to the capsule were carried out with resorbable sutures.

Lyophilized transplants which were easy to handle and store were used whenever a well suited deep frozen graft was not available. A total of 23 operations were carried out between May 1984 and December 1986. In 17 cases the lyophilized allografts were used and in 6 cases deep-frozen allografts were inserted.

MRI has failed so far as a tool for the assessment of healing after meniscus repair [14]. MRI is even more difficult to interpret after meniscus replacement. Perhaps further enhancement in MRI technique and understanding of MRI pictures will make this test a future tool for evaluation.

All patients were seen regularly in our outpatient clinic and the average follow-up was 36 months with a range from 24 to 50 months. Two year results were compared for three groups of patients. All had ACL replacement with bone-tendon-bone patellar tendon autografts. The groups that were studied are as follows:

group I, meniscus transplantation group;
group II control group with both menisci intact;
group III was a second control group of meniscectomized patients who refused a meniscus transplantation.

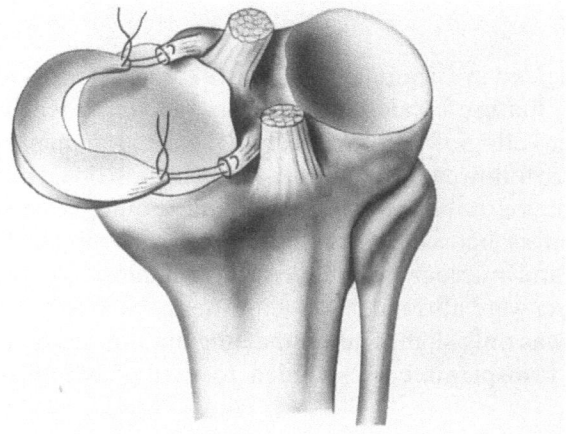

Fig. 1. Fixation of the graft to the remnants of the tibial insertion ligaments according to Milachowski et al., 1989 (27)

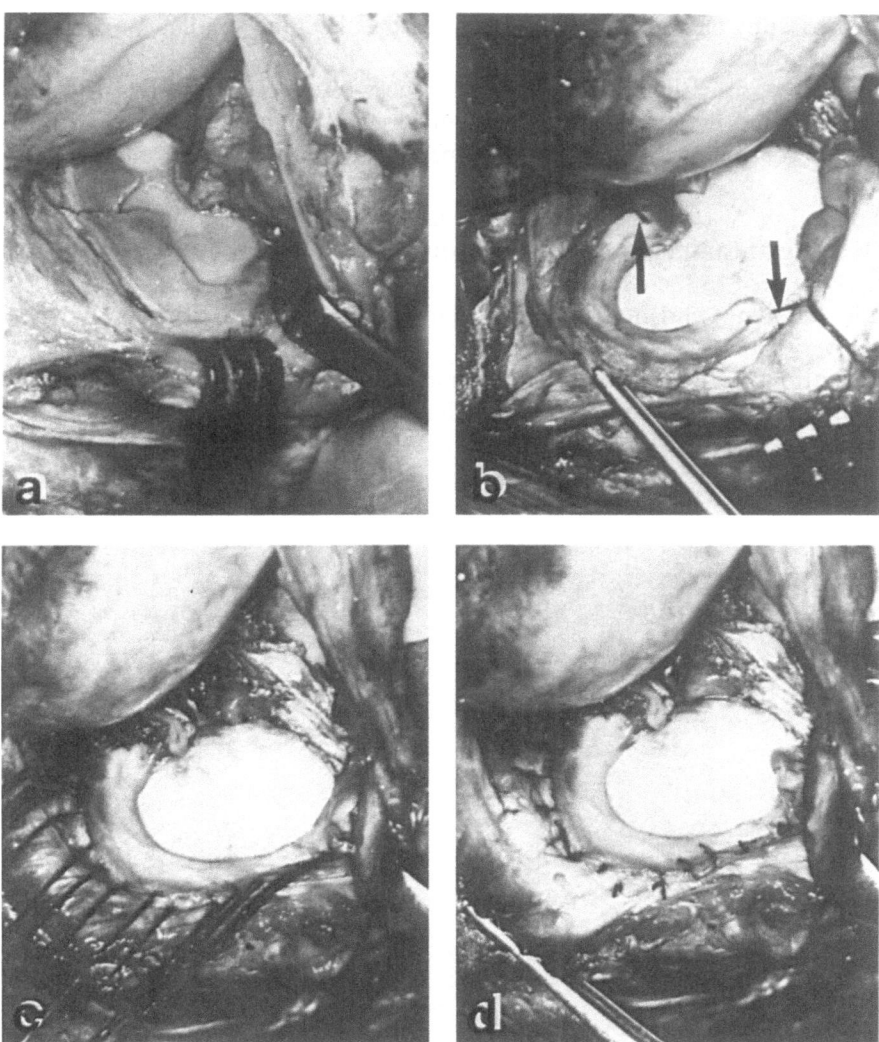

Fig. 2. Four steps during medial meniscus transplantation. **a** Removal of a completely torn medial meniscus. **b** Insertion of a meniscus allograft and fixation to the remnants of the tibial insertion ligaments. Arrows mark tag sutures. **c** The allograft is additionally fixed to the capsule. **d** The medial compartment is ready for repositioning (From Wirth et al.)

No significant differences could be shown between these groups according to the mean Lysholm scores.

Eighteen out of our 23 patients had agreed to follow-up arthroscopy at the time of hardware removal. Five of them had received deep frozen meniscal allografts and 13 had lyophilized menisci. In deep-frozen meniscal transplants arthroscopy was carried out in five of six patients at an average of 3.4 years after operation. In three cases the meniscus was normal in size, but in two cases it was smaller. In one patient arthroscoped at 18 months the meniscus was one third of its normal size.

In the lyophilized meniscal transplants arthroscopy was done at an average of 2 years after operation in 13 patients. In the first patient the meniscus was reduced by one third of its size at 10 months; at 23 months the transplant was completely destroyed. In the other cases, arthroscopy showed that the meniscus had become smaller, particularly after more than one year.

In five cases in this group the transplanted meniscus was reduced in size by two thirds after more than 15 months, and in a further four cases it was reduced by one third. Arthroscopy showed a normal apperance of the meniscus after more than one year only in one patient.

Histocompatibility testing was performed in 9 of 22 meniscal transplantation recipients [30]. A significant immune response could be detected in only one recipient, but it was not correlated to the clinical result.

In summary, we did not find any intact transplants after a follow-up of more than two years. After this period of time, all allografts that were examined were reduced in size and were soft to palpation. Because of the increasing awareness of the AIDS problem, our patients were increasingly reluctant to accept allografts in the late eighties. This fact together with the only fair medium-term results lead to our reason to stop the series and abandon allograft meniscal replacement.

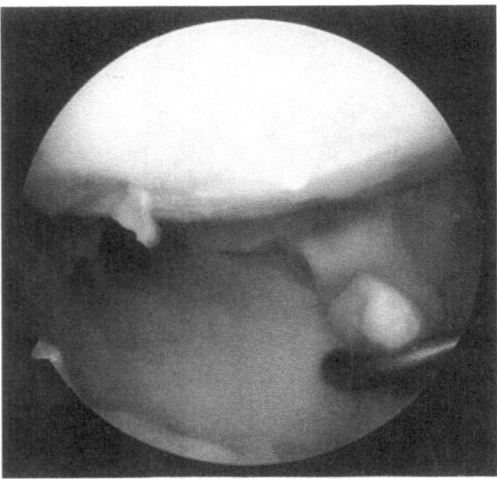

Fig. 3. Failure of anterior horn fixation one year after medial meniscus transplantation

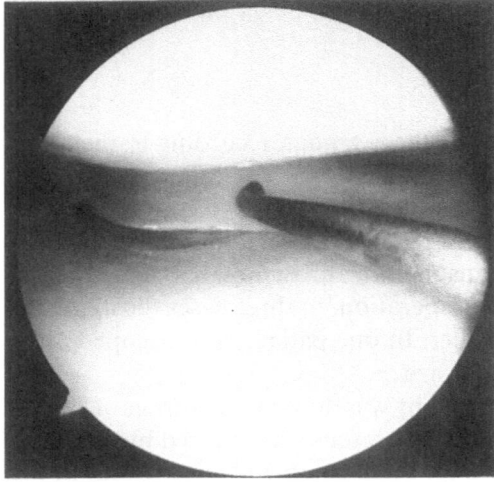

Fig. 4. Posterior horn of a meniscus allograft, well fixed and intact one year after insertion

Future Perspectives

The question whether the transplant has any influence on the further progress of degeneration of the joint surfaces is not yet known. There is a considerable frequency of degenerative meniscal lesions in the elderly population [1]. Therefore, allografts must be taken from young donors younger than 30 years of age. Donor and recipient should be of the same age or preferably, the donor should be younger than the recipient.

The question as to which graft type is suited best for meniscal transplantation has not been answered so far and different options are under investigation [6, 9, 12, 19, 22, 38, 39]. Frozen meniscal allografts have worked well clinically in some patients [37] and in animal experiments [13]. Our own clinical experience showed that the use of freeze-dried meniscal allografts cannot be recommended in all cases with predictable favorable results.

Proper function of the menisci in energy absorption and load distribution is dependent on the circular integrity of the meniscal structure that allows the creation of a hoop stress when the knee is loaded [7, 8, 16, 17, 35, 36]. Fixation of the posterior horn was a problem in some of our cases and a possible cause for failure [30]. The problem of fixation of the anterior and posterior horn of a meniscal allograft is not resolved at the present time. Soft tissue fixation avoids the risk of the use of allograft bone but requires more precision. The soft tissue techniques reported so far had a tendency of fail [25, 31], whereas bony fixation seems secure [18]. The challenge of pretensioning the graft around the condyle has not been met to date in allograft meniscal transplantation.

Disease transmission has not been reported so far in connection with meniscal transplantation [19]. However, the overall number of meniscal transplantations is still small and the risk will increase if the procedure gets more widely accepted. The situation of a young and otherwise healthy person as a possible recipient of a meniscal allograft is not comparable to that of a tumor patient who will undergo limb sparing tumor resection and receive an osteochondral allograft. For the tumor patient the benefit of the allograft procedure is enormous and almost always predictable. This cannot be said at present for the recipient of a meniscus. Consequently, the possibility of disease transmission weighs heavily against meniscal transplantation. We are intensively looking at the possibility of autologous meniscal replacement. This has the potential to avoid hygienic and immunological problems and make the procedure more acceptable for the patient [26, 27].

References

1. American Academy of Orthopaedic Surgeons (1989) Recommendations for the prevention of human immunodeficiency virus (HIV) transmission in the practice of orthopaedic surgery, Chicago, AAOS
2. Ahmed AM, Burke DL (1983) In vitro measurements of static pressure distribution in synovial joints. Part I: Tibial surface of the knee. J Biomech Eng 105: 216–225
3. Allen PR, Denham RA, Swan AV (1984) Late degenerative changes after meniscectomy: factors affecting the knee after operation. J Bone Joint Surg 66-Br: 666–671
4. Appel H (1970) Late results after meniscectomy in the knee joint: A clinical and roentgenologic follow-up investigation. Acta Orthop Scand [Suppl] 133: 1–111
5. Arnoczky SP, Adams ME, Mow V, et al (1988) The meniscus. In: Buckwalter JA, Woo SL-Y (eds) The injury and repair of muscoskeletal soft tissue. Park Ridge, IL: American Academy of Orthopaedic Surgeons, pp 487–537
6. Arnoczky SP, Warren RF, McDevitt CA (1990) Meniscal replacement using a cryopreserved allograft. Clin Orthop 252: 121–128

7. Beaupré A, Choukroun R, Guidoin R, et al (1986) Knee menisci. Clin Orthop 208: 72–75

8. Beaupré A, Choukroun R, Guidouin R, et al (1981) Les ménisques du genou. Rev Chir Orthop 67: 713–719

9. DeBoer HH, Koudstaal J (1991) The fate of meniscus cartilage after transplantation of cryopreserved non tissue-antigen-matched allograft. Clin Orthop 266: 145–151

10. Bullough PG, Munera L, Murphy J, et al (1970) The strength of the menisci of the knee as it relates to their fine structure. J Bone Joint Surg 52-B: 564–570

11. Brown TD, Shaw DT (1984) In vitro contact stress distributions on the femoral condyles. J Orthop Res 2: 190–199

12. Canham W, Stanish W (1986) A study of the biological behavior of the meniscus as a transplant in the medial compartment of a dog's knee. Am J Sports Med 14: 376–379

13. Canham W, Stanish W (1986) A study of the biological behavior of the meniscus as a transplant in the medial compartment of a dog's knee. Am J Sports Med 14: 376–379

14. Cannon WD (1991) Arthroscopic meniscus repair. In: McGinty J (ed) Operative arthroscopy. New York: Raven Press, pp 237–251

15. Coventry MB (1979) Upper tibial osteotomy for gonarthrosis. The evolution of the operation in the last 18 years and long-term results. Orthop Clin North Amer 10: 191–210

16. Fairbank TJ (1948) Knee joint changes after meniscectomy. J Bone Joint Surg 30B: 664–670

17. Fithian DC, Kelly MA, van Mow C (1990) Material properties and structure-function relationships in the menisci. Clin Orthop 252: 19–31

18. Garret JC (1991) Meniscal transplantation in the human knee: A preliminary report. Arthroscopy 7: 57–62

19. Garrett JC (1992) Meniscal transplantation. In: Aichroth PM, Cannon WD, Patel DV (eds) Knee surgery, current practice. Köln: Deutscher Ärzteverlag, pp 95–103

20. Huckell JR (1965) Is meniscectomy a benign procedure? A long-term follow-up study. Can J Surg 8: 254–260

21. Jackson JP (1968) Degenerative changes in the knee after meniscectomy. Br Med J 2: 525–527

22. Jackson DW, McDevitt CA, Simon TM, et al (1992) Meniscal transplantation using fresh and cryopreserved allografts. An experimental study in goats. Am J Sports Med 20: 644–656

23. Johnson RJ, Kettelkamp DB, Clark W, et al (1974) Factors affecting late results after meniscectomy. J Bone Joint Surg 56-A: 719–729

24. Jorgensen U, Sonne-Holm S, Lauridsen F, et al (1987) Long-term follow-up of meniscectomy in athletes: A prospective lingitudinal study. J Bone Joint Surg 69-B: 80–83

25. Keene GCR, Paterson RS, Teague DC (1987) Advances in arthroscopic surgery. Clin Orthop 224: 64–7015

26. Kohn D, Wirth CJ, Reiss G, et al (1992) Medial meniscus replacement by a tendon autograft. Experiments in sheep. J Bone Joint Surg 74-B: 910–917

27. Kohn D (1993) Autograft meniscus replacement: experimental and clinical results. Knee Surg Sports Traumatol Arthroscopy 1: 123–125

28. Lynch MA, Henning CE, Glick KRjr (1983) Knee joint surface changes: Long-term follow-up meniscus tear treatment in stable anterior cruciate ligament reconstructions. Clin Orthop 172: 148–153

29. Medlar RC, Mandlberg JJ, Lyne ED (1980) Meniscectomies in children: Report of long-term results (mean 8, 3 years) of 26 children. Am J Sports Med 8: 87–92

30. Milachowski KA, Weismeier K, Erhard W, et al (1987) Die Meniskustransplantation. Tierexperimentelle Untersuchung. Sportverletzung—Sportschaden 1: 20–24

31. Milachowski KA, Weismeler K, Wirth CJ (1989) Homologous meniscus transplantation. Experimental and clinical results. Int Orthop 13: 1–11

32. Mow VC, Ratcliffe A, Chern KY, et al (1992) Structure and function relationships of the menisci of the knee. In: Mow VC, Arnoczky SP, Jackson DW (eds) Knee meniscus. Basic and clinical foundations. New York: Raven Press, pp 37–58

33. Pinkowski IL, Reimann PR, Suio-Ling C (1989) Human lymphocyte reaction to freeze-dried allograft and xenograft ligamentous tissue. Am J Sports Med 17: 595–600

34. Scuderi GR, Insall JN (1992) Total knee arthroplasty—Current clinical perspectives. Clin Orthop 276: 26–32

35. Seedhom BB, Dowson D, Wright V (1974) Functions of the menisci: A preliminary study. J Bone Joint Surg 56-B: 381–382
36. Shrive NG, O'Connor JJ, Goodfellow JW (1978) Load-bearing in the knee joint. Clin Orthop 131: 279–287
37. Wirth CJ, Milachowski KA, Weismeier K (1986) Meniscus transplantation in animal experiments and initial clinical results. Z Orthop 124: 508–512
38. Wirth CJ, Rodriguez M, Milachowski KA (1988) Meniskusnaht, Meniskusersatz. Stuttgart, New York: Thieme
39. Zukor DJ, Rubins JM, Daigle MR, et al (1991) Allotransplantation of frozen irradiated menisci in rabbits [Abstract]. J Bone Joint Surg 73-B [Suppl 1]: 45

Authors' address: Prof. Dr. med. D. Kohn, Direktor der Orthopädischen Universitätsklinik, Postfach, D-66424 Homburg (Saar), Federal Republic of Germany.

Viable Meniscal Transplantation

R. Verdonk[1], P. Van Daele[1], B. Claus[1], K. Van Den Abbeele[1], P. Desmet[1], G. Verbruggen[2], E. M. Veys[2], and H. Claessens[1]

[1]Department of Physical Medicine and Orthopaedic Surgery, [2]Department of Rheumatology, Gent University Hospital, Gent, Belgium

Summary

It is postulated that restoring the normal congruency between femur and tibia with normal menisci could be a solution to many mechanical knee problems.

Good functional results have been achieved with the transplantation of menisci in compartmental meniscal degeneration. However, this type of chondroprotection can only be evaluated after 10 to 20 years of follow-up.

Satisfactory incorporation of meniscal transplants has been obtained with fresh allografts, but availability remains a problem with this method of meniscal substitution.

Incorporation and ingrowth of fibroblasts have been shown in freeze-dried and deep-frozen meniscal allografts. In a small number of transplants shrinking has been observed on repeat arthroscopy.

Viable meniscal allograft implantation has been initiated in a series of 25 patients. The value of this method has been studied. With the use of a semisynthetic medium the semilunar cartilages can be kept viable without apparent loss of fibrochondroblast cell activity. During this incubation period the appropriate recipient can be selected and prepared. There is sufficient time to conduct laboratory screening and to evaluate the culture results and disease transmission factors. In this way, live transplant hazards can be avoided which results in a higher success rate.

It should be kept in mind that the knee is a weightbearing joint. The patient himself is responsible for mechanical loading, and medical control of these conditions is not always possible.

The intensity of loading thus remains an aspect that cannot always be determined scientifically and must be considered in pathology.

In view of the promising results obtained with tendon allografts and with meniscal allografts in sheep [5], meniscus transplantation in humans has become an attractive treatment option, while the outcome of synthetic meniscus replacement has been rather disappointing. Meniscal transplantation involves the necessity to store and preserve meniscal material.

Meniscal Culture

Harvesting of Human Donor Menisci

Donor menisci are removed in the operating room under strict aseptic conditions, mainly in conjunction with the procurement of other organs [heartbeating (multiple organ donors) or non-heartbeating donors]. Cold ischaemia must not exceed 12 hours. During this period meniscal viability remains intact.

Both menisci of each knee are removed with a small synovial rim for manipulation. The meniscus itself is treated in a strictly atraumatic manner.

In vitro Culture

The menisci are placed in culture medium immediately after harvesting. The medium consists of DMEM (Dulbecco's modified Eagle's medium) with 0.002 M L-glutamine, 1/1000 antibiotic-antimycotic suspension (streptomycin 10 μg/ml, penicillin 10 U/ml, fungizone 0.025 μg/ml) and 20% fetal calf serum (FCS). The recipient's serum is used for clinical applications.

The menisci are stored in a plastic container (DANCON, Teknunc − 4000 Roskilde, Denmark). Seventy ml of incubation medium are added. The containers are placed in an incubation chamber (modular incubation chamber, Flow Laboratories—Del Mar, CA U.S.A.) at a constant temperature of 37°C and under continuous air flow (95% air and 5% CO_2).

Humidity is controlled by placing an open receptacle filled with sterile water in the incubation chamber. The incubation media are replaced every three days [3].

Meniscal Metabolism

To study the metabolic function of the cells, proteoglycan (PG) metabolism was examined. The collagen fibres were not studied.

Metabolism and Topography

To determine the influence of the site of harvesting on PG-metabolism, 4 menisci were sliced anteroposteriorly into 5 fragments. The anterior and posterior horns were removed.

There was no difference in ^{35}S PG-production between the 5 fragments (anterior → posterior). Moreover, the production rates apparently were more dependent on the menisci than on the location (anterior → posterior). No difference was found in the produced percentage of ^{35}S PG-aggregates between the anterior and posterior horns.

If comparisons are to be made regarding the effect of incubation time on PG-production, one should always start with material from the same meniscus. Furthermore, the quality is not affected by the location in the meniscus, and is also preferably studied using the same meniscus. A difference up to 10% with regard to aggregate production in the same meniscus is considered an acceptable biological variation.

Two menisci, and in a later experiment three menisci, were sliced laterolaterally into four fragments. ^{35}S PG-production in the extract was higher at the inner margin of the meniscus than in the rest of the meniscus. This can be due either to the higher methodological extractability of these smaller fragments or to their higher intrinsic PG-production.

There was no difference in the produced percentage of ^{35}S PG-aggregates, monomers and small PGs, between the medial and lateral fragments of the meniscus. The extractability of the ^{35}S PGs was significantly higher in the medial fragments. This can be explained by either a greater intrinsic extractability or an increased local production.

No significant difference in water content according to the anatomical location was observed.

Effect of Culture Time on Meniscus PG-Metabolism

The effect of culture time on meniscus PG-metabolism and meniscus structure was studied using DMEM without FCS in the prelabelling period.

A distinct peak production of PGs was seen in the second week of culture, which in the third week tended to fall to bottom values inferior to those observed in the first week of culture.

There was also a progressive increase of the relative amount of PGs in the medium, which was a parameter for catabolism or for immobilization throughout the culture period.

The extractability of the PGs increased slightly with the time spent in culture. With an increasing culture time the original meniscus structure became less capable of retaining the glycosaminoglycans (GAGs), so that increasing amounts of these diffused to the medium (Fig. 1).

The water content increased during the first two weeks.

It can thus be stated that the meniscus degenerates rapidly when the specimens are cultured in FCS-free medium.

Because of this degeneration, medium continuously supplemented with 20% FCS was used in further experiments.

Values of total de novo PG-production were optimal in the second week of culture. Consequently, the immobilization of de novo produced PGs was highest or the catabolic influence minor during this week. After three weeks of culture total de novo PG-production decreased and after four weeks it fell to levels inferior to the initial de novo PG-production.

De novo PG-production was ten times higher in the culture medium continuously supplemented with 20% FCS than in the medium without 20% FCS in the prelabelling period (Fig. 2).

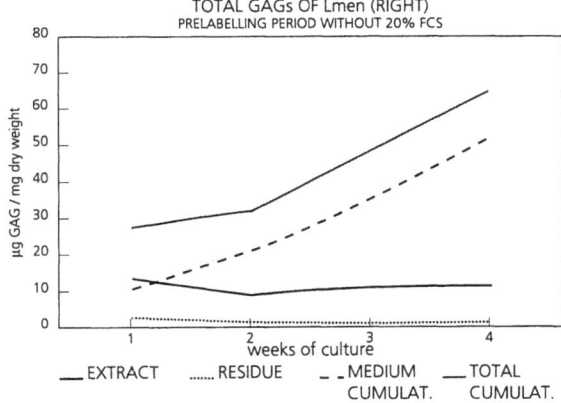

Fig. 1. Cumulative amounts of GAG in extract, residue and medium during the four weeks of culture. Four fragments of the same meniscus (n°19) were studied. GAG values are expressed as μg/mg dry weight in extract, residue and medium

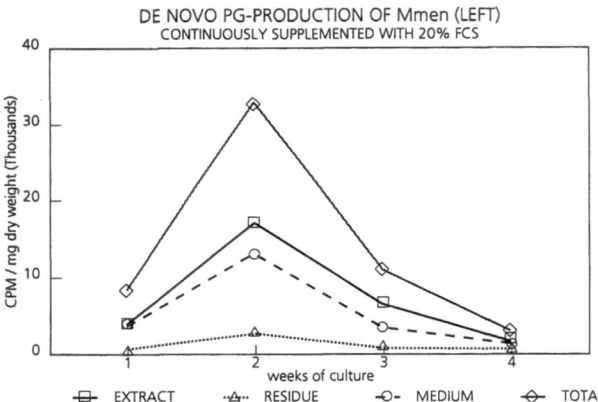

Fig. 2. ^{35}S incorporation in proteoglycans in residue, extract and medium during the four weeks of culture. Four fragments of the same meniscus (Lmen.left n°20) were studied. ^{35}S values are expressed as CPM/mg dry weight for extract, residue and medium

It can be stated that the quality of the de novo synthesized PGs was optimal during the first week of culture.

After 4 weeks of culture in medium supplemented with 20% FCS the original meniscal structure had remained fairly intact as compared to culture in medium not continuously supplemented with FCS.

Clinical Experience

Material and Methods

Since the beginning (January 1989) of our clinical experience, 36 patients underwent viable meniscal allografting. The first 25 patients were included in the present study running from January 1989 to September 1993. The duration of follow-up ranged between 4 years 8 months and 1 year (mean: 2 years 11 months). There were 23 men (92%) and 2 women (8%). Eleven left knees (44%) and 14 right knees (56%) were operated upon. The majority of patients underwent transplantation of the medial meniscus (18 cases, i.e. 72%). In 7 patients (28%) the lateral meniscus was transplanted. Mean age at the time of surgery was 33 years 4 months (range: 23 years 5 months to 48 years 2 months). Mean age at the last follow-up examination was 36 years 3 months (range: 27 years 2 months to 52 years 2 months). A solitary viable meniscal transplantation was performed 16 times. Transplantation was combined with a valgus osteotomy in 6 cases, and with an intraarticular ACL reconstruction using a tendon allograft in 3 cases [1].

Operative Technique

Epidural anesthesia is induced. In case of a medial meniscal transplant anterior and posteromedial incisions are performed. After inspection of the joint the medial meniscal remnant is removed. The meniscal allograft is implanted from posterior to anterior, threaded with 5 or 6 × 2.0 poly-dioxanone (PDS) sutures mounted on a dual needle (Ethicon, Ethnor J.J. – Neuilly, France).

In case of a lateral meniscal transplant a parapatellar arthrotomy incision is made, allowing the resection of the lateral meniscal remnant. An osteotomy of the proximal insertion of the lateral collateral ligament is performed, allowing for widening of the lateral joint line. The threaded allograft is inserted from posterior to anterior after which the bony insertion of the lateral collateral ligament is firmly attached with a screw.

In the first 10 cases a plaster cast was used as postoperative immobilization, which has been abandoned. A brace is now used, allowing for progressive mobilization. After 6 weeks partial weightbearing is allowed.

Clinical Evaluation

It is best – but not always easy – to use an objective rating system to evaluate the results of viable meniscal allografting.

Since meniscal transplantation, performed as an isolated or combined procedure, is in essence comparable to an arthroplasty, the "Hospital for Special Surgery (HSS)" knee rating system [2] has been used, which considers pain, stability and function. Flexion and extension contractures, malalignment and the use of crutches represent minus points.

In order to come to valid conclusions, imaging of the intra-articular status is of paramount importance. Magnetic resonance imaging (MRI) of the meniscal bodies is able to confirm ingrowth of the allografted material into the synovial wall. MR-images also provide information on cartilage quality and ligament reconstruction. All 25 patients in this clinical study were followed-up by means of MRI, but the procedure was not performed at regular intervals.

Because MRI gives very accurate information, an arthroscopic evaluation is only performed to obtain material for histological studies and to assess the appearance and firmness of meniscal fixation.

Complications

1. Synovitis
Four patients had transient synovitis. Three cases presented with mechanical cell count. One inflammatory synovitis eventually regained normal function of the knee joint. Infectious parameters also returned to normal levels.

2. Range of motion
Manipulation under anesthesia was necessary in three cases including in combined procedures with a valgus osteotomy and intraarticular ligamentoplasty for ACL deficiency.

3. Infection
Clinical evidence of osteomyelitis or arthritis was not seen. One patient developed an inflammatory joint effusion, but cultures yielded no growth. The evolution was uneventful.

Results and Discussion

Young patients with mechanical complaints, who had already undergone one or more meniscectomies, were considered for inclusion in this series. The medial compartment of the knee joint was predominantly involved (72%) and to a lesser extent the lateral compartment (28%).

A number of patients also complained of knee instability due to ACL-deficiency (3 cases). In some other patients the mechanical complaints could be ascribed to obvious axial malalignment (6 cases).

Scoring systems were not systematically used preoperatively in the evaluation of the 25 cases, since the patient population was too diverse. The constant factor in all cases was a medial or lateral meniscectomy. Several other elements were combined, e.g. axial malalignment, ligamentous laxity.

Ultimately, intractable pain not responding to analgesics was the principal reason for instituting treatment. Based on the experiments of Wirth, Milachowski and Weismeier [5], and of Zukor et al. [6, 7] meniscal transplantation was considered. The work of Verbruggen [3] and Verbruggen et al. [4] on cartilage metabolism and cartilage cell structures enabled us to culture the harvested semilunar cartilages in toto so that viable material could be implanted.

No major clinical complications were encountered in our series of 25 patients, although the population was fairly heterogeneous as far as the operative procedures were concerned.

Repeat arthroscopies were performed on 8 patients at different points of time postsurgery and always showed viable meniscal tissue, both macroscopically and microscopically (Fig. 3).

Some arthroscopies were performed shortly after viable meniscal allografting (4 months), others after more than 2 years (24 months). It may thus be assumed that the viability of the meniscal allografts is intact.

These findings were confirmed on MRI. No major differences were seen with various imaging techniques.

Over the years (maximum duration of follow-up: 4 years 8 months) the mean HSS score decreased slowly and slightly.

In the first year, an arbitrarily chosen score of more than 175 was achieved in 72% of the cases. After 4 years, only 60% of the patients still scored higher than 174 (Fig. 4). One patient underwent a total knee arthroplasty 4 years after viable medial meniscus transplantation; the meniscal transplant was found to be well preserved, but the lateral compartment showed severe degenerative changes, which had been the reason for knee joint replacement.

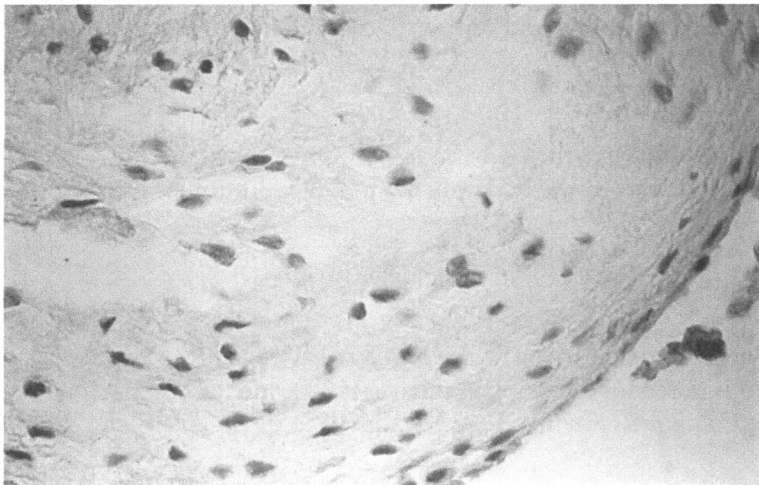

Fig. 3. Viable cells are present in the anterior horn 4 months postoperatively. Some fibrin covering is observed (H&E; × 400)

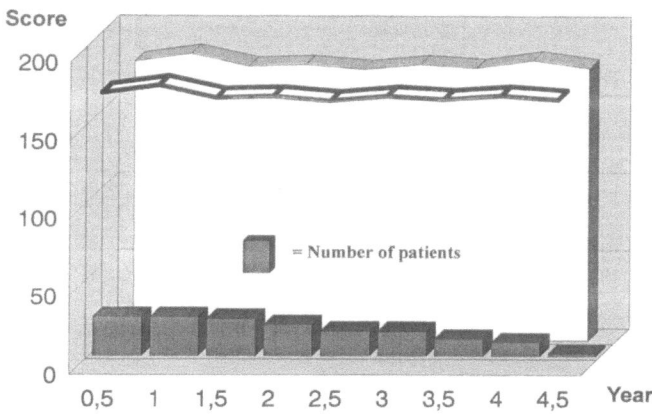

Fig. 4. Patient scores at 0 to 4 years of follow-up. Over the years, the mean HSS score decreases slowly and slightly

Although a favourable effect of the associated corrective osteotomy could be anticipated, these scores were considered in the overall results.

Our initial intention was indeed to determine whether ingrowth of viable meniscal material can achieved in the long run, and whether the allograft would be subject to rejection, shrinking or synovialization.

It remains an open question whether viability, of which histological evidence was obtained in 8 patients, has any effect on the long-term functional results.

The postoperative follow-up is far too short to allow any strong conclusions to be drawn. From a technical viewpoint, however, allografting has no negative effect on the clinical results.

References

1. Arnauw G, Verdonk R, Harth A, Moerman J, Vorlat P, Bataillie F, Claessens H (1991) Prosthetic versus tendon allograft replacement of ACL-deficient knees. Acta Orthop Belg 57 (Suppl II): 67–74
2. Insall JN, Dorr LD, Scott RD, Scott WN (1989) Rationale of the Knee Society clinical rating system. Clin Orthop 248: 13–14
3. Verbruggen G (1990) Reparatieprocessen en katabole fenomenen in humaan articulair kraakbeen. Proefschrift tot het verkrijgen van de graad van geaggregeerde voor het hoger onderwijs, Gent.
4. Verbruggen G, Veys EM, Malfait AM, Cochez P, Schatteman L, Wieme N, Heynen G, Broddelez C (1989) Proteoglycan metabolism in tissue cultured human articular cartilage. Influence of piroxicam. J Rheumatol 16: 355–362
5. Wirth CJ, Milachowski KA, Weismeier K (1986) Die Meniskustransplantation im Tierexperiment und erste klinische Ergebnisse. Z Orthop 124: 508–512
6. Zukor DJ, Cameron JC, Brooks PJ, Oakeshott RD, Farine I, Rudan JF, Gross AE (1990) The fate of human meniscal allografts. In: Ewing JW (ed) Articular cartilage and knee joint function: basic science and arthroscopy. New York: Raven Press, pp 147–152
7. Zukor DJ, Cameron JC, Brooks PJ, Oakeshott RD, Gross AE (1988) The fate of human meniscal allografts. Orthop Trans 12: 658

Authors' addresses: R. Verdonk, M.D., MS, P. Van Daele, M.D., B. Claus, M.D., K. Van den Abbeele, M.D., P. Desmet, M.D., H. Claessens, M.D., MS (Professor Emeritus) Department of Physical Medicine and Orthopaedic Surgery, Gent University Hospital, De Pintelaan 185, B-9000 Gent, Belgium; G. Verbruggen, M.D., Ph.D., E.M. Veys, M.D., Ph.D., Department of Rheumatology, Gent University Hospital, De Pintelaan 185, B-9000 Gent, Belgium.

Articular Cartilage Cryopreservation and Transplantation

W. W. Tomford, C. Ohlendorf, and H. J. Mankin

Orthopaedic Research Laboratories, Massachusetts General Hospital, Boston, Massachusetts, U.S.A.

Introduction

Although advances in joint replacement have significantly improved the treatment of articular cartilage degeneration in elderly individuals, the treatment of articular cartilage loss by the use of prosthetic devices has not been as successful in young people. Joint replacement implants loosen and plastic bearing surfaces wear out prematurely in young people. For this reason, the use of biological substitutes to replace and resurface articular cartilage defects in younger age groups remains a popular and worthwhile endeavor.

The most extensive experience in biological replacement of articular cartilage in young people has been reported from the experience of bone tumor surgeons. In their cases, frozen or cryopreserved osteoarticular grafts have been used as transplants because these types of grafts can be banked to provide different sized grafts for different individuals. The surgical use of these types of articulating grafts has provided a unique opportunity for the evaluation of the fate of transplanted frozen articular cartilage. This paper will review the results of transplantation of frozen and cryopreserved articular cartilage allografts and current and future research in cryopreservation of articular cartilage.

Clinical Transplantation

Although Lexer reported results of the first large series of osteoarticular transplants, most of his grafts were fresh [8, 9]. Ottolenghi reported the earliest extensive experience with transplantation of frozen cartilage [21, 22, 23]. Following transplantation of over fifty osteoarticular allografts, Ottolenghi noted signs of aseptic necrosis in the subchondral area of the grafts within two years of transplantation. He believed that a lack of joint innervation led to abnormal forces across the joint with destruction of cartilage which was ultimately responsible for necrosis of the joint surface. He found that although subchondral collapse occurred, the function of the joint frequently remained reasonable and did not require surgery for several years thereafter.

Following Ottolenghi's reports, Parrish reported the fate of twenty-one patients who received massive frozen osteoarticular allografts [24, 25]. Like Ottolenghi, Parrish noted bone resorption in the subchondral area with subsequent degenerative joint

Work in this paper supported in part by NIH Grant AR21896.

changes. Parrish however noted that patients had to have either fusion or amputation following extensive degenerative joint changes.

Following Parrish's efforts, Mankin began transplantation of frozen osteoarticular allografts for the treatment of bone tumors in the early 1970's [14]. Mankin began attempts at cryopreservation of the articular cartilage of these types of allografts based upon Audrey Smith's pioneering work in this field [29]. Mankin found that about 15% to 20% of the transplanted cryopreserved osteoarticular grafts developed subchondral collapse and fatigue fractures which led to deterioration and destruction of the articular cartilage [13]. Mankin noted, as did Ottolenghi and Parrish, that excessive bone turnover in the metaphyseal area frequently resulted in weakening of the local cancellous bone and subsequent joint destruction [15]. In a study by Waber, approximately 10% of the osteoarticular grafts in Mankin's series required prosthetic replacement at three years after transplantation due to subchondral collapse and joint deterioration [36]. Mankin has published data to suggest that, at least in the hip joint, it is preferable to perform a primary joint (bipolar) replacement rather than rely on the fate of a frozen osteoarticular allograft [6]. Nonetheless, osteoarticular allografts are still used in his patients if the fit or articulation with the normal side of the joint is good. Flynn recently reviewed seventeen patients who received a cryopreserved osteoarticular allograft femoral condyle for treatment of osteonecrosis [4]. He found that 12 of the 17 patients reviewed had a good or excellent result and concluded that treatment of unicondylar osteonecrosis using this method was as successful as treatment with a unicondylar prosthesis.

Historically, several investigators have concluded that frozen or cryopreserved osteoarticular allografts provide a reasonable replacement of joint cartilage in short term results (2 to 5 years) but deteriorate over longer times [1, 17, 19, 34, 35], and recent reports have confirmed these findings. Zatsepin and Burdygin in 1994 published their experience with frozen (− 30 degrees to − 70 degrees C.) allografts [37]. They found that the most frequent long-term complication was joint deterioration. Virtually all of their patients with distal femoral allografts and a little more than half of their patients with proximal tibial allografts eventually developed arthrosis. Mnaymneh et al. has reported that up to 10% of recipients of distal femoral allografts cryopreserved with glycerol developed articular cartilage deterioration after two to five years postoperatively [16]. Brien et al. recently compared the fate of recipients of osteoarticular allografts with that of recipients of endoprosthetic devices [2]. They found that frozen allografts with cartilage cryopreserved with glycerol provided joints that initially endured as well as the artificial joints.

In conclusion, clinical results of preservation of joint mechanics and function following frozen or cryopreserved osteoarticular allograft transplantation are initially good. However, long term the cartilage deterioration necessitates joint replacement or arthrodesis.

Research in Cryopreservation

Research continues in the field of cryopreservation of cartilage in attempts to maintain the survival of chondrocytes in osteoarticular cartilage after transplantation in order to preserve joint function. Several authors have reported results of methods of cryopreservation of articular cartilage. Most of the early studies concentrated on preservation of isolated cells [7, 10, 32]. These studies showed that isolated cells could be cryoprotected with preservation of up to 85% chondrocyte viability. Unfortunately, similar viability rates have not been achieved with chondrocytes in an intact cartilage matrix. Tomford found that viability rates up to 40% were possible but that results were variable [31], and Malinin has reported similar results [12]. Recently, two studies have shown that a major problem in achieving high viability in intact cartilage is related to the fact that there is a lack of uniform preservation of cells throughout the matrix. Muldrew et al. showed with the use of a model which employed plugs of osteoarticular cartilage that the major area of loss of chondrocyte viability following cryopreservative treatment with dimethyl sulfoxide (DMSO) and freezing is in the central portion of the cartilage plug [18]. In a more recent study, Ohlendorf reported a visual study of the location of viable cells following freezing of an osteoarticular graft in which chondrocytes survive only on the surface of the cartilage [20]. In Ohlendorf's experiments, intact osteoarticular cartilage was exposed to and frozen in phosphate buffered saline (PBS) and DMSO. Following thawing, viable cells were confined to the superficial layer of the cartilage matrix. DMSO appeared to increase the number of viable cells in the surface area in which chondrocyte survival occurred but no viable cells were noted in the middle or deep layers of the cartilage.

Research efforts in the evaluation of transplanted cryopreserved articular cartilage have included several animal models. Herndon and Chase published a classic study in 1952 in which they found that frozen (−20 degrees Centigrade) cartilage degenerated within a few month in a dog whole joint transplant model [5]. Seligman et al. in 1972 also found no cartilage survival in a whole joint trasplant model in the dog [28]. They noted that the femoral articular surface deteriorated faster and worse than the corresponding tibial plateau. They also noted replacement of dead cartilage by fibrocartilage. Schachar reported a study in felines in which cryopreserved cartilage degeneration appeared to be related more to ligament and joint stability failure than to lack of survival of chondrocytes [27]. The author reported a series of transplants of cryopreserved osteoarticular allografts of the proximal radius in outbred cats [33]. At six month follow-up, fresh autograft cartilage retained a normal appearance, but frozen allograft cartilage showed loss of cells in the basal and middle layers of the cartilage. Of interest is the similar finding in the recent in vitro study by Ohlendorf in which the only surviving cells following freezing were the cells in the surface layer [20]. Stevenson noted in a study of proximal radius transplants that the cartilage from frozen, cryopreserved grafts did not fare well [30]. Few chondrocytes survived, and the cartilage in frozen grafts had significantly less glycosaminoglycan compared to that of fresh allografts. Malinin reported recently that the cartilage in joint transplants in baboons showed degenerative changes over five years that were similar to those which he has observed in cryopreserved human osteoarticular transplants [11].

An important study of retrieved human allografts was reported by Enneking and Mindell in 1991 [3]. They observed that no chondrocytes survived transplantation but that the necrotic cartilage functioned well for several years, perhaps because it was covered by fibrovascular reparative tissue. This finding was echoed by Lexer's reports [8,9] and is similar to the findings reported in research reports on the fate of transplanted cartilage.

One of the major problems involved in the longevity of osteochondral allograft transplants is the importance of proper fit and size on survival of the cartilage [26]. For example, if there is an incongruity in the joint in which the transplant is performed, this incongruity will result in rapid wear of the articular surfaces. Therefore, regardless of the fact that cartilage cells are cryopreserved, the transplanted joint must have a normal or near normal congruency.

In summary, frozen or cryopreserved articular cartilage appears to provide a functional joint for several years after transplantation provided the fit or size match of the allograft is satisfactory. Research in the area of cryopreservation shows that surface cells seem to be able to survive the process of freezing but that all of these cells may not survive several years after transplantation. Future progress in transplantation of frozen articular cartilage will depend upon advances in cryopreservation as well as in achieving anatomic replacements.

References

1. Alho A, Karaharju EO, Karkaoa O, Laasonan EM, Holmstrom T, Muller C (1989) Allogeneic grafts for bone tumors. Twenty-one cases of osteoarticular and segmental grafts. Acta Orthop Scand 60: 143–153
2. Brien EW, Terek RM, Healey JH, Lane JM (1994) Allograft reconstruction after proximal tibial resection for bone tumors: an analysis of function and outcome comparing allograft and prosthetic reconstructions. Clin Orthop 303: 116–127
3. Enneking WF, Mindell ER (1991) Observations on massive retrieved human allografts. J Bone Joint Surg 73A: 1123–1156
4. Flynn JM, Springfield DS, Mankin HJ (1994) Osteoarticular allografts to treat distal femoral osteonecrosis. Clin Orthop 303: 38–43
5. Herndon CH, Chase SW (1952) Experimental studies in the transplantation of whole joints. J Bone Joint Surg 34A: 564–578
6. Jofe MH, Gebhardt MC, Tomford WW, Mankin HJ (1988) Reconstruction for defects of the proximal part of the femur using allografts. J Bone Joint Surg 70A: 507–516
7. Kiefer GN, Sundy K, McAllister D, Shrive NG, Franc CB, Lam T, Schachar NS (1989) The effect of cryopreservation on the biomechanical behavior of bovine articular cartilage. J Orthop Res 7: 494
8. Lexer E (1925) Joint transplantation in arthroplasty. Surg Gynecol Obstet 40: 782–809
9. Lexer E (1908) Substitution of whole or half joints from freshly amputated extremities by free-plastic operation. Surg Gynecol Obstet 6: 601–607
10. Lowe AC, Smith AU (1975) Isolation, freezing, and storage of rabbit growth plate chondrocytes. Laboratory Practice 24: 511–513
11. Malinin TI, Mnaymneh W, Lo HK, Hinkle DK (1994) Cryopreservation of articular cartilage: ultrastructural observations and long terms results of experimental distal femoral transplantation. Clin Orthop 303: 18–32
12. Malinin TI, Wagner JL, Pita TC, Lo H (1985) Hypothermic storage and cryopreservation of cartilage: an experimental study. Clin Orthop 197: 15–26
13. Mankin HJ, Doppelt SH, Tomford WW (1983) Clinical experience with allograft implantation: the first ten years. Clin Orthop 174: 69–83
14. Mankin HJ, Fogelson FS, Thrasher AZ, et al (1976) Massive resection and allograft transplantation in the treatment of malignant bone tumors. N Engl J Med 294: 1247–1255
15. Mankin HJ, Gebhardt MC, Tomford WW (1987) The use of frozen cadaveric allografts in the management of patients with bone tumors of the extremities. Orthop Clin North Am 18: 275–287
16. Mnaymneh W, Malinin TI, Lackman RD, Hornicek FJ, Ghandur-Mnaymneh L (1994) Massive distal femoral osteoarticular allografts after resection of bone tumors. Clin Orthop 303: 103–115
17. Mnaymneh W, Malinin TI, Makley JT, Dick H (1985) Massive osteoarticular allografts in the reconstruction of extremities following resection of tumors not requiring chemotherapy and radiation. Clin Orthop 197: 76–87
18. Muldrew K, Hurtig M, Novak K, Schachar N, McGann LE (1994) Localization of freezing injury in articular cartilage. Cryobiology 31: 31–38
19. Muscolo DL, Petracchi LJ, Ayerza MA, Calabrese ME (1992) Massive femoral allografts followed for 22–36 years. J Bone Joint Surg 74B: 887
20. Ohlendorf C, Tomford WW, Mankin HJ (1996) Chondrocytes are viable in cryopreserved osteochondral articular cartilage. J Orthop Res (in press)
21. Ottolenghi GE (1972) Massive osteo and osteo-articular bone grafts: technique and results of 62 cases. Clin Orthop 87: 156–164

22. Ottolenghi CE (1966) Massive osteo-articular bone grafts: transplants of the whole femur. J Bone Joint Surg 48B: 646
23. Ottolenghi CE, Muscolo DL, Maenza R (1988) Bone defect reconstruction by massive allograft: technique and results of 51 cases followed for 5–32 years. In: Straub LR, Wilson PD (eds) Clinical transient orthopaedics. New York: Thieme-Stratton, p 171
24. Parrish FF (1973) Allograft replacement of all or part of the end of a long bone following excision of a tumor. J Bone Joint Surg 55A: 1–22
25. Parrish FF (1976) Total and partial half joint resection followed by allograft replacement in neoplasms involving ends of long bones. Transplant Proc 8 [Suppl 1]: 77
26. Rodrigo JJ, Salsovich L, Travist C, et al (1978) Osteocartilaginous allografts as compared with autografts in the treatment of free joint osteocartilaginous defects in dogs. Clin Orthop 134: 342–349
27. Schachar NS, Henry WB Jr, Wadsworth P, Mankin HJ (1983) Fate of massive osteochondral allografts in a feline model. In: Friedlander GE, Mankin HJ, Sell KW (eds) Osteochondral allografts. Boston: Little Brown and Co, pp 81–101
28. Seligman GM, George E, Yablon I, et al (1972) Transplantation of whole knee joints in the dog. Clin Orthop 87: 332–344
29. Smith AU (1976) Cartilage. In: Karow AM Jr, Abouna AJM, Humphreys AL Jr (eds) Organ preservation for transplantation. Boston: Little Brown and Co, p 214
30. Stevenson S, Dannucci GA, Sharkey NA, Pool RR (1989) The fate of articular cartilage after transplantation of fresh and cryopreserved tissue-antigen-matched and mismatched osteochondral allografts in dogs. J Bone Joint Surg 71A: 1297–1307
31. Tomford WW, Fredericks GR, Mankin HJ (1972) Cryopreservation of intact articular cartilage. Trans Orthop Res Soc 7: 176
32. Tomford WW, Fredericks GR, Mankin HJ (1984) Studies in cryopreservation of articular cartilage chondrocytes. J Bone Joint Surg 66A: 253–259
33. Tomford WW, Henry WB Jr, Trahan CA, et al (1984) The fate of allograft articular cartilage: fresh and frozen. Trans Orthop Res Soc 9: 217
34. Volkov M (1970) Allotransplantation of joints. J Bone Joint Surg 52B: 49
35. Volkov MV, Imamaliyev AS (1976) Use of allogenous articular bone implants as substitutes for autotransplants in adult patients. Clin Orthop 114: 192–202
36. Waber BA, Tomford WW, Mankin HJ, et al (1989) Long term results of osteoarticular allografts in weight bearing joints. In: Aebi M, Regazzoni P (eds) Bone transplantation. Berlin: Springer, pp 210–218
37. Zatsepin ST, Burdygin VN (1994) Replacement of the distal femur and proximal tibia with frozen allografts. Clin Orthop 303: 95–102

Authors' address: William W. Tomford, M.D., Christian Ohlendorf and Henry J. Mankin, Orthopaedic Research Laboratories, Massachusetts General Hospital, Boston, MA 02114, Massachusetts, U.S.A.

Surface Repair of Osteochondral Defects: Allografts Versus Substitute Materials

G. Bentley

Institute of Orthopaedics, University College London, United Kingdom

Surface replacement for articular cartilage defects has assumed greater importance in recent years because of two factors. The first is the increasing longevity of the population throughout the world which is leading to a higher incidence of osteoarthritis, initiated in some cases by early injury to the joints, and the second is the increased incidence of joint injuries caused by sporting and other accidents in the younger population.

The central problem with articular cartilage is that it is a unique tissue composed of a type II collagen spongy network which is packed with proteoglycans which are responsible for maintaining the water content and the turgor and resilience. Articular cartilage also is unique in so far as it has no nerve fibres and therefore gives the patient no warning when it is injured and also because it has little or no repair capacity. Without going into the details of the structure of articular cartilage and its metabolic activity, it is generally true to say that there is no turnover of collagen in articular cartilage and the proteoglycan content can increase to a limited extent only in response to trauma or other adverse conditions which lead to depletion of the proteoglycan content of the matrix.

In early osteoarthritis there is loss of matrix staining in the superficial zone of the cartilage together with some cell death and with slight fibrillation of the collagen meshwork at the surface. This may be a repairable state. However at the stage when most patients present for treatment there is extensive damage to the articular cartilage which has no prospect of repair.

It is therefore appropriate to consider the breakdown of articular cartilage in three stages pathologically and to consider the repair available at each stage.

1) Grade 1 – Intrinsic cartilage damage is the stage when there is damage to the cartilage only and no involvement of the subchondral bone. Work in our laboratory has shown that there is some capacity for repair in early articular cartilage damage but this is very limited indeed in the human [1]. It may be augmented by the use of non-steroidal anti-inflammatory drugs and also by growth factors but neither of these has proved useful in the clinical situation.

2) In grade 2 damage of the articular cartilage there is exposure of the subchondral bone but no deformation. At this stage the only repair that is available is the formation of fibro-cartilage from the subchondral marrow which occurs naturally but may be augmented by drilling of the articular surface or by stimulating the circulation of the subchondral bone by, for example, juxta-articular osteotomy. Although such procedures which include abrasion arthroplasty can produce some fibrocartilage on the surface of the joint, such repair tissue is rapidly destroyed and does not form a long-

lasting surface layer. This is because it lacks type II collagen and the normal proteoglycans necessary to give the normal resilience and weight-bearing capacity of articular cartilage.

3) Grade 3 is the stage of joint destruction and at this stage the only methods available for treatment are either arthrodesis of the joint or replacement joint arthroplasty. Whilst arthroplasty has improved greatly over the last 15 years there is still a fundamental problem of wear of high density polyethylene and thus better materials or new designs avoiding point loading are required to increase the longevity of such implants.

There is therefore the need for joint allografts to give an articular surface which is made up of normal articular cartilage especially in young people in whom joint replacement is not acceptable from the point of view of the longevity and stability of the prosthesis and the complications that will occur in a vigorous young person who places high stresses on the joint.

The earliest work with osteochondral allografts began in 1908 with Lexer [2] and Judet [3] but over the years it has been generally found that osteochondral allografts undergo slow rejection. This is because of the bony component of the graft which is necessary to secure the cartilage to the host. Despite methods of preparing the graft this has been their general fate.

Because of this some years ago in our laboratory we developed the technique of isolation of chondrocytes from the matrix by enzymatic digestion and subsequently culture of that cartilage for storage purposes. Storage produces increased numbers of cells and we demonstrated by immuno-fluorescence that these cells, if maintained in high density in culture, will produce normal type II collagen.

We then transplanted preparations of intact cartilage and cultured chondrocytes as allografts into the knee joint of rabbits and followed these up for one year. We found high success rates with both cultured and intact cartilage grafts and established firmly that cartilage could be transplanted as an allograft alone without great difficulty [4] (Fig. 1).

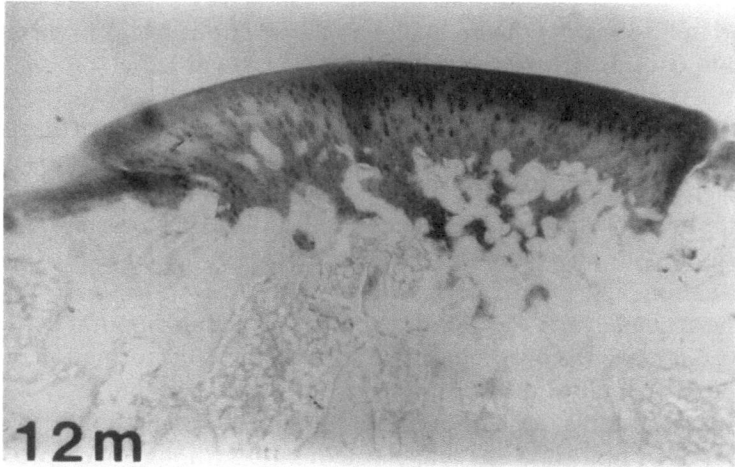

Fig. 1. Filling of an osteochondral defect by an intact plug of allograft articular cartilage in the rabbit knee. There is complete incorporation of the graft and no sign of rejection after 12 months (Toludine blue × 90)

However there is a problem in the supply of material available for this type of allograft, particularly in humans where, although culture of chondrocytes is possible, the number of cells that can be grown is much less than in animals.

At present xenografts do not seem to be feasible.

In 1986 Langer and Gross [5] published their 8 year follow-up of osteochondral allografts transplanted from renal transplant donor patients and placed in the recipient within 24 hours of death of the donor. They found a high success rate despite the fact that the patients were not immunologically matched. This led to a renewed interest in osteochondral allografts and our unit was involved in this work also. We employed osteochondral allografts for the treatment of post-traumatic articular cartilage defects, osteochondritis, and osteoarthritis. Our first case was a severe case of osteoarthritis with valgus deformity in which we corrected the deformity by an osteochondral allograft of the femoral condyle and of the tibial condyle together with its attached meniscus. Unfortunately the loading on this graft was too great and the graft disintegrated and collapsed after 12 months. Following on this experience where necessary we have carried out realignment of the knee before carrying out an osteochondral allograft. Practical experience has been in 7 cases of which 3 were osteochondritis, one was post-traumatic, and 2 were osteoarthritis. The results of the patients with osteochondritis and post-traumatic defects have been successful over 3–7 years (Figs. 2, 3), compared with the 2 cases for osteoarthritis both of which required later knee replacement operations.

It thus seems that for success with osteochondral allografts it is necessary to have certain biomechanical and possibly immunological criteria. The biological criteria are a young disease free donor and a fresh graft. The biomechanical factors are correct

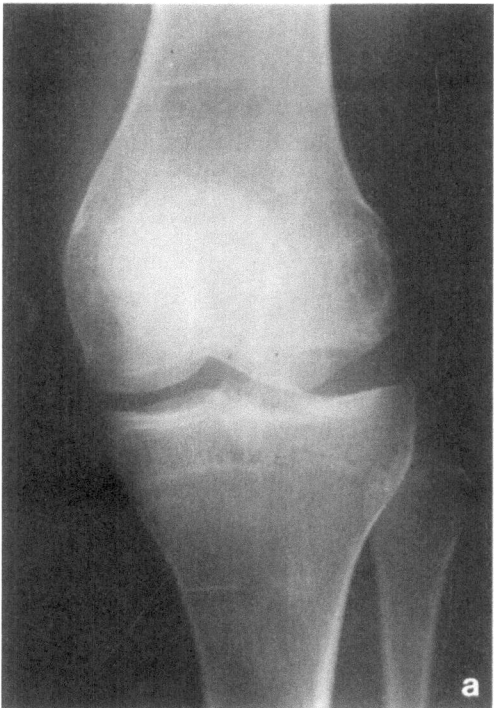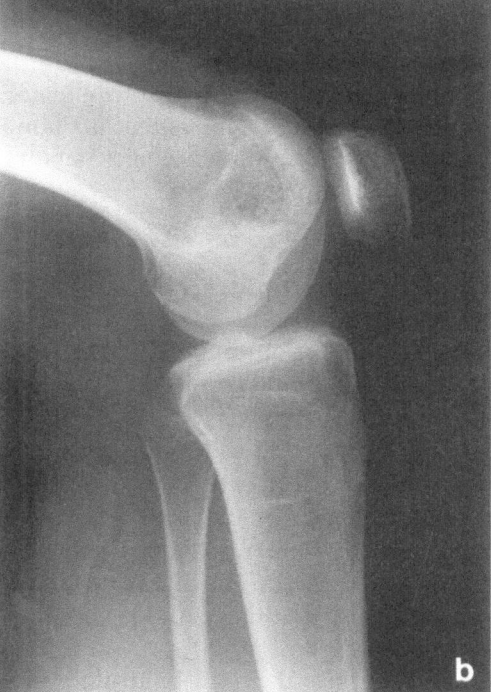

Fig. 2. Pre-operative antero-posterior (**a**) and lateral (**b**) radiograph of an osteochondral post-traumatic defect in the knee of a 16 year old girl

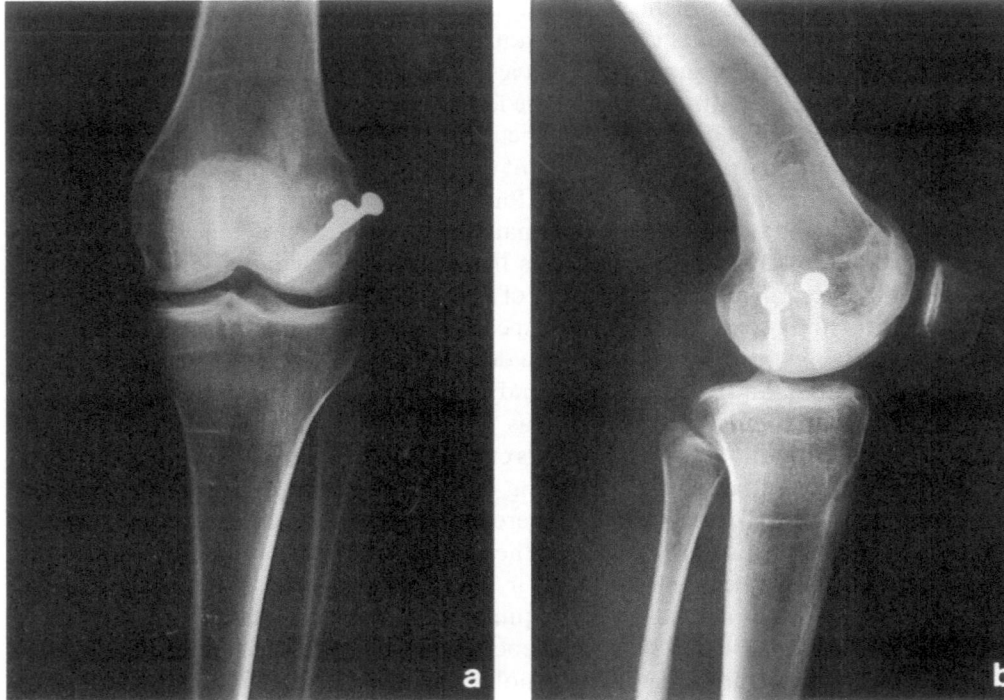

Fig. 3. Post-operative antero-posterior (**a**) and lateral (**b**) radiograph at 3 years showing complete osteochondral allograft incorporation

alignment of the knee, slight prominence of the graft to ensure that it is subjected to normal forces in the joint, and a subchondral bone fragment of at last 1 cm thickness to avoid fracture. The immunological factors required are unknown but may include more precise tissue typing.

The Matrix Support Prosthesis

This is a concept of re-inforcing the repair tissue produced on the surface of joints by drilling, by the implantation of a meshwork of carbon fibre or rods of carbon fibre to support the fibrocartilage formed from the subchondral marrow. This technique was first used by Muckle and Minns [6] and was initially used by them for the treatment of osteochondritis and early osteoarthritis (Fig. 4).

We performed an independent review of 96 cases followed for a period of 1–5 years. Both subjective and objective criteria were used for this retrospective assessment and the results showed that 71% of patients had an excellent or good result [7]. This of course does not mean that the method is perfect but certainly the results are better than that of a placebo response of 30–40% and have never been surpassed by any operation to simply resurface the joint by drilling or abrasion (Figs. 4, 5). We therefore decided to pursue this method in a prospective study which is still under way. We have assessed the first 30 patients of whom 17 had chondromalacia of the patella and 13 had osteochondritis of the medial or lateral femoral condyle [8]. The patients had been monitored

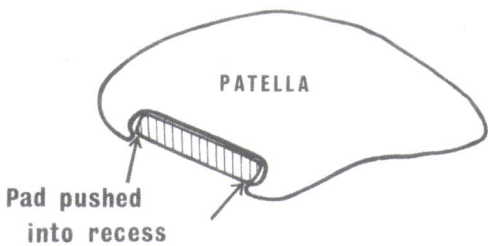

Fig. 4. Diagram to illustrate the principle of the matrix support prosthesis. Osteochondral bone is carefully drilled to achieve a suitable bed for the carbon fibre matrix which is then a support for the repair fibrocartilage formed from the bone

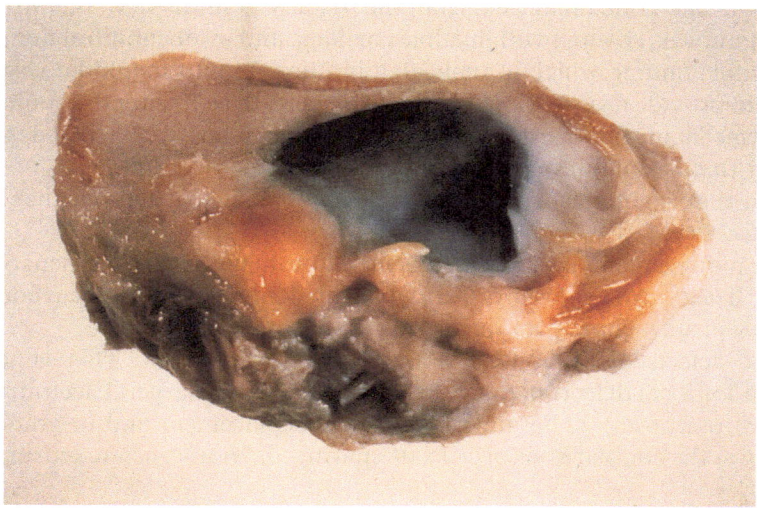

Fig. 5. Macroscopic appearance of a patella removed 3 years after implantation of carbon fibre matrix. The smooth fibrocartilaginous repair tissue is obvious on the surface of the carbon fibre

clinically and arthroscopically at one year intervals and the results are as yet incomplete. A total of 72 patients are in the study.

So far the early results show only 40% satisfactory results for chondromalacia patellae but 90% satisfactory results for osteochondritis dissecans. This is at a follow-up period of 2 years. It appears that the results for chondromalacia patellae are unsatisfactory if there is a large defect since the mechanical demands of the patello-femoral joint are much greater than those of the main femoro-tibial joint.

These studies have led us into further research to try to find methods of improving the quality of repair material in joint surface defects. A number of materials are being tested but in addition we have pursued the concept of supplementing the carbon fibre meshwork with implants of viable chondrocytes in order to produce a more normal type of composite graft of carbon fibre and living chondrocytes.

In the laboratory, rabbit chondrocytes have been grown for 3 weeks in a carbon fibre mesh and the cells grow without difficulty in the carbon mesh and immunofluorescent studies show that there is normal type II collagen and normal proteoglycan (chondroitin 4 sulphate, chondroitin 6 sulphate and keratan sulphate) in the cultures after 3 weeks. Following this finding the cultures were transplanted as composite grafts into the articular surface of mature rabbit knees and the animals were sacrificed at 3 months. The immunofluorescent study shows that there is also type II collagen and normal proteoglycan in the transplanted material after 3 months.

Thus this experiment showed that the hyaline cartilage phenotype was maintained in these cultures for 3 weeks and also for 3 months after transplantation into the articular surface. However it is notable that the defect in the articular surface is deeper than the surrounding articular cartilage and therefore physically softer. Hence a material that would encourage formation of hyaline cartilage but also of a subchondral bone plate would seem to be an advantage.

In an attempt to find a suitable biocompatible bone cement as a carrier material, experiments were being carried out on a polymer THM-PMMA in this laboratory. It was observed after 8 weeks of implantation of this material into the femoral condyle of a rabbit that not only was the bone unaffected from the toxicity point of view, but also that the surface of the joint was covered with hyaline cartilage and a subchondral bone plate. This is a remarkable finding which, if replicated in human joints, could be very important since it would provide a surface of hyaline cartilage with a subchondral bone plate which has similar mechanical properties to normal cartilage. Thus it is likely to last and to bear load better than carbon fibre reinforced fibrocartilage.

Thus it can be seen that this aspect of joint treatment for early articular cartilage damage is slowly being solved [9].

Our program of the management of osteoarthritis therefore includes the treatment of early articular cartilage defects up to the size of 3 cm which are treated by a pad of carbon fibre and clinical trials will start shortly on the use of the new material.

In larger stage one defects osteochondral allografts are carried out. This same treatment is carried out for focal defects of grade 2 damage. Of course larger defects are still dealt with by tibial osteotomy or by unicompartment replacement and in grade 3 disease we are looking at the comparisons of cruciate sparing and non-cruciate sparing total knee replacement.

In the future it appears that osteochondral allografts are definitely established for the treatment of post-traumatic defects and for osteochondritis dissecans but their role in chondromalacia patellae and early osteoarthritis seems less certain. It is possible that in these situations the use of carbon fibre or some other matrix support type of material may be feasible in the more difficult cases of early articular cartilage damage.

References

1. Bentley G (1985) Articular cartilage changes in chondromalacia patellae. J Bone Joint Surg 67B: 769
2. Lexer E (1908) Die Verwendung der freien Knochenplastik nebst Versuchen über Gelenkversteifung und Gelenktransplantation. Arch Klin Chir 86: 939
3. Judet H (1908) Essai sur la greffe des tissues articulaires. Comp Rend Acad Sci 146: 193
4. Aston JE, Bentley G (1986) Repair of normal and arthritic articular surfaces by allografts of articular and growth-plate cartilage. J Bone Joint Surg 67B: 29
5. Langer F, Gross AE, West M, Urowitz ER (1978) The immunogenicity of allograft knee joint transplants. Clin Orthop 132: 155
6. Muckle DS, Minns RJ (1979) The use of filamentous carbon fibre for the repair of osteoarthritic articular cartilage. J Bone Joint Surg 61B: 381
7. Pongor P, Betts J, Muckle DS, Bentley G (1992) Woven carbon surface replacement: independent clinical review. Biomaterials 13 (15): 1070
8. Bentley G, Cobb AG, Hemmen B, Archer C (1992) The cartilage matrix support prosthesis. An experimental and clinical study. J Bone Joint Surg 74B [Suppl III]: 267
9. Bentley G (1992) Articular tissue grafts. Ann Rheum Dis 51 (3): 292–296

Author's address: Prof. George Bentley, ChM, FRCS, Institute of Orthopaedics, Royal National Orthopaedic Hospital, Stanmore Middx, HA7 4LP, U.K.

The Use of Fresh Osteochondral Allografts to Replace Traumatic Joint Defects

A.E. Gross[1], R.J. Beaver[2], D.J. Zukor[3], A. Czitrom[4], and M.T. Ghazavi[1]

[1]Division of Orthopaedic Surgery, Mount Sinai Hospital, Toronto, Ontario, Canada
[2]Royal Perth Hospital, Perth, Western Australia
[3]Department of Orthopaedic Surgery, Jewish General Hospital, McGill University, Montreal, PQ
[4]Orthopaedic Center of Dallas, Dallas, Texas U.S.A.

The scientific rationale for utilizing fresh rather than preserved osteochondral allografts is as follows. Cartilage harvested without a blood supply within 24 hours of the death of the donor is 100% viable and can be preserved for up to 4 days at 40° C. This has been shown both experimentally and clinically [4, 8, 12, 27, 29, 30, 32, 33, 42, 6, 37, 47, 11, 28, 9, 23]. The bone whether fresh or preserved, is not viable because of its inability to survive without immediate vascularization, but remains structurally intact and mechanically strong until it is replaced by host bone by creeping substitution [3, 11, 28, 30] or weakened and absorbed by invasion of granulation tissue. Freezing on the other hand kills the cartilage [39]. Even with cryopreservation, the best viability rates that could be achieved varied from 15 to 50% using glycerol or DMSO (dimethyl sulfoxide) and controlled rates of freezing and thawing [5, 40, 44, 45, 38, 19]. It has also been shown that freezing decreases the immunogenicity of the bone, but does not ablate it completely [13]. Fresh bone is more immunogenic than frozen bone, but there is not enough of a difference to affect the clinical outcome [13]. It has been shown that chondrocytes are immunogenic [14] but when surrounded by matrix they are isolated from the immunocompetent cells and do not sensitize the host.

The indications for fresh osteochondral allografts do not justify the use of immunosuppressive drugs and we therefore felt that surgical vascularization of these grafts should not be carried out.

We hoped that fresh osteochondral allografts would provide viable cartilage with the potential to survive transplantation and bone that although dead, would remain structurally intact until host bone replaced it. Immediate surgical vascularization was not carried out and immunosuppression was not used.

The clinical rationale for this program which was started after the immunology was worked out [13, 14] was that fresh osteochondral allografts could be performed in younger higher demand patients where implants were not desirable and arthrodesis not acceptable.

The clinical program started in 1972 at Mount Sinai Hospital, University of Toronto and as of September 1, 1994, 221 fresh grafts have been performed. Initially these grafts were performed for unicompartmental osteoarthritis, spontaneous osteonecrosis of the knee, steroid induced osteonecrosis of the knee, osteochondritis dissecans and most commonly traumatic defects. A review of our first 100 cases revealed that the best indication was for traumatic defects in young patients [26].

Based on this review [26] we now perform primarily unicompartmental, unipolar fresh osteochondral allografts for traumatic joint defects about the knee in young people (under 50).

Graft Procurement, Handling and Operative Technique

Donors are located by the Multiple Organ Retrieval and Exchange program of Toronto and to be suitable, must meet the criteria outlined by the American Association of Tissue Banks [43]. They must also be less than 30 years old (and preferably younger) to provide healthy, viable cartilage. Graft procurement is carried out within twenty-four hours of death under strict aseptic conditions with the specimen consisting of the entire knee joint with the capsule intact. After taking appropriate cultures the graft is stored in one litre of sterile Ringer's Lactate at 4°C with added Cefazoline (1 gm.), and Bacitracin (50,000 u). Tissue typing is no longer performed and no attempt is made to match donor and recipient other than on the basis of size. No immunosuppression is used.

The recipient patient is notified as soon as a donor has been located and immediately makes his or her way to the hospital as prearranged. Implantation is usually achieved by twelve hours and always within twenty-four hours. This schedule can be adhered to despite the fact that many of the patients come from diverse parts of the United States and Canada.

The transplantation procedure is usually performed in a clean-air room with the operating team wearing body exhaust suits. The patients routinely receive pre and post operative prophylactic antibiotics (Cefazolin if no allergy exists). The favored surgical approach is direct midline which allows easy access for both the transplant and either proximal tibial or distal femoral osteotomy if indicated. Should later salvage procedures by necessary the same approach is used with little risk of skin complications. Following arthrotomy, the involved damaged articular surface is resected to a good bleeding cancellous bone surface. The donor tissue is then cut to appropriate size and implanted aiming for a tight fit with accurate reproduction of normal anatomy. Fixation is augmented by cancellous screws. If the meniscus is irreparably damaged or has previously been excised it is replaced by an allograft meniscus which is sutured to the capsule of the recipient.

Some changes in technique have evolved since this procedure was last reported. The graft itself is no longer used to correct alignment. This is achieved by osteotomy either prior to or at the time of allograft implantation. This decision depends on whether the graft involves the same side of the joint as the osteotomy or not. For example a lateral tibial plateau graft can be done simultaneously with a distal femoral varus osteotomy (Figs. 1, 2 Case 1) and a medial femoral condyle graft can be accompanied by a high tibial valgus osteotomy (Figs. 3, 4, Case 2).

The preference is to perform either distal femoral varus or proximal tibial valgus osteotomies. If the realignment procedures involves the same side of the joint as the graft, it should be carried out several months after or prior to transplantation to allow sufficient time for revascularization of host bone. As well this obviates the technical difficulties of performing these two procedures at the same site. The two most common surgical procedures are illustrated in Figs. 1 to 4.

Post-operatively the limbs are no longer immobilized but started immediately in the recovery room on continuous passive motion (C.P.M.) in order to maximize cartilage nutrition and prevent stiffness. The machines have been specially modified to allow positioning in either varus or valgus alignment.

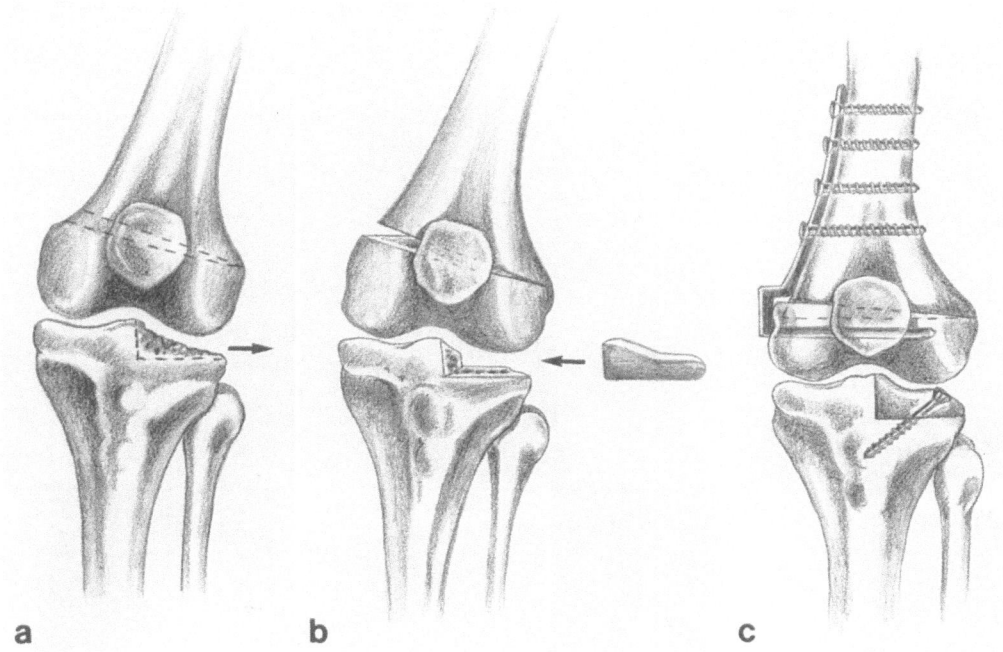

Fig. 1. Illustration of lateral tibial plateau allograft and distal femoral varus osteotomy. **a** Old lateral plateau fracture with depression of plateau and an associated valgus deformity. Dotted line in femur outlines osteotomy. Dotted line in lateral tibial plateau outlines planned resection; **b** Lateral plateau has been resected to a horizontal bed of healthy cancellous bone and the osteochondral allograft is shown ready for insertion; **c** The allograft is inserted and the distal femoral varus osteotomy performed to correct the deformity. The allograft is fixed with small cancellous screws and the osteotomy with an offset 90° condylar hip plate

Patients are protected from full weight bearing for approximately one year by a long leg brace with an ischial ring.

Clinical Material

Between January 1, 1972 and January 1, 1992, 126 fresh osteocartilaginous allografts have been performed for post-traumatic knee joint defects. A recent follow-up study of fifty-five grafts included fifty-one patients that had follow-up greater than two years. All patients were followed prospectively, clinically, and radiographically. A rating score was calculated using a point protocol. This includes both subjective and objective data and was previously reported by McDermott [26].

Radiographs were carefully scrutinized. Factors examined included joint alignment, fit and fixation of the graft, bone union, graft collapse and fragmentation, preservation of cartilage space, and development of osteoarthritis. Pre- and postoperative antero-posterior, lateral, oblique and skyline views and weight bearing films were utilized for this analysis.

The average age was 17.8 years (range 10–70) with average follow-up of 5.3 years (range 2–16.5 years). Thirty-three patients were male and eighteen female. The average interval from injury to grafting was 3.9 years (range 2 months – 27 years).

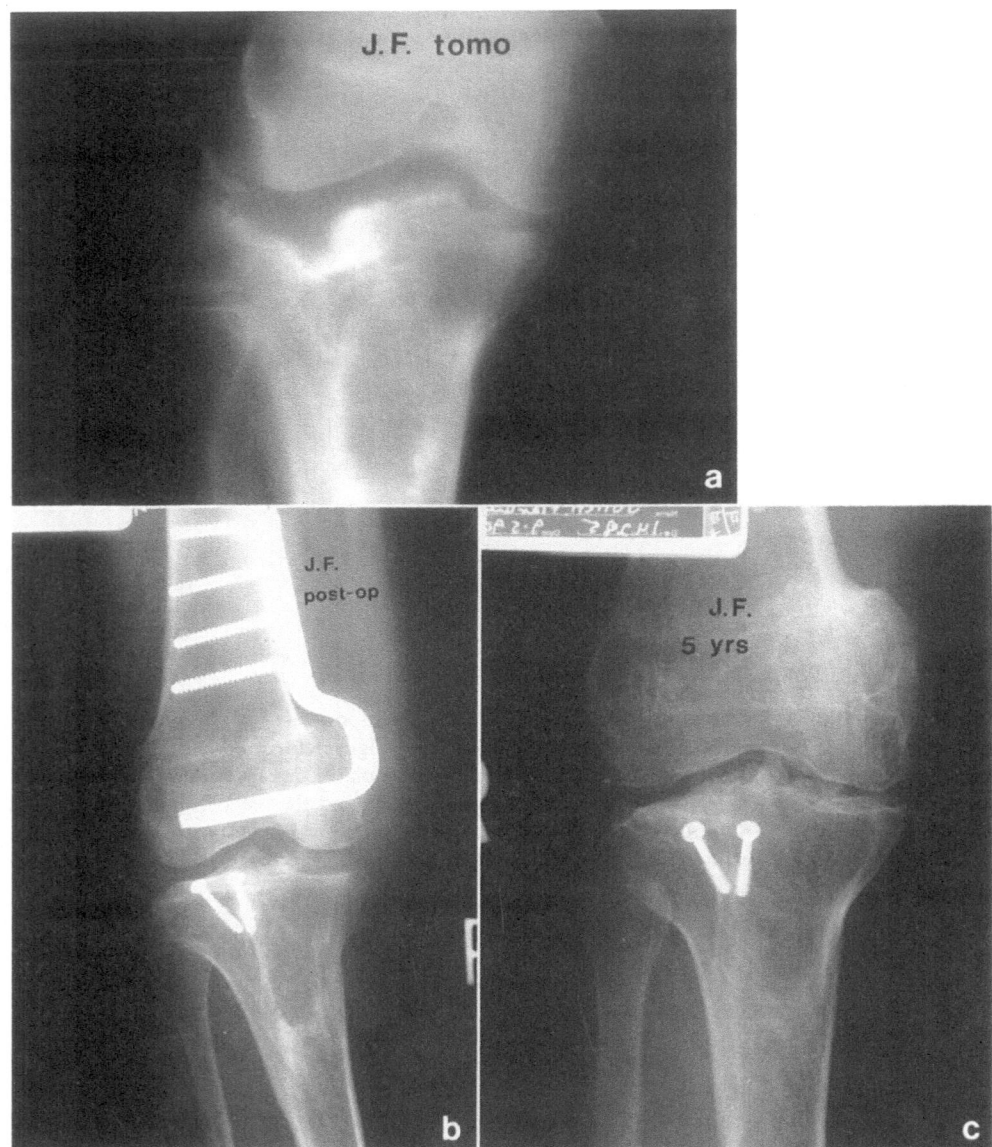

Fig. 2. CASE 1: Fractured lateral tibial plateau. **a** AP x-ray tomogram of the right knee in a 30 year old female who had suffered a lateral tibial plateau fracture 2 years earlier; **b** AP x-ray 2 years after reconstruction of the right knee with a fresh lateral tibial plateau allograft and a distal femoral varus osteotomy; **c** AP X-ray 5 years past transplant. There has been minimal collapse of the graft but joint space is well maintained and the knee is well aligned

Of the fifty-five allografts, the majority (thirty-three) were of the tibial plateau with five medial and twenty-eight lateral. Seventeen involved the femoral condyle with eight medial and nine lateral. Four involved both femoral condyle and tibial plateau of the same compartment and were termed unicompartmental bipolar grafts. One of these was medial and the other three lateral. One graft was used to resurface the patella.

Twenty realignment osteotomies were carried out in nineteen patients who received transplants. Distal femoral osteotomies were performed in ten patients to achieve varus

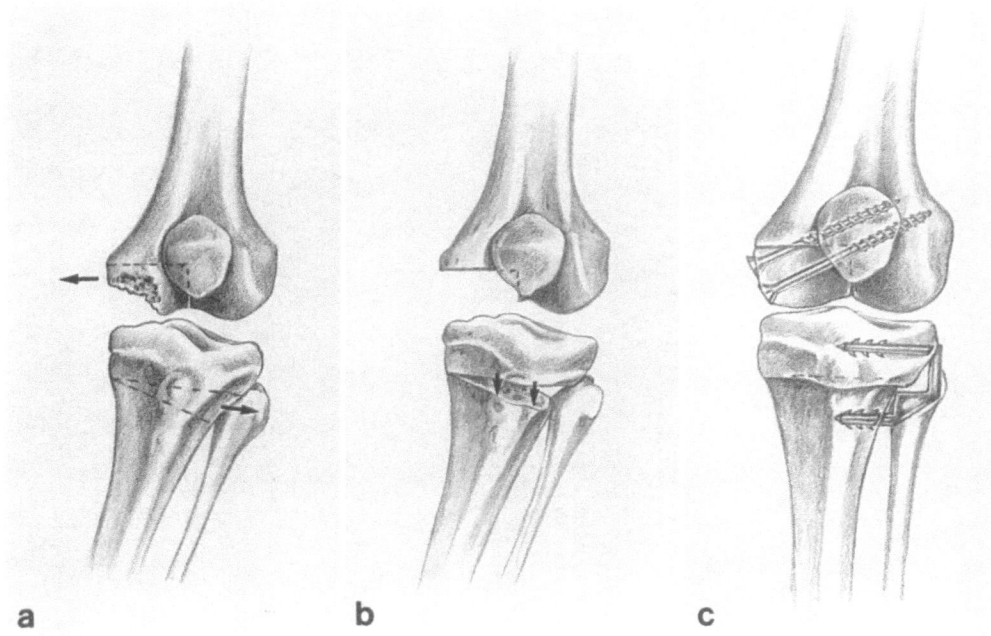

Fig. 3. Illustration of medial femoral condyle allograft and high tibial osteotomy; **a** Traumatic loss of medial femoral condyle with secondary varus deformity. Dotted line in femur indicates line of resection in preparation for allograft. Dotted line in tibia indicates valgus osteotomy; **b** Diseased condyle has been resected and high tibial valgus osteotomy performed; **c** Osteochondral allograft has been inserted and held with two cancellous screws. Osteotomy is held with 2 staples

and twice to achieve valgus alignment. High tibial valgus osteotomies were performed in seven patients and varus tibial osteotomy in one. Of the twenty osteotomies nine were carried out prior to or simultaneous with allograft implantation. This practice increased in frequency towards the end of the series.

Menisci were included with twenty-eight of the grafts. Twenty-one were left attached to their corresponding lateral tibial plateau allograft at time of implantation and five to the medial plateau. Two were actual "free" meniscal allografts at the time of replacement of the lateral femoral condyle.

Results

Clinical Analysis

Patients were rated either as successes or as failures. A successful result required improvement of the rating score by at least ten points or maintenance of a score of seventy-five points or higher. Patients were rated as failures if there was any decrease in the rating score or if subsequent salvage surgery was necessary.

Overall forty-two of the fifty-five grafts or 76% were successful. These had an average pre-operative score of 66.5 (range 31–93) and an average post-operative score of ninety-one (range 68–100).

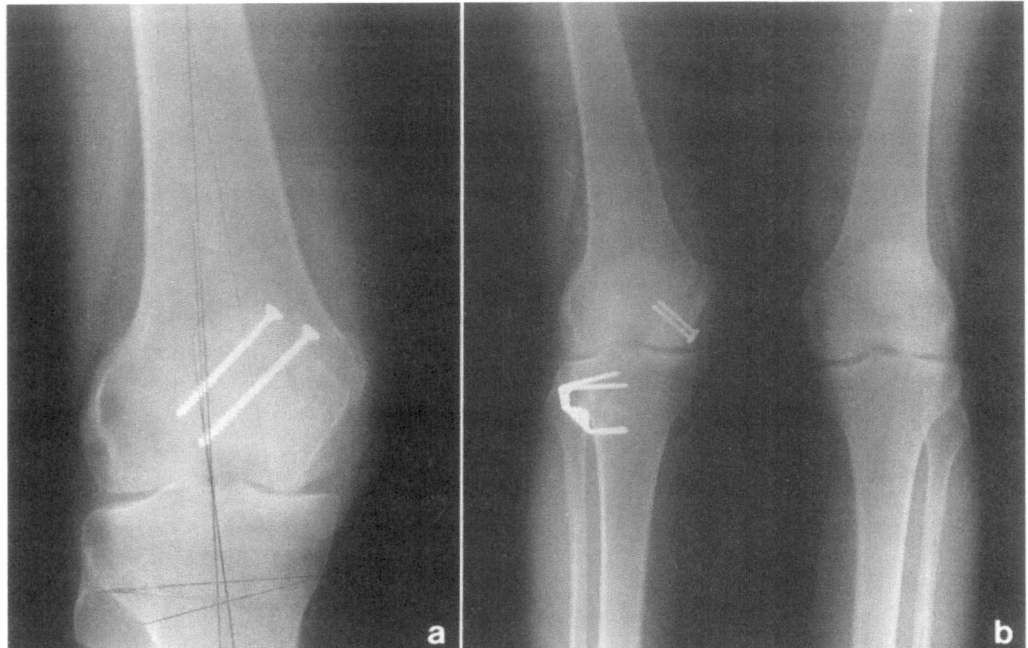

Fig. 4. CASE 2: Post traumatic osteonecrosis medial femoral condyle. **a** AP x-ray right of the knee of 30 year old female with traumatic loss of part of medial femoral condyle. The screws are holding a fractured patella; **b** AP x-ray right knee 6 years following fresh osteochondral allograft to replace the damaged part of the medial condyle. A valgus osteotomy of the tibia was performed to correct the varus deformity

Of the thirteen failures four were unicompartmental bipolar grafts, eight were lateral plateau replacements and one was a medial plateau graft. Four patients have undergone salvage procedures – one arthrodesis at eight years, and three total knee replacement at two, four and six years respectively. The other nine grafts were still functioning but were considered failures because of varying degrees of pain or stiffness.

The seventeen femoral condyle replacements and the single patellar graft were successful as were four of the five medial plateau grafts and twenty of the twenty-eight lateral plateau replacements. All four bipolar grafts failed. Of the nineteen patients who had osteotomies, only four had an unsuccessful result. Of the twenty-eight patients who received meniscal allografts, twenty-one were successful. However, seven of the thirteen failures had an associated meniscal allograft.

Radiographic Review

Every attempt was made to standardize technique but it was obvious during the course of this analysis that perfectly comparable views were the exception rather than the rule. This affects serial measurements of parameters such as height of the bone or cartilage.

Radiographic union was defined as establishment of structural continuity between host bone and allograft. Union occurred in all of the fifty-five grafts. This was usually present by nine to twelve months. Restoration of normal bone density (of the allograft) was usually evident within two to four years.

Adequate X-rays for assessment of bone collapse and cartilage space were available for fifty-four of the grafts.

The joint space was seen to be well preserved in thirty patients, decreased in ten patients and absent or arthritic in fourteen patients. Virtually all the grafts were seen to settle at least 1–3 mm, and the majority did not collapse further. Fifteen grafts had evidence of collapse greater than 4–5 mm. One graft collapsed completely.

No actual fractures of grafts were seen. However, six grafts were fragmented adjacent to their articular surface. Whether this represents microfractures or mechanically induced degeneration remains unresolved. Alignment of the knees was assessed on weight bearing radiographs of the entire lower extremities. Forty-four patients had adequate X-rays for this. For a lateral compartment graft ideal alignment is considered to be a femoral-tibial axis of zero to a few degrees of varus. Conversely for a medial compartment replacement ideal alignment is ten degrees or more of femoral-tibial valgus.

Sixteen patients were seen to be ideally aligned, eight of these by osteotomy.

In twenty-eight patients alignment was judged to be suboptimal. Nine had undergone osteotomy with inadequate correction.

Of the sixteen well-aligned patients, there were three failures. Only one of these three had had an osteotomy. Eliminating the other two early in the series where alignment correction was achieved by graft height alone, only one out of fourteen patients with ideal alignment failed.

Of the twenty-eight poorly aligned patients, there were six failures. Only two of these six had had an osteotomy. One osteotomy was performed three years after allograft implantation and the other one year after grafting with failure to adequately correct alignment.

No composite graft failed because of problems with the meniscal allograft. No meniscal allografts have been excised in isolation. Another study looked at the long term survival of fresh small fragment osteochondral allografts for traumatic defects of the knee. The study was comprised of 92 allografts in 91 patients. These patients have been followed prospectively since 1972. At review, a Kaplan-Meier survivorship analysis was performed on the cases. The results demonstrated that fresh osteochondral allografts when performed for post traumatic defects had an overall survival rate of 73% at 5 years and 58% at 10 years. The unipolar grafts had a 77% survival at 5 years, 69% survival at 10 years, and a 67% survival at 14 years. The bipolar grafts had a 57% survival at 5 years, 19% survival at 10 years, and a 19% survival at 14 years. The unipolar grafts had a significantly lower failure rate than the bipolar grafts at all time periods. Therefore, we no longer advocate the use of bipolar grafts. We currently recommend unipolar grafts for major post traumatic osteochondral defects in the knees of young, high demand patients. Careful patient selection and correction of joint malalignment are essential for best results [2].

Complications

Nine complications occurred in eight patients. Three knees required manipulations for stiffness early in the series when post-operative immobilization for 14–21 days was still being used. This complication was not seen following the introduction of C.P.M. One of these three patients was later diagnosed as reflex sympathetic dystrophy. Other complications included one wound hematoma which required evacuation and one intra-operative rupture of an already frayed patellar tendon, which was successfully repaired immediately.

Three patients had complications related to the respiratory system. No documented deep vein thrombosis or pulmonary emboli occurred. There were no infections. There were two late deaths unrelated to surgery.

Discussion

Long-term results of fresh, small fragment osteochondral allografts are encouraging. The best indication is late reconstruction following traumatic loss of a joint segment [26, 18, 48]. However, patient selection remains a vital consideration. Best results have been seen in highly motivated patients who have no evidence of degenerative arthritis prior to allografting.

In our original group of 100 patients, 24 grafts were performed for osteoarthritis with a clinical success rate of only 42% [26]. This was felt to be due to the necessity for bipolar grafts (unicompartmental), obesity, and deformity. These patients were slightly older and did not tolerate post-operative bracing. The same factors applied to the 11 patients with spontaneous osteonecrosis of the knee where only 3 obtained a successful result. Grafts were also performed for 3 patients with steroid induced osteonecrosis with all 3 failing probably due to poor host bone related to blood supply and steroids. Based on our early experience we therefore felt that the best patient for this procedure was young, and had traumatic loss of one pole (a condyle or a plateau).

The rationale for using fresh rather than stored allografts is based on clinical and experimental evidence supporting the maintenance of viability and function of chondrocytes after fresh transplantation [7]. Currently, experimental work on cryopreservation techniques indicates that relatively high percentages of chondrocytes (50%) survive after freezing and thawing of cartilage in animal models [44, 45, 38, 19]. However, as yet, there is little objective evidence of prolonged survival of preserved cartilage following implantation in humans. Few reports with histological evidence appear in the literature, and while these are often biopsies of failed cases, the cartilage is usually described as severely degenerated and "distinctly abnormal" [20, 24, 21].

However, even in twelve out of eighteen failed cases reported by Oakeshott et al. [28] hyaline cartilage survival and matrix production, as late as 9.5 years following transplantation of fresh grafts was seen. This was demonstrated by staining techniques and electron microscopy. It is likely that in successful cases cartilage survival is even better.

While intact cartilage is considered immunoprivileged [30] the bony component of the graft is known to be immunogenic [3, 13, 15]. Antigenicity has been shown to be decreased significantly, though not eliminated completely, by freezing and freeze drying (both of which adversely affect the cartilage) [13]. A definite immune response following transplantation of fresh, frozen or freeze-dried bone has been well documented [29, 13, 15]. However, neither the presence nor the magnitude of this response correlates with clinical success or failure of the graft [15, 34, 39]. Previous reviews of fresh bone and cartilage transplants have failed to reveal evidence of clinically significant or histologically detectable rejection [1, 4, 10, 11, 16, 17, 22].

In the literature, only the series of Volkov [46] reported the phenomenon of rejection and this was with frozen grafts. However, clinical rejection has not been identified in fourteen years of experience with over 130 fresh grafts at this institution.

Many authors have stated that the fate of the allograft depends heavily on mechanical factors [45, 24, 46, 8, 36, 25]. Analysis of failed grafts from this center revealed a high association of failure with poorly sized grafts, grafts less than 1 cm in thickness (resulting in fragmentation and fracture) and grafts where internal fixation was not used [28].

The present series illustrates the success of unipolar grafts in the knee. Though only a small number of bipolar grafts [27] are presented, they were all failures.

The role of osteotomy to realign the joint, especially in weight-bearing extremities, cannot be overemphasized. Of the nineteen patients who underwent osteotomy even when performed late – only four were in the failed group. The preferred realignment procedure to correct valgus deformity is distal femoral varus osteotomy [25]. Proximal tibial valgus osteotomy is used to correct varus deformity. Joint surface obliquity and site of the allograft must be taken into consideration. In the present series only one out of fourteen grafts in well aligned extremities failed. Best results can be achieved by adhering to the principles described including correct sizing, realignment and fixation to achieve ideal mechanical conditions along with prompt implantation of fresh, healthy cartilage to maximize cell viability.

Grafts should be "decompressed" by realignment osteotomy either at the time of or prior to transplantations. Perhaps consideration should be given to extending the period of protected weight bearing beyond one year (the interval currently used), to two or three years or until the bony portions returns to iso-density. Many of the early cases were performed prior to the recognition of the importance of these factors. Thus, long term objective assessment of patients treated by adherence to the above principles is of considerable interest and part of an ongoing study.

Complications in this series were relatively minor. As this is a relatively conservative procedure involving minimal bone resection, no "bridges are burned". Subsequent salvage surgery (i.e. arthroplasty, or arthrodesis) certainly is not compromised and conversely may even be facilitated because deficient bone stock has been replaced.

We are presently doing 10–20 fresh osteochondral allografts per year for traumatic defects about the knee. This group of patients is young with unipolar osteochondral deficits rather than just pure chondral lesion. Thus far we have been able to meet the needs of patients referred to us from all over North America. A program of fresh grafts for dealing with chondral lesions of the knee is under way in Atlanta [9]. The fresh osteochondral allograft program in San Diego dealt with defects around the knee and hip [23].

Summary

Long term follow-up of fresh, small fragment osteochondral allograft reconstruction of traumatic joint surface defects of the knee revealed 76% to be clinically successful. Best results can be achieved by adhering to the principles described including correct sizing, realignment and internal fixation to achieve ideal mechanical conditions along with prompt implantation of fresh, healthy cartilage to maximize cell viability. Mechanical factors seem to be more important than immunological factors in determining the fate of the grafts. Correct alignment should be achieved by osteotomy rather than by the graft. Bipolar grafts should be avoided if possible. We have achieved encouraging results with these grafts for unipolar traumatic defects about the knee. We have also been pleased with a very small series of grafts for traumatic defects of the talus.

Conclusions and Recommendations

1. Traumatic loss of a joint segment is the best indication for fresh osteochondral allografts.

2. Patient selection is a vital consideration.
3. Mechanical conditions seem more important to successful results than immunological factors.
4. Ideal alignment of the extremity to "unload" the graft is an absolute requirement and if necessary should be achieved by osteotomy prior to or simultaneous with allograft implantation.
5. Internal fixation of the allograft should be used.
6. Bipolar allografts should be avoided if at all possible.
7. Menisci can be implanted if the recipient's meniscus is absent or irreparably damaged.
8. C.P.M. is a useful post-operative adjunct.
9. Fresh, small fragment osteochondral allografts can be successfully used to reconstruct joint surfaces following traumatic segmental loss.

References

1. Aston J, Bentley G (1986) Repair of articular surfaces by allografts of articular and growth-plane cartilage. J Bone Joint Surg 68B(1): 29–35
2. Beaver RJ, Mahomed M, Backstein D, Davis A, Zukor DJ, Gross AE (1992) Fresh osteochondral allografts: post traumatic defects in the knee, a survivorship analysis. J Bone Joint Surg 74-B: 105–110
3. Burchardt H (1983) The biology of bone graft repair. C.O.O.R. 174: 28–42
4. Campbell CJ, Ishida H, Takahashi H, Kelly F (1963) The transplantation of articular cartilage. An experimental study in dogs. J Bone Joint Surg 45-A: 1579–1592
5. Chesterman PJ, Smith AU (1968) Homotransplantation of articular cartilage and isolated chondrocytes: an experimental study in rabbits. J Bone Joint Surg 50-B: 184
6. Craigmyle MBL (1958) An autoradiographic and histochemical study of long-term cartilage grafts in the rabbit. J Anat 92: 467–472
7. Czitrom A, Keating S, Gross A (1990) The viability of articular cartilage in fresh osteochondral allografts after clinical transplantation. J Bone Joint Surg 72-A: 574
8. DePalma AF, Tsaltas TT, Mauler GG (1963) Viability of osteochondral grafts as determined by uptake of S^{35}. J Bone Joint Surg 45-A: 1565–1578
9. Garret J (1987) Osteochondral allografts for treatment of chondral defects of the femoral condyles: early results. Proceedings of the Knee Society. Am J Sports Med 14: 4, 387
10. Goldberg VM, Porter BB, Lance EM (1980) Transplantation of the canine knee joint on a vascular pedicle. J Bone Joint Surg 62-A: 414
11. Kandel RA, Gross AE, Gavel A, McDermott AGP, Langer F, Pritzker KPH (1985) Histopathology of failed osteoarticular shell allografts. Clin Orthop Rel Res 197: 103–110
12. Lance EM, Fisher RL (1970) Transplantation of the rabbit's patella. J Bone Joint Surg 52-A: 145–156
13. Langer F, Czitrom AA, Pritzker KP, Gross AE (1975) The immunogenicity of fresh and frozen allogeneic bone. J Bone Joint Surg 57-A: 216
14. Langer F, Gross AE (1974) Immunogenicity of allograft articular cartilage. J Bone Joint Surg 56-A: 297
15. Langer F, Gross AE, West M, Urovitz EP (1978) The immunogenicity of allograft knee joint transplants. Clin Orthop 132: 155
16. Lexer E (1908) Substitution of joints from amputated extremities. Surg Gynecol Obstet 6: 601
17. Lexer E (1925) Joint transplantation and arthroplasty. Surg Gynecol Obstet 40: 782
18. Locht RC, Gross AE, Langer F (1984) Late osteochondral allograft resurfacing for tibial plateau fractures. J Bone Joint Surg 66-A: 328
19. Malinin TI, Wagner JL, Pita JC, Lo H (1985) Hypothermic storage and cryopreservation of cartilage. Clin Orthop 197: 15–26
20. Mankin HJ, Doppelt S, Tomford WW: Clinical experience with allograft implantation. Clin Orthop 174: 69–86

21. Mankin HJ, Doppelt SH, Sullivan TR, Tomford WW (1982) Osteoarticular and intercalary allograft transplantation in the management of malignant tumours of bone. Cancer 50: 613

22. Meyers MH: Resurfacing of the femoral head with fresh osteochondral allografts. Clin Orthop 197: 111–114

23. Meyers M, Akeson W, Convery R (1989) Resurfacing of the knee with fresh osteochondral allografts. JBJS 71-A(5): 704–713

24. Mnaymneh W, Malinin TI, Makley JT, Dick HM (1985) Massive osteoarticular allografts in the reconstruction of extremities following resection of tumors not requiring chemotherapy and radiation. Clin Orthop 197: 76–87

25. McDermott AGP, Finkelstein JA, Farine I, Boynton EL, MacIntosh DL, Gross AE (1988) Distal femoral varus osteotomy for valgus deformity of the knee. JBJS 70-A(1): 110

26. McDermott AGP, Langer F, Pritzker KPH, Gross AE (1985) Fresh small fragment osteochondral allografts. Clin Orthop 197: 96–102

27. McKibbin B (1971) Immature joint cartilage and the homograft reaction. J Bone Joint Surg 53-B(1): 123–135

28. Oakeshott RD, Farine I, Pritzker KPH, Langer F, Gross AE (1988) A clinical and histologic analysis of failed fresh osteochondral allografts. Clin Orthop Rel Res 233: 283–294

29. Paccola CAJ, Xavier CAM, Goncalves RP (1979) Fresh immature articular cartilage allografts. A study on the integration of chondral and osteochondral grafts both in normal and in papain-treated knee joints of rabbit. Arch Orthop Traumat Surg 93: 253–259

30. Pap K, Krompecher S (1961) Arthroplasty of the knee. Experimental and clinical experiences. J Bone Joint Surg 43-A: 523–537

31. Pelker RR, Friedlaender GE, Markham TC (1983) Biomechanical properties of bone allografts. COOR 174: 54–57

32. Porter BB, Lance EM (1974) Limb and joint transplantation. A review of research and clinical experience. Clin Orthop 104: 249–274

33. Pritzker KPH, Gross AE, Langer F, Luk SC, Houpt JB (1977) Articular cartilage transplantation. Hum Pathol 8: 635–651

34. Prolo DI, Rodrigo JJ (1985) Contemporary bone graft physiology and surgery. Clin Orthop 200: 322

35. Rodrigo JJ, Sakovich L, Travis C, Smith G (1978) Osteocartilaginous allograft as compared with autografts in the treatment of knee joint osteocartilaginous defects in dogs. Clin Orthop 134: 342

36. Rodrigo JJ, Block N, Thompson EC (1978) Joint transplantation. Vet Clin North America 8: 523

37. Rodrigo J, Thompson E, Travis C (1980) 4°C Preservation of avascular osteocartilaginous shell allografts in Rats. Transact Orthop Res Soc 5: 72

38. Schachar NS, McGann LE (1986) Investigations of low-temperature storage of articular cartilage for transplantation. Clin Orthop 208: 146–150

39. Sedgewick AD, Moore AR, All-Duaij AY, Edwards JCW, Willoughby DA (1985) Studies into the influence of carrageenan induced inflammation on articular cartilage degradation using implantation into air pouches. Br J Exp Pathol 66: 445

40. Simon W, Richardson S, Herman W, Parsons R, Lane J (1976) Long-term effects of chondrocyte death on rabbit articular cartilage in vivo. J Bone Joint Surg 58-A(4): 517–526

41. Smith AU (1965) Survival of frozen chondrocytes isolated from cartilage of adult mammals. Nature 205: 782

42. Thomas V, Jimenez S, Brighton C, Brown N (1984) Sequential changes in the mechanical properties of viable articular cartilage stored in vitro. J Orthop Res 2: 55–60

43. Tissue Banking: In: Fawcett KJ, Barr HR (eds) Arlington, V.A.: American Association of Blood Banks, pp 97–107

44. Tomford WW, Dugg GP, Mankin HJ (1985) Experimental freeze-preservation of chondrocytes. Clin Orthop 197: 11–14

45. Tomford WW, Mankin HJ (1983) Investigational approaches to articular cartilage preservation. Clin Orthop 174: 22–27

46. Volkov M (1970) Allotransplantation of joints. J Bone Joint Surg 52-B: 49

47. Wiley AM, Kosinka E (1974) Experimental and clinical aspects of transplantation of entire hyaline cartilage surfaces. J Am Geriatr Soc 25: 547
48. Zukor D, Oakeshott R, Gross A (1989) Osteochondral allograft reconstruction of the knee. Part 2. Experience with successful and failed fresh osteochondral allografts. Am J Knee Surg 2(4): 182–191

Authors' addresses: A.E. Gross, M.D., FRCS(C) and M.T. Ghazavi, M.D., Division of Orthopaedic Surgery, Mount Sinai Hospital, 600 University Avenue, Suite 476A, Toronto, ONT M5G IX5, U.S.A.; R.J. Beaver, MB, BS, FRCS(C), Royal Perth Hospital, Perth, Western Australia; D.J. Zukor, M.D., FRCS(C), Department of Orthopaedic Surgery, Jewish General Hospital, McGill University, Montrael; A. Czitrom, M.D., FRCS(C), Ph.D., Orthopaedic Surgery and Orthopaedic Oncology, Orthopaedic Center of Dallas, U.S.A.

Subject Index

SpringerMedicine

Henry V. Crock

A Short Practice of Spinal Surgery

Second, revised edition
1993. 278 partly colored figures. XVI, 338 pages.
Cloth DM 228,–, öS 1596,–
ISBN 3-211-82351-4

The dramatic developments in imaging technology and surgical techniques that have revolutionized spinal surgery in the last decade are expertly covered in this clear, concise working manual, ideal for both beginners and experienced practitioners. You'll find helpful guidelines for recognizing and treating disc prolapse and other disabling forms of disc disease and injury, an important review of surgical anatomy in relation to such pathological problems as spinal stenosis and cervical myelopathy, step-by-step surgical techniques integrated with applied anatomy, documented results of new procedures, advice on how to handle failed operations, the medical management of spinal surgery patients, and much more. Here is a useful, practical and safe surgical guide, full of valuable tips and recommendations, and providing a unique framework for diagnosing and treating lesions of the neck, thorax and lower back. Beautifully illustrated, written by a world-renowned specialist and teacher, and covering the most important new developments in the field, it is essential for all who perform spinal surgery.

"I would recommend this book for an in-depth analysis of the lumbar spine and its degenerative states. ... extremely beneficial for the resident early in training as he or she attempts to correlate the complex anatomy of the lumbosacral region with associated pathological states."

Journal of Neurosurgery

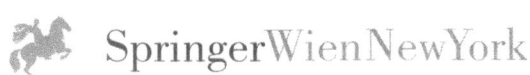
SpringerWienNewYork

P.O.Box 89, A-1201 Wien • New York, NY 10010, 175 Fifth Avenue
Heidelberger Platz 3, D-14197 Berlin • Tokyo 113, 3-13, Hongo 3-chome, Bunkyo-ku